Communication Sciences and Disorders

From Science to Clinical Practice

Communication Sciences
and
Disorders

From Science to Clinical Practice

Ronald B. Gillam, Ph.D.

Associate Professor
Department of Communication Sciences and Disorders
The University of Texas at Austin

Thomas P. Marquardt, Ph.D.

Professor
Department of Communication Sciences and Disorders
The University of Texas at Austin

Frederick N. Martin, Ph.D.

Professor
Department of Communication Sciences and Disorders
The University of Texas at Austin

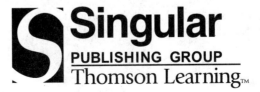

S Singular
PUBLISHING GROUP
Thomson Learning™

GOVERNORS STATE UNIVERSITY
UNIVERSITY PARK
IL 60466

Communication sciences
and disorders : from

Singular Publishing Group
Thomson Learning
401 West A Street, Suite 325
San Diego, California 92101-7904

Singular Publishing Group publishes textbooks, clinical manuals, clinical reference books, journals, videos, and multimedia materials on speech-language pathology, audiology, otorhinolaryngology, special education, early childhood, aging, occupational therapy, physical therapy, rehabilitation, counseling, mental health, and voice. For your convenience, our entire catalog can be accessed on our website at **http//www.singpub.com.** Our mission to provide you with materials to meet the daily challenges of the everchanging health care/educational environment will remain on course if we are in touch with you. In that spirit, we welcome your feedback on our products. Please telephone **(1-800-521-8545)**, fax **(1-800-774-8398)**, or e-mail **(singpub@singpub.com)** your comments and requests to us.

Library of Congress Cataloging-in-Publication Data

Communication sciences and disorders : from science to clinical practice / [edited by] Ronald B. Gillam, Thomas P. Marquardt, Frederick N. Martin].
    p. cm.
Includes bibliographical references and index.
ISBN 0-7693-0040-5 (soft cover : alk. paper)
  1. Communicative disorders. I. Gillam, Ronald B. (Ronald Bradley, 1955-
II. Marquardt, Thomas P. III. Martin, Frederick N.

RC423.C647 2000
616.85'5—dc21   99-054168

Contents

Preface

This book was written for undergraduate students who are enrolled in their first course in communication sciences and disorders. We wrote it with two important assumptions in mind. First, we assumed that the students who read this book would have relatively little prior knowledge about the scientific study of communication, the nature of communication disorders, or the professions of audiology and speech-language pathology. Second, we assumed that if students found the content of this book to be interesting, they would enroll in courses that would reexamine in much greater depth most of the topics that are included in this book.

Given these assumptions, we focused on providing the reader with a wide-angle view of communication sciences and disorders. We wanted to show the considerable forest that is communication sciences and disorders without having to focus on too many individual trees. Whenever possible, we aimed for width rather than depth. We want readers to have a sense of the variety of topics that speech, language, and hearing scientists study and the variety of individuals that audiologists and speech-language pathologists treat. Like many introductory texts, we provide basic information about hearing disorders that cause conductive and sensorineural hearing losses; speech disorders that are related to impairments in articulation, voice, and fluency; and language disorders in children and adults. Unlike many introductory texts, this book provides readers with basic information about hearing, speech, *and* language sciences. We also include basic information about the applied assessment and intervention practices that make speech, language, and hearing professionals invaluable members of the medical and educational communities. Finally, readers will be happy to note that this book includes chapters on multicultural issues, deafness, dysarthria, and dysphagia.

We did not want to tell readers everything we know about each topic. To this end, only the most critical concepts are described in detail, many examples are provided, and only seminal works are cited. If we have selected our topics wisely and have explained them well, the content of this book will provide students with the background knowledge they need to get the most out of subsequent undergraduate and graduate courses.

Finally, we have provided students with a means for seeing and hearing the human communication disorders they are reading about. Most professors present case studies of individuals with communication disorders in class via a combination of videotape, slides, audiotape, and text. Each of the authors of this book has struggled with the difficulties of setting up and using a variety of media in classroom contexts and the problems associated with a lack of student access to case study information outside the classroom. To begin to overcome these difficulties, we put digitized video and audio of individuals with communication disorders on a two-volume CD-ROM set that is included with each book. The CD-ROMs will enable professors to provide information about common or unusual cases in a single, highly accessible format, and it will enable students to watch the segments many times over in order to make the most of the enhanced learning opportunities they provide.

Acknowledgments

There are many people who contributed to the creation of this book. Marie Linvill saw the potential in the idea of an introductory book with an accompanying CD-ROM and gave us a great deal of encouragement and support along the way. Kristin Banach and Brad Bielawski have been patient and helpful as they shepherded the book to press. Special thanks to Ann Hillis, Ken Logan, LaVae Hoffman, Maria Muñoz, and two anonymous reviewers for their editorial comments about earlier versions of the chapters, and to Janet Pegues for her assistance with the glossaries.

A number of people assisted us in creating the CD-ROMs. First, and foremost, LaVae Hoffman endured the hardship of working for many masters, none of whom understood the intricacies of multimedia development. Without her loyalty, ingenuity, and hard work, this project would not have been possible. We thank many of our colleagues and students who agreed to appear in the video segments including Tracy Clark, Valerie Stahl, Rhonda Reese, Sam Gumpert, Regina Edwards, Maria Muñoz, Janet Pegues, Stephanie Echeverri, Alicia Gratton, Sarah Harper, Kathi Henion, Laura Jackson, Jeff Martin, Erin Moore, and Liza Sánchez. The authors wish to express their appreciation to Dr. Paul Burns, an otorhinolaryngologist with the Austin Ear, Nose and Throat Clinic, for his assistance in creating the endoscopy movies. Grateful appreciation is extended to Mr. Chad Smiddy who created the embryologic morphing sequence of the human face. Thanks to the Cochlear Corporation and Michael McKay who loaned a device for photographs. Finally, special thanks to Juan Diaz of the College of Communication Faculty Production Studio and Christopher Blandy of the ACITS program at The University of Texas at Austin who provided technical advice that served to improve the quality of the video and audio segments.

Finally, the editors and authors thank those individuals with communication disorders and their family members who allowed their images and words to be included on the CD-ROMs. We applaud their continuing struggle to compensate or overcome their communication disorders, and we share their hope that their appearance on the CD-ROMs will contribute to the education of the next generation of audiologists, speech-language pathologists, and deaf educators.

Contributors

Lisa M. Bedore, Ph.D., is an Assistant Professor of Communication Sciences and Disorders at The University of Texas at Austin where she teaches courses on articulation and language disorders in children. Dr. Bedore has research interests in the areas of child language and phonological development and disorders with a special interest in Spanish-speaking children. Her current research projects focus on morphological development in Spanish-speaking children with specific language impairment and in typically developing children. She has published in journals such as *Clinical Linguistics and Phonetics; Journal of Speech, Language, and Hearing Research;* and the *American Journal of Speech-Langugage Pathology.* Dr. Bedore serves as an editorial consultant in the area of language for the *Journal of Speech, Language, and Hearing Research* and for the *American Journal of Speech-Language Pathology.* Prior to pursuing doctoral studies, she supervised and taught in the area of speech-language pathology in Mexico City.

Mark E. Bernstein, Ed.D., is an Associate Professor of Communication Sciences and Disorders at The University of Texas at Austin. He has been a classroom teacher of deaf children, and his degree is in the area of applied psycholinguistics and child language acquisition. Dr. Bernstein's scholarly interests range from techniques for speech development in the deaf, to working with parents of hearing impaired children, to descriptive studies of the use of simultaneous communication, to language categories and lexical acquisition in children. Dr. Bernstein has published in *Applied Psycholinguistics, Sign Language Studies, The American Annals of the Deaf,* and the *Journal of Child Language,* among others. He serves on the editorial boards of *The American Annals of the Deaf* and the *Journal of Learning Disabilities* and has been a reviewer for *Language, Speech, and Hearing Services in Schools.* Dr. Bernstein was the recipient of the 1990–1991 College of Communication Teaching Excellence Award and the 1997–1998 Texas Excellence Teaching Award.

Craig A. Champlin, Ph.D., is an Associate Professor of Communication Sciences and Disorders at The University of Texas at Austin where he teaches courses in hearing science, instrumentation, electrophysiological audiometry, and hearing conservation. As a member of the Institute for Neuroscience, he also team-teaches a course that covers the principles of neuroscience. Dr.

Champlin's research focuses on physiological correlates of auditory perception, the effects of noise on hearing, temporal processing of sound, and otoacoustic emissions. He has received numerous research grants, most of which have targeted the study of auditory evoked potentials in humans. Dr. Champlin has published research articles in the *Journal of the Acoustical Society of America, Hearing Research,* the *Journal of Speech and Hearing Research,* and others. In addition, Dr. Champlin has been a consultant on projects dealing with community noise issues, hearing conservation education in children, and infant hearing screening.

Rodger M. Dalston, Ph.D., is the Amon G. Carter Jr. Professor of Communication Sciences and Disorders and Chair of the Department at The University of Texas at Austin. He is a Fellow of the American Speech-Language-Hearing Association and past President of the American Cleft Palate-Craniofacial Association. Dr. Dalston currently serves as an editorial consultant for the *Cleft Palate Journal* and the *American Journal of Orthodontics and Dentofacial Orthopedics.* He teaches courses in voice, research, and craniofacial anomalies. His research concerning the impact of craniofacial anomalies on communicative interactions has appeared in a number of journals, including *Journal of Plastic and Reconstructive Surgery, Journal of Prosthetic Dentistry, Folia Phoniatrica, Journal of Speech and Hearing Research, Cleft Palate Journal,* and the *Journal of Computer Uses in Speech Language Pathology.* Prior to joining the faculty in 1994, Dr. Dalston served on the faculty at Northwestern University for 11 years and subsequently held the position of Director of Speech and Language Pathology at the University of North Carolina Craniofacial Center for 15 years. He has received awards for teaching excellence at both institutions.

Barbara L. Davis, Ph.D., is an Associate Professor of Communication Sciences and Disorders at The University of Texas at Austin. Her major area of research involvement is acquisition of speech motor control in normally developing infants. She is co-principal investigator of an NIH grant to study early speech development in normally developing, hearing impaired, and speech delayed infants. Her other research interests include developmental apraxia and communication assessment with multicultural populations. Her research has appeared in journals such as *Journal of Speech, Language, and Hearing Research; Applied Psycholinguistics; Clinical Linguistics;* and *Phonetica.* Dr. Davis' teaching interests include phonological development and disorders, acoustic and perceptual phonetics, and infant-toddler intervention. She has won the Texas Excellence Teaching award, one of the most prestigious offered by the university.

Ronald B. Gillam, Ph.D., is an Associate Professor of Communication Sciences and Disorders at The University of Texas at Austin where he teaches courses in language development, language assessment and intervention, cognition, research methods, and language disorders in school-age children. His research concerns relationships among memory, phonological representation, and language development in school-age children with specific language impairments. He has also studied literacy development, language assessment practices, language intervention approaches, and narrative development. His research has been funded by the U.S. Department of Education and the National Institute on Deafness and Other Communication Disorders and has been published in the *Journal of Speech, Language, and Hearing Research;* the *American Journal of Speech-Language Pathology; Language, Speech, and Hearing Services in Schools;* the *Journal of Research in Childhood Education;* and the *Journal of Childhood Communication Disorders.* Dr. Gillam has edited two issues of *Topics in Language Disorders* that concerned memory, and he was an Associate Editor of the *American Journal of Speech-Language Pathology.*

Dena Granof, Ph.D., holds the position of lecturer in the Department of Communication Sciences and Disorders at The University of Texas at Austin where she teaches courses on dysphagia, multihandicapped populations, and language intervention. Prior to joining the faculty at the University of Texas, she was Director of Speech, Language and Cognitive Therapy for the Starbright Pediatric Rehabilitation Institute.

LaVae M. Hoffman, M.A., is a doctoral candidate and Sparrgrove Fellow at The University of Texas at Austin. She specializes in the design and production of multimedia software to support instructional objectives. Her research activities are related to information processing in children with language impairment, technologically based intervention, and pedagogical issues in communication sciences and disorders. Prior to her doctoral studies, she was a practicing speech-language pathologist for 12 years, a state and local educational program specialist, and a university clinical supervisor. Ms. Hoffman has produced and co-authored *Case Studies in Communication Sciences and Disorders,* an award-winning multimedia CD-ROM set highlighting language differences and disorders in children. Her primary clinical interests include preschool-age children with language impairments and developmentally appropriate practices in service delivery.

Janice E. Jackson, Ph.D., is an Assistant Professor of Communication Sciences and Disorders at The University of Texas at Austin where she teaches courses in language acquisition, multicultural assessment, and multicultural research. She recently completed a doctoral degree at the University of Massachusetts at Amherst and a postdoctoral appointment at Vanderbilt University. Her research focuses on child language development and disorders in African-American children. She has extensive experience as a speech-language pathologist in California, Georgia, and Massachusetts.

Thomas P. Marquardt, Ph.D., is the Ben F. Love Professor in Communication Sciences and Disorders at The University of Texas at Austin where he teaches courses in aphasia, dysarthria, differential diagnosis of communication disorders, and introduction to communication sciences and disorders. Dr. Marquardt's primary research interests are in developmental and acquired apraxia of speech and differential diagnosis of speech and language disorders subsequent to brain damage. The author of *Neurogenic Communication Disorders* and co-author of *Appraisal and Diagnosis of Speech and Language Disorders,* he has published articles in the *Journal of Speech and Hearing Research, Cortex,* and *Brain and Language* on topics such as compensatory articulation in Broca's aphasia, the effects of linguistic factors on speech errors in acquired apraxia, syntax in developmental apraxia, and intelligibility of voice output communication aids.

Frederick N. Martin, Ph.D., is the Lillie Hage Jamail Centennial Professor in Communication Sciences and Disorders. He has served on the faculty for more than 30 years. His publications include 14 single-authored books, 16 edited books, 19 book chapters, 114 journal articles, 100 conference and convention papers, and several monographs. Dr. Martin has won the Teaching Excellence Award of the College of Communication, the Graduate Teaching Award, and the

Texas Excellence Award for Academic Advising of the Ex-Students' Association, in addition to being the second-prize winner of the Beltone Award for Outstanding Teaching in Audiology. He is a Fellow of the American Speech-Language-Hearing Association and the American Academy of Audiology, from which he received the "Career Award in Hearing" in 1997. His research interests revolve around theories of bone conduction, pediatric diagnosis, and patient and parent counseling.

John A. Nelson, Ph.D., is an Assistant Professor of Communication Sciences and Disorders at The University of Texas at Austin. His research interests are in hearing aids, cochlear implants, digital signal processing, and temporal auditory processing. During his doctoral training, Dr. Nelson received the Student Investigator Award from the American Academy of Audiology to study auditory processing of temporal modulations. Dr. Nelson's research has been published in the *American Journal of Audiology, Journal of the American Academy of Audiology,* and the *Journal of Rehabilitation Research and Development.* He teaches undergraduate and graduate courses in amplification, auditory habilitation, and auditory rehabilitation. Prior to his doctoral studies, he had a clinical and research position with the Veterans Affairs Medical Center in Augusta, Georgia, and he worked in private practice in South Carolina.

Elizabeth D. Peña, Ph.D., holds the rank of Assistant Professor. Her expertise is in the area of assessment and assessment bias. Dr. Peña's research is in the area of dynamic assessment applied to bilingual (Spanish/English) preschool children. She is Co-Principal Investigator of a project funded by the National Institute of Deafness and Other Communicative Disorders to develop and validate a language test for Hispanic children speaking nonstandard English and Spanish. She was recently awarded the Mentored Clinical Scientist Development Award from the National Institutes of Health (NIDCD) to investigate the nature and measurement of modifiability in children.

Gene R. Powers, Ph.D., is Professor Emeritus at The University of Texas at Austin where he served as Director of the Program in Communication Sciences and Disorders. He was at the University of Connecticut for 13 years prior to joining the faculty at The University of Texas at Austin in 1974. During his academic career, Dr. Powers taught many courses including the introductory course, which he taught to several thousand students from 1961 until his retirement in 1993. Dr. Powers' research and publications were primarily in the areas of professional concerns and communication problems associated with cleft palate. He has been active in a number of professional organizations and was named Fellow in the American Speech-Language-Hearing Association (ASHA). He has served on a variety of ASHA committees and boards including the Ethical Practices Board. He was chair of the Education and Training Board, the predecessor of the Council on Academic Accreditation, and he chaired the American Boards of Examiners in Speech Pathology and Audiology, which is now called the Professional Standards Council. Dr. Powers served as a member of the Texas State Board of Examiners in Speech-Language Pathology and Audiology from 1990–1996 and served as chairman from 1994–1996.

CD-ROM: Volumes 1 and 2

Authored and Produced by LaVae M. Hoffman

There are two multimedia CD-ROMs that accompany this book. The highlights of the CD-ROMs include:

- A movie of an audiological evaluation
- Pictures of the ossicular chain and hearing aids that the student can manipulate using the mouse
- Demonstrations of hearing with and without amplification
- Video segments of individuals with articulation disorders, developmental language disorders, fluency disorders, aphasia, and dysarthria.
- A morphing sequence showing the development of the face and skull.
- Movies of an endoscopic evaluation.
- An adult with cerebral palsy communicating with an augmentative system.
- Video fluoroscopic images of normal and disordered swallows.

The system requirements for running the CD-ROMs are summarized in the following list. These CDs will run on Power Macintosh computers running MAC OS 7.1.2 (or later versions) or PC computers running Windows 95, Windows 98, or Windows NT system software. Users should be aware that the multimedia segments on these CDs require more memory than most other computer applications. Because the memory requirements of multimedia CD-ROMs are high, the CD-ROMs should only be run on computers that meet the minimum requirements listed. Because the memory requirements of multimedia CD-ROMs are high, the CD-ROMs may run slowly in computers with older operating systems or less memory. As a general rule, faster machines with more memory will run the program with less waiting time and better video and audio quality. Best results will be obtained if you listen to the segments through headphones or amplified external speakers. If students do not own the kinds of computers that are required to play the CD-ROMs, we hope more advanced computers will be available in computer labs at the college or university they attend.

Macintosh Operating System

A Power PC computer running at a minimum of 166 MHz (200 MHz or higher is recommended).

Windows Operating System

A computer that contains at least a Pentium I processor (Pentium Pro, Pentium II with MMX, or

Macintosh OS 7.1.2 or later.

A minimum of 32 MB of installed RAM (at least 64 MB of RAM is recommended).
An 8x CD-ROM drive or better.

At least 12 MB of available hard-disk space.
External speakers or headphones.

Pentium III processors are preferable) or equivalent running at a minimum of 166 MHz (200 MHz or higher is recommended).
Windows 95, Windows 98, or Windows NT 4.0 with Service Pack 3 or later system software.
A minimum of 32 MB of installed RAM (at least 64 MB of RAM is recommended).
An 8x CD-ROM drive or better.
Direct X version 3.0 or later.
At least 14 MB of available hard-disk space.
External speakers or headphones.
A SoundBlaster or compatible sound card.

The shaded boxes in the text refer the reader to segments on the CD-ROMs that illustrate or highlight information in the book. Students may want to play the CD-ROMs as they are reading, or they may want to read a chapter in its entirety before they view any of the segments. In either case, students should view the CD-ROM segments multiple times in order to better understand the examples that are provided.

 CD-ROM

CD-ROM Volumes 1 and 2

Volume 1 of the CD-ROM contains media that supports the information contained in Chapters 1 through 11. Volume 2 contains media that supports the information contained in Chapters 12 through 19.

Before You Start the CD-ROM

• Quit all other applications.

• If you have a Power Macintosh computer, turn the virtual memory off.

• Install Acrobat Reader.

For computers running **Mac OS:** Open the "Acrobat Reader 4.0" folder. Then double click on the "Reader Installer" file. Follow the instructions contained in the dialog boxes to complete the installation.

For computers running **Windows:** Open the "Acrobat4" folder. Then double click on the "ar40eng.exe" file. Follow the instructions contained in the dialog boxes to complete the installation.

• Install QuickTime 4.

For computers running **Mac OS:** Open the "QuickTime 4" folder. Double click on the "QuickTime 4 Installer" file. Follow the instructions contained in the dialog boxes to complete the installation. When prompted to choose installation type, select the "Full" installation. Where it asks for a Registration Number, leave the box blank. Restart your computer.

For computers running **Windows:** Open the "QT402" folder. Double click on the "QT4Inst.exe" file. Follow the instructions contained in the dialog boxes to complete the installation. Restart your computer.

Start the CD-ROM

• Double-click on the icon named, "CSD Vol. 1" or "CSD Vol. 2."

• Double-click on the icon for the chapter you are reading.

• Double-click on the movie icon that matches the number of the CD-ROM shaded box you are looking at (e.g., Ch.02.01). Some of the titles end with .mov and others end with .pdf. These letters designate whether the file is a QuickTime movie document (.mov) or an Acrobat Reader document (.pdf). If you install the QuickTime and Acrobat Reader applications onto your hard drive before you try to view the documents, the appropriate program should open when you double click on either type of file.

To Play Segments on the CD-ROMs

When you open the CD-ROMs, you will see a list of files and folders. Each chapter in the book that has corresponding media will have a folder on the CD-ROMs. There are some chapters, like Chapter 1, that do not have accompanying segments on the CD-ROMs. When you open the folder for a chapter, you will see a list of segments. Some of these segments are movies with video and audio, and some segments contain pictures but no sound. Simply double click on the segment you want to play, and it will open in QuickTime 4 or Adobe Acrobat Reader 4.0.

You can increase the size of the movies on your screen. When QuickTime 4 opens, click and hold the arrow in the bottom right corner of the QuickTime television set. Drag until the television set is the size you want. You can also double the size of the movie. When QuickTime 4 opens, go to the "Movie" menu and select "Double Size." The amount of information in the file does not change even though the size of the movie screen doubles. As a result, you will notice that the movies are "sharper" when you play them at the normal size. If you step back from the screen a little, even the larger-sized movies will look relatively sharp and clear.

Remember, the movies will play and sound a little differently on different types of computers. For example, we have found that the video looks darker on some computers than it does on others.

If the QuickTime player is not capable of accommodating the data requirements for a video, it will respond by maintaining the audio portion and dropping (or skipping) video frames. As a result, the movie will appear jerky or out of synch with the audio. The most likely cause of this situation is playing the movies on a computer that doesn't have adequate memory available or the appropriate processor speed. If your computer has not been restarted for a while, it may have less available memory. Be certain to restart your computer occasionally for this reason.

If your computer is not capable of reading the data fast enough, it may be helpful to copy the movie to the hard drive and play it from there. To conserve space, the movie should be deleted from the hard drive when you are finished playing it.

We recommend that you open and play only one movie at a time. This will maximize the memory and processing capabilities of your computer. If multiple movies are open at the same time, you will likely experience a degradation in visual quality and playback performance.

We hope you enjoy these movies and learn as much from them as we have.

Dedication

To the memory of Tracy Clark and Jennifer Sparrgrove,
two of our favorite students who would be two of our favorite
colleagues had their lives not ended much too early.

1

GENERAL CONSIDERATIONS

1

Communication Sciences and Disorders: The Discipline

Gene R. Powers

1 To understand the discipline of communication sciences and disorders.

2 To learn the evolution and history of the discipline and the professions of speech, language, and hearing science; speech-language pathology; and audiology, and to project the kinds of changes in these professions that might be expected in the future.

3 To learn about the educational background and professional activities of speech, language, and hearing scientists; speech-language pathologists; and audiologists.

4 To understand the regulation of the professions of audiology and speech-language pathology by state agencies and professional organizations.

---

5 To learn about the Code of Ethics and how ethics are enforced for the professions in communication sciences and disorders.

THE DISCIPLINE

There are many children and adults who have difficulties speaking and hearing. In fact, in the United States today, there are approximately 46 million people who have some type of a communication disorder (National Institute of Deafness and Other Communication Disorders, 1995). Some of these individuals were born with conditions like deafness (an inability to hear sounds), or cleft palate (a large opening in the roof of the mouth). Others acquired their difficulties as a result of diseases (like meningitis) or accidents. Fortunately, there are specialists who can offer help to people with communication disorders and their families. These specialists are called audiologists; speech-language pathologists; and speech, language, and hearing scientists. These are professions within the discipline of communication sciences and disorders.

A **discipline** is a unique area of study, but a **profession** is an area of practice. The discipline of **communication sciences and disorders (CSD)** encompasses the study of human communication processes, breakdowns in those processes (referred to as communication differences and disorders), and the efficacy of practices involved in assessing and assisting individuals with communication differences and disorders. The major components of the discipline are speech, language, and hearing sciences; audiology; and speech-language pathology. Deafness studies (studies of communication processes among individuals who are deaf) and deaf education (education and rehabilitation of individuals with severe to profound hearing impairments) are related areas that are included in this textbook. These components are not mutually exclusive since some professionals may be engaged in activities related to one, two, or even all five of these interest areas.

There are many factors that justify the need for CSD, and there are many beneficiaries of the research and practices that occur within the discipline. Research in human communication processes can add greatly to our understanding of how people interact with one another, solve problems, and process information. Individuals with impairments in language, speech, or hearing can benefit substantially from the services provided by audiologists, speech-language pathologists, and deaf educators.

Communication sciences and disorders is a relatively new field of study and practice. Earlier in the 20th century, this area was completely unknown. Even now, many people are unfamiliar with the discipline, the professions of audiology and speech-language pathology, and the terminology related to communication disorders.

Evolution and History of the Discipline

The widespread use of the descriptor, communication sciences and disorders, to identify the discipline is quite recent—probably no more than 15 or 20 years. The terms *speech pathology* and *audiology* have longer histories. Even these terms, however, are recent in comparison to professional titles such as psychologist, sociologist, journalist, architect, teacher, and lawyer. According to Moeller (1976), the first use of the term speech pathology occurred in the 1920s and appeared for perhaps the first time in print in a University of Iowa catalogue for the 1924–1925 academic year. The term was used by Lee Edward Travis (1931) in a course description for clinical psychology of speech. The addition of *language* to form the word speech-language pathology occurred later when it became obvious that professionals were dealing with much more than just the process of speech production.

The word *audiology* was coined during World War II by Drs. Ray Carhart and Norton Canfield to describe a new science that focused on the aural rehabilitation of individuals who suffered war-related hearing loss (Newby, 1958). World War II was a catalyst for the advancement of the field of audiology, and it fostered a union of audiology and speech pathology. Both professions began conducting research and providing clinical services to service personnel during that period.

Early leaders in the field, such as Travis, stressed the importance of basing treatment on sound research. The early emphasis on scientific problem solving in the laboratory, the classroom, and the clinical setting has become a hallmark of the discipline of communication sciences and disorders. Like Travis, we believe it is critical that all assessment and treatment decisions should be based on sound scientific principles and research findings. There are times when it appears that professional concerns dealing with service delivery obscure the importance of basic and applied research in the discipline. A critical concern for the discipline is that there has been a dramatic increase in the number of practitioners within the professions, but the number of individuals engaged in research in human communication and its disorders has failed to keep pace. We hope students who read this book will become fascinated with the discipline and will seriously consider pursuing research careers.

CHARACTERISTICS OF THE DISCIPLINE

The discipline of communication sciences and disorders has drawn heavily from a number of other fields such as psychology, medicine, linguistics, education, rehabilitation, anatomy, and physiology. These disciplines have contributed significantly to our understanding of human communication and have served as the basis for thinking about communication disorders. Research in communication sciences and disorders is conducted in a variety of locations. Diversity is also reflected in the settings in which speech-language pathologists practice, which include schools, preschools, hospitals, rehabilitation agencies, and nursing homes. The diversity adds to the intrigue of the field and makes it an attractive career choice for individuals with widely varied interests.

THE PROFESSIONS

The American Speech-Language-Hearing Association (ASHA) is the primary scholarly and professional organization for individuals in the field of communication sciences and disorders. ASHA considers communication sciences and disorders to be a single discipline with two separate professions: audiology and speech-language pathology. It seems reasonable, however, to consider speech, language, and hearing sciences as another professional entity even though direct service delivery in not a part of this endeavor. Those involved in education of the deaf or hearing impaired represent another important professional constituency. Since these individuals are not usually a part of CSD programs, however, they will not be included in this discussion.

Speech, Language, and Hearing Sciences

Communication sciences would logically encompass more than just the study of human communication processes. For example, studies in mass communication and in engineering relating to transmission and transfer of signals clearly fall in the realm of communication sciences. For our purposes, we will consider speech, language, and hearing sciences as the investigation of anatomical, physiological, and perceptual factors that form the bases of and contribute to the production and comprehension of speech and language. Obviously, some of the research would be directed to exploring phenomena other than speech and language, per se. For example, learning more about how humans process auditory, visual, and other stimuli of all kinds is likely to shed light on how we communicate.

Speech, language, and hearing scientists come from a variety of educational backgrounds. Some individuals are primarily speech scientists, others are hearing scientists, and others are language scientists. Because of this diversity, it is difficult, if not impossible, to define the limits of CSD scientists. Suffice it to say, however, that the majority have strong backgrounds in the sciences and hold advanced degrees, most often a Ph.D. (Doctor of Philosophy). The degrees may be awarded in areas such as acoustics, anatomy and physiology, biological sciences, communication sciences and disorders, education, linguistics, physics, psychology, or speech communication. Because speech, language, and hearing scientists are so diverse, it is almost impossible to trace the history of this area of study. Clearly, research on human communication processes occurred long before the professions of audiology and speech-language pathology existed and before courses entitled speech science or hearing science were offered in any university.

The majority of people engaged in speech, language, and hearing sciences work in university settings. However, some scientists in CSD work for governmental agencies like the Veterans Administration or for independent operations such as Bell Telephone and Haskins Laboratories. The primary activity of these scientists is research and teaching. Some are engaged in research that deals exclusively with the normal processes of communication. Others conduct research on both normal and disordered communication (Figure 1–1).

The goals and objectives of the speech, language, and/or hearing scientist focus on discovering and better understanding human communication processes. Regardless of the underlying objectives, however, basic research about communication will undoubtedly be of value to professionals in speech-language pathology and audiology and individuals with communication differences and disorders who they serve.

It is vital that the practicing professional stay abreast of current research results in order to provide the best possible services. There has been general

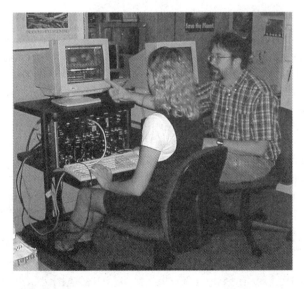

Figure 1–1. Two hearing scientists preparing stimuli for a study of speech perception.

agreement within our discipline that a firm grounding in normal communication processes is necessary in order to pursue any of the professions. As a result, a course of study emphasizing science is an integral part of the curriculum in CSD. Coursework with titles such as hearing science, speech science, language science, language acquisition, neurolinguistics, psychoacoustics, and psycholinguistics are regular offerings in CSD departments and programs. Many of these courses occur early in the academic program so that students will have the prerequisite knowledge they need in order to understand breakdowns in communication, ways to analyze those breakdowns, and ways to help individuals with communication breakdowns.

Speech-Language Pathology

Speech-language pathology is practiced in a variety of work environments. It is estimated that there were more than 100,000 professional speech-language pathologists in 1999. It is amazing that there were fewer than 5,000 such practitioners 50 years ago. These professionals assess and treat a variety of individuals with speech and/or language disorders. Speech disorders include problems in speech sound production or articulation, fluency, and voice, whereas language disorders are characterized by difficulties in the use or comprehension of the symbolic aspects of communication. Chapter 4 provides a brief overview of these disorders, and later chapters summarize what is known about communication disorders and the principal ways of assessing and treating them.

History of the Profession

Speech-language pathology developed from interests in disorders of speech, particularly stuttering. Much of the early research was aimed at discovering the causes of stuttering, but soon attention was directed to providing remedial services to individuals with various types of speech problems. As early as the 1920s, academic courses in "speech correction" were offered in some universities. Clinical sites for providing services to individuals with problems in speech and language, however, were limited. Initially, the vast majority of such services were provided at college and university clinics that were developed primarily as training facilities. Increasingly, however, service programs were developed in medical settings and the public schools.

Speech-language pathology professionals who practiced in the medical environment were usually called speech therapists; those who practiced in the public school setting were often called speech correctionists or speech teachers. Malone (1979) reported that speech-language pathologists (SLPs) have been identified by nearly 100 different titles. Although the term speech pathologist was introduced early in the development of the field and was widely used by those in the profession for many years, the term, speech therapist, is probably the title that is most often used by the general public. Some believe that this label is unfortunate since other professionals such as physicians often prescribe the activities of a therapist. Speech-language pathologists (SLPs) do not work under a physician's orders. We conduct our own evaluations, determine who is and who is not eligible for intervention, prescribe our own treatment, and deliver our own services.

The title, speech-language pathologist, was adopted by the American Speech and Hearing Association in 1976. The term *language* was added to the official title because much of the work being done by CSD professionals covered the areas of symbolic language (what is said and understood) and speech production (how it is said). The term *pathologist* was selected to emphasize that CSD professionals prescribe and deliver their own treatment. Thus, although rather cumbersome, the designator of choice has become speech-language pathologist, which is often shortened to SLP.

Work Settings and Populations Served

Speech-language pathology (SLP) services are provided in ever-widening work settings, with a resultant increase in the variety of patient populations served. Elementary and secondary school systems continue to be the largest employer of SLPs, although the number of professionals employed in other settings is rising quickly. Increasingly, SLP services are being conducted in infant and early childhood programs housed in state agencies and public schools. Medical settings that employ SLPs include hospitals, rehabilitation centers, and freestanding speech and hearing centers. Nursing homes and home health care units also provide employment opportunities for the SLP. One of the most dramatic increases in work settings for SLPs in the last two or three decades has been in the area of private practice. The way private practice is carried out is variable and offers many possibilities to the practitioner. Given the variety of environments in which SLPs work, it should not be surprising that the age ranges of individuals served by SLPs extend from birth to old age. Of course, individuals from all ethnic groups and economic levels receive speech and language services (Figure 1–2). Further characteristics of the individuals who are served by SLPs are considered in more detail in Chapter 4.

Academic Preparation

It is ASHA's official policy that a master's degree should be the minimum qualification for working as a speech-language pathologist. Many states have licensure laws that make it illegal for individuals who do not have a master's degree to call themselves speech-language pathologists. Licensure and required credentials for professional practice are considered in greater detail later in this chapter.

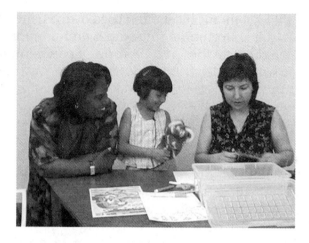

Figure 1–2. Two speech-language pathologists collecting a language sample from a child.

Scope of Practice

The term, *scope of practice,* refers to the types of activities that SLPs should engage in. Given the diversity of settings where SLPs work, it should not be surprising that their scope of practice is broad and varied. Initially, much of the practice in the area of speech-language pathology was directed toward individuals with disorders of speech. For many years, SLPs have also provided services to individuals with language problems resulting from brain damage from strokes or accidents. In recent decades, there has been a dramatic shift to treating developmental language delays and disorders in children. This change is due, in part, to the fact that numerous subtle language problems, particularly among children, previously went undetected until children went to school. The scope of practice has also been expanded to include cognitive training and treatment of swallowing disorders in elderly individuals. Both of these areas may be included in the scope of practice of other professions such as neuropsychology or occupational therapy. At the other end of the age continuum, the scope of practice has expanded to include language stimulation and assisting parents of high-risk infants and toddlers. For those of us who have been in the field for many years, the expanded scopes of practice are truly remarkable.

Audiology

Audiology is a widely recognized profession that is practiced in many different work environments. Audiologists are professionals who study, assess, and treat individuals who have hearing impairments. Some are engaged in evaluation and diagnosis of hearing loss; others provide educational and/or rehabilitative services. The number of professional audiologists has increased significantly in the past 50 years, but there are far fewer audiologists than SLPs. It has been estimated that there are between 15,000 and 20,000 practicing audiologists in the United States today.

History of the Profession

Audiology was first identified as an area of scientific study and professional practice during World War II. According to Newby (1958), audiology grew out of the merging of speech pathology and otology during World War II in what were called aural rehabilitation centers. **Otology** is the medical specialty that deals with ear disease and the peripheral hearing mechanism. Obviously, there were professionals working with the hearing impaired prior to the 1940s, most notably those who specialized in the education of the deaf and hearing impaired, but the professional field of audiology was not in existence before that time. Early in its development, audiology related more to speech pathology than it did to otology. As a result, academic training, research, and clinical activities encompassing both audiology and speech pathology were initiated. For example, in 1947, the American Speech Correction Association became the American Speech and Hearing Association, and the *Journal of Speech Disorders* became the *Journal of Speech and Hearing Disorders*.

Work Settings and Populations Served

Since the beginning of the profession, most audiologists have been employed in medical environments such as physician's offices, hospitals, and rehabilitation centers. Other audiologists, sometimes referred to as educational or habilitative audiologists, are employed in educational facilities such as public schools or schools for the deaf or hearing impaired. Increasing numbers of audiologists own private practices where they dispense hearing aids and other devices. The activities of audiologists are influenced by their employment setting. For example, audiologists employed by physicians spend most of their time evaluating patients to determine the nature and extent of hearing loss and the potential benefits of amplification. Audiologists employed in educational or rehabilitation centers are more likely to provide both assessment and rehabilitative services.

The populations served by audiologists vary in age from the newborn to the very elderly. The audiologist may evaluate and/or provide remediation to such divergent individuals as those who have mild, perhaps temporary, hearing losses to those with profound, permanent hearing losses. People with no hearing impairment are often tested by audiologists. You have probably received a hearing test at some point in your life, and the examiner may well have been an audiologist (Figure 1–3).

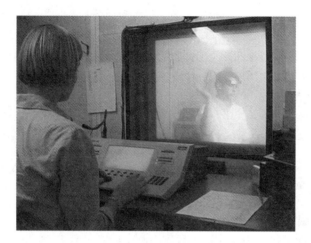

Figure 1–3. An audiologist administers a hearing test.

Academic Preparation

Just as in speech-language pathology, the policy of ASHA is that a master's degree in audiology is the minimal level of education for an individual to practice as an independent professional. Satisfactory completion of specified coursework and clinical practice as part of the degree is also necessary. Other requirements to qualify for professional credentials exist and will be considered later in this chapter.

Currently, plans are underway to require a clinical doctorate in audiology (called the AuD) as the minimum criterion for entry into the profession. This requirement is set to take effect in the year 2012. Many hurdles remain before these plans can be implemented, and it is difficult to predict with any certainty when, how, and if the changes in the entry criterion will occur.

Scope of Practice

Audiologists have traditionally been engaged in the evaluation of the extent and type of hearing loss, assessment of the benefits of amplification, and habilitation and rehabilitation of those who exhibit hearing deficiencies. Early in the history of the profession, there were limitations as to what activities could be used to accomplish assessment and treatment objectives. For example, it was once considered unethical for audiologists to sell or dispense hearing aids or other amplification devices. This ethical position has changed and, presently, dispensing of hearing aids is a major part of audiological practice.

Another recent change in an audiologist's scope of practice relates to infant hearing screening. Several states have enacted legislation requiring universal auditory screening of newborn infants. The legislation will probably be expanded to many other states in the coming years. As a result of new legis-lation and the development of more sophisticated auditory tests for infants and other difficult-to-test clients, more audiologists are engaging in newborn and high-risk infant testing.

An important scope-of-practice issue for audiology has to do with what physicians stake out as exclusively within their own scope of practice. For example, it has long been the position of the American Medical Association that invasive intrusions into the body or any body cavity for diagnostic or treatment purposes is limited to the physician. This position has created dif-ficulties, at times, for audiologists when they are doing certain types of hear-ing testing. Cerumen (ear wax) that is impacted in the ear canal can interfere with hearing testing. If the audiologist is unable to remove the cerumen be-cause its removal is considered an invasive procedure, the result would be an unnecessary referral to a physician for a minor procedure that could easily be accomplished by the audiologist. As a result, many states now include ceru-men management as part of the legal scope of practice for audiologists.

Another new activity that is included within the scope of audiological practice relates to testing balance disorders that may be caused, in part, by inner ear problems. Without a doubt, the scope of practice for audiology will continue to expand as new needs are identified and new technology is developed.

REGULATION OF THE PROFESSIONS

Consumers want to know that persons who present themselves as physicians, lawyers, speech-language pathologists, or audiologists (to name just a few service-oriented professions) have received an appropriate level of training in their area. Just as you would not want to be operated on by a physician who failed medical school, you would not want to be fitted for a hearing aid by someone whose education and training consisted of a 10-page correspon-dence course on hearing aids from the Quickie School of Easy Degrees. Poor services by SLPs and audiologists can cause real harm. To protect the public interest, audiology and speech-language pathology must be regulated.

There are basically two ways in which individual professionals are regu-lated: **licensure** and **certification.** For the purposes of this discussion, li-censure will refer to fully credentialed speech-language pathologists and audiologists as defined by an individual state. In the case of licensure, a state government passes an act (a law) that creates a set of minimum criteria for practicing as a professional in that state. Most licensure acts also create state-funded licensure boards of examiners who manage the law through writing implementation rules and monitoring the process and the licensees.

State licensure of speech-language pathology and audiology is relatively new. Florida adopted the first licensure act for speech-language pathology and audiology in 1969. Since that time there has been a steady increase in the number of states that regulate speech-language pathology and audiology. Presently, there are 41 states that license both SLPs and audiologists. Several other states regulate speech-language pathology or audiology, but not both.

Certification is somewhat different from licensure in that the standards are developed and administered by professional organizations or state agencies. In the case of speech-language pathology and audiology, this function is assumed by standards boards affiliated with ASHA. These boards also set criteria and monitor **accreditation** of academic programs and facilities providing clinical services in communication sciences and disorders.

Licensure and Certification Standards

The American Speech-Language-Hearing Association (ASHA) developed a standards program to certify individuals in speech-language pathology and audiology at a time when there were no state regulations and no licensure laws related to these professions. Had there been appropriate licensing in each state, it would have been less important for ASHA to develop standards. As it turned out, the certification standards ASHA adopted have became the model for most licensure laws. A person may be certified by ASHA and licensed in a state (or multiple states) in either speech-language pathology or audiology. It is also possible to obtain dual certification (both speech-language pathology and audiology) and/or licensure.

Speech-language pathologists can obtain the **Certificate of Clinical Competence (CCC)** in either profession from ASHA. To obtain the Certificate of Clinical Competence (CCC), the applicant must have earned a master's degree or a higher degree with a major emphasis in speech-language pathology, audiology, or both. The content areas of coursework are specified, and it is further required that students satisfactorily complete supervised clinical practice during their education. Both credentials require that the applicants obtain a passing score on a national, standardized examination and that they complete a 9-month internship or clinical fellowship year (CFY) under supervision.

It is important for practicing SLPs and audiologists to have the Certificate of Clinical Competence (CCC) as well as a state license. These credentials assure the consumer that the professional has met appropriate educational and practical prerequisites. In addition, professionals who provide speech-language pathology or audiology services often need to have the CCC in order to be reimbursed for their services. Federal laws and regulations have been adopted that require that all Medicare or Medicaid speech-language pathology or audiology services must be provided or supervised by a person holding the CCC. A number of insurance carriers who reimburse for these services have adopted similar requirements. Agencies, including public school programs, that receive reimbursement for these services must assure that they are provided by qualified personnel as defined by the regulations. These regulations have a major impact on funding and are a strong incentive for agencies to hire qualified personnel.

Although similar in most major aspects, there are a number of areas where the specific requirements for state licensure and the CCC differ. For example, at present ASHA does not require **continuing education units (CEUs)** to maintain the CCC. However, many states require that continuing education units (CEUs) be completed annually before a license can be renewed. Renewal of the ASHA certificate is automatic if the dues and fees are paid. On the other hand, state licenses are issued on an annual basis in most cases and thus must be renewed each year. In those states that require continuing education, the renewal application must include evidence of the satisfactory completion of CEUs.

ETHICS

The principles of conduct governing an individual or a group are called **ethics.** Generally, we think of ethics as a measure of what is the moral or "right thing to do" whether or not it is legal. For those professionals who serve the public, one of the overriding considerations is that the activities engaged in are in the best interest of the consumer and not the provider. Obviously, there may be differences of opinion about what constitutes ethical behavior. Therefore, most professional groups, including ASHA, have developed official codes of ethics (American Speech-Language-Hearing Association, 1994). Table 1–1 summarizes the principles of ethics that have been adopted by ASHA.

Codes of ethics are subject to change as new issues arise or as views as to what constitutes ethical behavior are modified. For example, at one time it was considered unethical in many professions to advertise. In most instances, that view no longer holds, partly in response to consumer demands for more information about the professionals. Sometimes, there is a fine line as to what is in poor taste and what is unethical.

People may well have different beliefs as to what constitutes ethical and unethical behavior. Therefore, enforcement of ethical practices may be problematic. Among professional organizations, including ASHA, once a code of ethics has been adopted by the membership the organization must assume the responsibility of enforcing the code. The Ethical Practices Board (EPB) of ASHA is charged with enforcing the code of ethics. Once an individual member has been found to have violated the code, a number of disciplinary actions are available to the Ethical Practices Board (EPB). The most severe penalty open to the EPB is stripping the person of membership and certification. Once this penalty has been imposed, the individual may or may not continue to practice in the field, depending on the employer and whether or not the state where the practice is being conducted has a licensure law.

Table 1–1. Principles of Ethics and Representative Rules of Ethics From the Code of Ethics of the American Speech-Language-Hearing Association

Principle I—Individuals shall honor their responsibility to hold paramount the welfare of persons they serve professionally.

- Individuals shall provide all services competently

- Individuals shall use every resource, including referral, to ensure that high-quality services are provided.

- Individuals shall not discriminate on the delivery of professional services on the basis of race, sex, age, religion, national origin, sexual orientation, or handicapping condition.

- Individuals shall not reveal, without authorization, any professional or personal information about the person served professionally, unless required by law to do so or unless doing so is necessary to protect the welfare of the person or of the community.

Principle II—Individuals shall honor their responsibility to achieve and maintain the highest level of professional competence.

- Individuals shall engage in only those aspects of the professions that are within the scope of their competence considering their level of education, training, and experience.

- Individuals shall continue their professional development throughout their careers.

Principle III—Individuals shall honor their responsibility to the public by promoting public understanding of the professions, by supporting the development of services designed to fulfill the unmet needs of the public, and by providing accurate information in all communications involving any aspect of the professions.

- Individuals shall not misrepresent their credentials, competence, education, training, or experience.

- Individuals shall not misrepresent diagnostic information, services rendered, or products dispensed or engage in any scheme or artifice to defraud in connection with obtaining payment or reimbursement for such services or products.

Principle IV—Individuals shall honor their responsibilities to the professions and their relationships with colleagues, students, and members of allied professions. Individuals shall uphold the dignity and autonomy of the profession, maintain harmonious interprofessional and intraprofessional relationships, and accept the professions self-imposed standards.

- Individuals shall not engage in dishonesty, fraud, deceit, misrepresentation, or any form of conduct that adversely reflects on the professions or on the individual's fitness to serve persons professionally.

- Individuals' statements to colleagues about professional services, research results, and products shall adhere to prevailing professional standards and shall contain no misrepresentations.

- Individuals who have reason to believe that the Code of Ethics has been violated shall inform the Ethical Practice Board.

Source: From "Code of Ethics of the American Speech-Language-Hearing Association," 1994, *Asha,* (Supplement). Reprinted with permission.

Most states that have adopted licensure laws have included codes of ethics similar to the ASHA Code of Ethics. Furthermore, state boards of examiners have the authority to legally enforce the codes, which means that those found in violation may be unable to practice professionally in their state. Sharing of information among the states and with ASHA is critical to protect the public from unethical practitioners.

SUPPORT PERSONNEL

During the past decade, there have been concerns about the shortage of qualified professionals and the rising costs of delivery of health care services and educational services. Both of these concerns have created an impetus for the utilization of **support personnel** who are individuals with less training who perform some duties under the supervision of licensed and certified SLPs and audiologists. It has also been argued that many of the activities of professionals, including classroom teachers, physicians, nurses, physical therapists, as well as audiologists and speech-language pathologists, can be performed just as well by individuals with less formal training. Obviously, utilizing such individuals would result in cost saving and presumably more efficiency. As a result, there has been a proliferation of support personnel in many professions in recent years. Support personnel qualifications in some professions, such as nurse's aides, licensed practical nurses, and physical therapy assistants, are fairly uniform and well established across the United States. This is not the case in audiology and speech-language pathology, although much discussion in ASHA and at the state levels is occurring with regard to support personnel. In all probability, the use of support personnel in these professions will expand in the future.

Defining the roles and regulating support personnel is difficult, at best. If we are to serve clients in an optimal way, it is critical that support personnel engage only in activities for which they are fully qualified and that they are well supervised by competent professionals. Suffice it to say that the issue of support personnel in speech-language pathology and audiology is in a fluid state at the present time. ASHA has developed guidelines for speech-language pathology assistants (but not for audiology assistants) that specify an associate degree and certain coursework and clinical practice. Implementation of these guidelines is currently under study. Several states, including Kentucky, Louisiana, and Texas, have licensed speech-language pathology assistants and audiology assistants. These states require assistants to have a baccalaureate degree plus some experience. The specific requirements for support personnel may vary among states, and some licensure laws do not deal with support personnel at all. It behooves those interested in such positions to know what is required in the state in which they reside. It is likely that there will be many changes in this area in the coming years.

PROFESSIONAL AND SCHOLARLY ASSOCIATIONS

American Speech-Language-Hearing Association

The American Speech-Language-Hearing Association (ASHA) serves as the primary professional and scholarly home for speech, language, and hearing scientists; speech-language pathologists; and audiologists. ASHA is a large organization (approximately 100,000 members and growing) with headquarters in Rockville, Maryland, near the nation's capital. ASHA engages in numerous activities designed to serve the needs of its members as well as individuals with communication disorders. Some of these activities include research dissemination, public relations, and lobbying for CSD professionals and the public they serve.

Another useful function of ASHA is making information available to its members and other interested individuals, including students. There is a toll free number, 1-888-321-2724, for all kinds of information about the organization, the discipline, and the professions. ASHA also maintains a web site, <www.asha.org>, with a vast amount of data that are continually updated. ASHA also sponsors an annual convention and many local workshops that provide members and students with important information about new research results and clinical procedures.

Publications

One of the important functions of ASHA is to provide information to its members through research and professional publications. There are several scholarly and professional journals published by ASHA on a regular basis. These include the *Journal of Speech, Language and Hearing Research*, the *American Journal of Audiology*, the *American Journal of Speech-Language Pathology*, and *Language, Speech, and Hearing Services in the Schools*. In addition, there are a number of newsletters published regularly, including the *ASHA Leader*, that address many important issues.

The ASHA Standards Program

The association has long operated a standards program that certifies individuals within the professions, accredits academic programs and clinical facilities, and maintains a code of ethics. The principal purpose of the standards program is the protection of the consumer. The Council on Professional Standards, which is semiautonomous, administers the **certification** of individuals and the **accreditation** of clinical facilities. Recently, another somewhat independent council, the Council on Academic Accreditation in Speech-Language Pathology and Audiology, was established to accredit and monitor academic programs in speech-language pathology and audiology.

Accreditation of academic programs in the areas of speech-language pathology and audiology is an important consideration for students who are considering majoring in one of these areas. A student must graduate from an accredited academic program in order to be certified by ASHA or licensed in most states. Therefore, it is critical that potential applicants for graduate programs in speech-language pathology or audiology know the accreditation status of the colleges or universities they are interested in attending.

A department or program in CSD may be accredited in speech-language pathology and/or audiology. Accreditation applies only to the master's level programs, although undergraduate courses and experiences are taken into consideration. Currently, there is no accreditation of doctoral level programs in the discipline, and it is highly unlikely that there ever will be for Ph.D. programs or other research doctoral degrees. However, should the Doctor of Audiology (AuD) be adopted as the entry level degree for the professional audiologist, accreditation of AuD programs would probably follow.

American Academy of Audiology

There are several associations comprised almost exclusively of audiologists or that include subgroups of audiologists. Examples of those organizations are the Academy of Dispensing Audiologists, the Academy of Rehabilitative Audiologists, and the Educational Audiology Association. The American Academy of Audiology (AAA) was created to address the needs of all audiologists. The Academy has grown rapidly to 5,000 members since it was founded in 1994. The goal of the Acadamy is to provide an organization specifically for audiologists (Hood, 1994). Some of the activities in place or planned by AAA are also carried out by ASHA. Examples include approving and monitoring continuing education experiences for members and certifying audiologists. AAA also sponsors annual conventions and various publications.

OTHER RELATED ORGANIZATIONS

There are other professional and scholarly associations that serve the needs of individuals within the professions and the discipline. For example, many SLPs and audiologists who are active in the speech and hearing sciences participate in the American Acoustical Society. Other organizations, such as the American Cleft Palate-Craniofacial Association and the Academy of Aphasia, serve the needs of members of ASHA who specialize in certain areas of practice. All 50 states have associations that are affiliated with ASHA and that sponsor annual conventions and various publications. In addition, there are regional and local associations that can be an excellent source of information.

In 1999, there were over 30 organizations officially listed with the American Speech-Language-Hearing Association as Allied and Related Professional Organizations (RPOs). Many of these represent special interest groups, such as presidents of state associations or supervisors in school settings. One related professional organization that is of special interest to students is the National Student Speech-Language-Hearing Association (NSSLHA), founded in 1972. The association is open to both undergraduate and graduate students majoring in any of the areas of communication sciences and disorders. Many academic programs in CSD have local chapters of the National Student Speech-Language-Hearing Association (NSSLHA). Because the organization is officially recognized by ASHA, there are many advantages in being a member. Some of these advantages include receiving a special journal for the National Student Speech-Language-Hearing Association (NSSLHA) plus one other ASHA publication. Members of NSSLHA also are afforded reduced rates at annual conventions and have access to ASHA's Employment Referral Center.

A Look Into the Future

The development of the discipline of communication sciences and disorders and the professions of speech-language pathology; audiology; and the speech, language and hearing sciences has been so dramatic during the 20th century that is it difficult to predict what lies ahead for the 21st century. We have every reason to hope and expect that research into the basic human communication processes and disorders of communication will expand our knowledge in many areas. This new knowledge could be beneficial in the prevention, evaluation, and treatment of a myriad of disabilities. It is not unreasonable to expect that some conditions that contribute to communication disorders, such as cleft palate and spina bifida, may be successfully corrected in utero. Reversal of certain kinds of hearing loss and neurological problems are also strong possibilities. Clinical research may reveal far more efficient ways to treat a variety of problems of communication.

There seems little doubt that the scope of practice for both speech-language pathologists and audiologists will continue to expand. This may well lead to accelerated development of credentials in areas of specialization. Specialization, particularly in speech-language pathology, has been a reality for many years, and recognition and credentials for the specialist have been studied for most of that time. Nonetheless, a uniform and generally accepted method of recognizing the specialist has yet to be developed. In all probability, this need will be more fully addressed early in the 21st century.

We also can anticipate that there will be a continued expansion of services to underserved populations in both urban and remote areas. Support personnel, if used wisely, may be of great benefit in accomplishing these expanded services. Technology, such as variations of telemedicine and use of the Internet, will be useful in meeting the needs of clients in rural areas where there are shortages of qualified personnel. Distance learning also is likely to be utilized more often to alleviate some of the shortages in qualified practitioners.

The past development of the discipline of communication sciences and disorders has been impressive and has resulted in attracting outstanding people into the professions. As the public has become more aware of the contributions that professionals in this area can make, recruitment into the professions has accelerated. The future of the discipline of communication sciences and disorders and the professions it includes is bright indeed.

SUMMARY

Communication sciences and disorders (CSD) is a discipline that consists of three professions: audiology; speech-language pathology; and speech, language, and hearing sciences. These professionals study and treat individuals with a variety of disorders that affect speech, language, and hearing abilities.

Information about the professions in terms of scopes of practice, academic preparation, work settings, and populations served was provided. Speech, language, and hearing scientists study basic communication processes and the nature of speech, language, and/or hearing disorders. Most scientists work in university settings, although some work in hospitals as well. Speech-language pathologists (SLPs) assess and treat speech and language disorders in infants, toddlers, preschoolers, school-age children, and adults. They may work in medical or educational settings. Audiologists primarily test hearing and prescribe and fit hearing aids. Most audiologists work in medical settings, although many have established their own private practices.

SLPs and audiologists are regulated through certification by the American Speech-Language-Hearing Association (ASHA) and by state agencies. Professionals who obtain a master's degree, pass a national examination, and complete a Clinical Fellowship Year (CFY) are eligible for the Certificate of Clinical Competency (CCC) from ASHA. These same kinds of experiences are often required for obtaining a state license. Some services are provided by support personal, who have less formal training than certified and/or licensed SLPs and audiologists. Support personnel, including speech therapy assistants and audiology assistants, are not uniformly regulated across states.

ASHA is the primary scholarly and professional home for the discipline. It publishes journals that disseminate research findings, promotes the professions in the media, and lobbies for CSD professionals and the public they serve. The association also operates a standards program that certifies individuals within the professions, accredits academic programs and clinical facilities, and maintains a code of ethics. Students can also join other professional organizations such as the American Academy of Audiology (AAA) and the National Student Speech-Language-Hearing Association (NSSLHA).

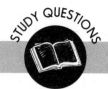

STUDY QUESTIONS

1 How does a discipline differ from a profession?

---

2 How do speech, language, and hearing scientists benefit from the professions of speech-language pathology and audiology?

---

3 What is meant by scope of practice as it relates to speech-language pathology and audiology?

---

4 How did World War II impact communication sciences and disorders?

---

5 What did Travis mean when he stated that the laboratory should precede the classroom and the clinic?

---

6 What are the different ways of regulating the professions of speech-language pathology and audiology?

---

7 What are the differences between certification and licensure?

---

8 How would you define ethical practice and how do you think it should be monitored?

---

9 What are the important functions of the American Speech-Language-Hearing Association?

REFERENCES

American Speech-Language-Hearing Association. (1994). Code of ethics. *Asha, 36* (March, Suppl. 13), 1–2.

Hood, L. J. (1994). The American Academy of Audiology: Unifying and working for the profession of audiology. *Audiology Today, 6*(3), 15.

Malone, R. L. (1979). Speech-language pathologist may be a mouthful but.... *Asha, 20,* 788.

Moeller, D. (1976). *Speech pathology and audiology: Iowa origins of a discipline.* Iowa City: University of Iowa Press.

National Institute on Deafness and Other Communication Disorders. (1995). *Research on human communication.* Bethesda, MD: Author.

Newby, H. (1958). *Audiology: Principles and practice.* New York: Appleton-Century Crofts.

Travis, L. E. (1931). *Speech pathology.* New York: D. Appleton-Century.

SUGGESTED READINGS

Moeller, D. (1976). *Speech pathology and audiology: Iowa origins of a discipline.* Iowa City: University of Iowa Press.

Paden, E. P. (1970). *A history of the American Speech and Hearing Association, 1925–1958.* Washington, DC: American Speech and Hearing Association.

Spahr, F., & Malone, R. (1998). The professions of speech-language pathology and audiology. In G. Shames, E. Wiig, & W. Secord (Eds.), *Human communication disorders* (5th Ed.). Boston: Allyn and Bacon.

Uffen, E. (1999). @ Your Service: The many face(t)s of ASHA's national office. *Asha, 41,* 28.

GLOSSARY

Accreditation: A procedure that recognizes educational institutions or facilities providing services to the public as maintaining and conforming to necessary standards.

Certification: A procedure by which an individual is affirmed as meeting a standard that is usually administered by a professional organization or a governmental agency.

Certificate of Clinical Competence (CCC): A certificate issued by the American Speech-Language-Hearing Association in either speech-language pathology or audiology that affirms the individual has met the minimal standards for practice in the profession.

Communication sciences and disorders: A discipline that consists of two professions (speech-language pathology and audiology). The professions are comprised of people who study the nature of communication and communication disorders and who assess and treat individuals with communication disorders.

Continuing Education Units (CEUs): Documentation that affirms a professional person has engaged in new learning related to their area of practice that is often required for renewal of a license.

Deaf education: Deaf educators teach academic subjects to children and adults with severe-to-profound hearing impairments.

Deafness studies: The common designation for academic programs and departments that contain scholars who study individuals who are Deaf.

Discipline: A unique field of study that is supplemented by research.

Ethics: The principles of conduct that govern an individual or a group. The American Speech-Language-Hearing Association has an official code of ethics, and members can be censured or they can lose their membership in the association for ethical violations.

Licensure: A procedure that grants *legal* permission for an individual to practice in a specific area, usually a profession, and affirms that standards have been met.

Profession: An area of practice requiring specialized knowledge and academic preparation.

Support personnel: Individuals with less training who perform some duties of audiologists and speech-language pathologists under the supervision of licensed and certified professionals.

2

Communication Across the Lifespan

Ronald B. Gillam and Lisa M. Bedore

LEARNING OBJECTIVES

1 To learn about the major processes in communication.

2 To know the definition of language.

3 To understand the processes and systems that underlie speech and language development.

4 To differentiate between language form, content, and use.

5 To learn about important changes in language development that occur during four major periods of development: infancy, the preschool years, the school-age years, and adulthood.

INTRODUCTION

Communication is any exchange of meaning between a sender and a receiver. This seemingly simple exchange is important because it is the primary means by which humans share their thoughts and feelings, express their identity, build relationships, pass on traditions, conduct business, teach, and learn. Some communication is intentional, as when you tell your friend about your course schedule. Some communication is unintentional, as when your friend interprets your facial expressions or your body language to indicate the feelings that you may have about another person you are talking to. Sometimes, a message that you intend to be understood in one way is actually understood in a different way by the person you are talking to. Such miscommunication can have negative consequences, such as when a friend takes an offhand comment or an e-mail message personally even though you did not intend for your statement to be an insult.

Most of the time, meaning is exchanged via a code, called language. **Language** is best defined as a standardized set of symbols and the knowledge about how to combine those symbols into words, sentences, and texts in order to convey ideas and feelings. Let's consider the parts of that definition more carefully.

Language is comprised of a set of symbols. This means that one thing (sounds, letters, or hand movements) represents or stands for something else (ideas, feelings, or objects). Groups of sounds, printed letters, or hand movements (as in the case of **American Sign Language**) do not have much intrinsic meaning in and of themselves. For example, all speakers of English agree that the sounds, *t–r–ee,* spoken in succession, represent a tall object with a trunk and leaves. We may not all have exactly the same type of tree in our minds when we hear the three sounds, *t–r–ee,* but nearly all speakers of English share the same general concept. This is because language is stan-

 CD-ROM

CD-ROM Summary

Volume 1 of the CD-ROM that accompanies this book contains a folder marked, Chapter 02. There are three movies in this folder. The first movie (Ch.02.01) shows children of various ages telling a story. We refer to various segments of this movie to demonstrate changes in language development over time. The second and third movies (Ch.02.02 and Ch.02.03) show a 2-year-old boy playing with a graduate student in speech-language pathology. These segments illustrate preverbal and early verbal communication.

dardized. The speakers of any particular language share reasonably similar meanings for certain groups of sounds, letters, or hand movements.

Languages need more than just words. Many of our thoughts are so complex that we cannot express them adequately with single words; groups of words are needed. Another important aspect of language is the conventions for grouping words together. For there to be meaningful communication, speakers need to agree not only on word meanings, but also on meanings that are inherent in word order. For example, if I said, "Mary helped Billy," we would all agree that Mary was the helper and Billy was the person who was helped. That isn't the same thing as "Billy helped Mary" even though the words themselves did not change. Our knowledge of the word-order conventions of our language makes it possible for us to use word sequences to express precise ideas about our environment.

THE PROCESS OF LANGUAGE PRODUCTION AND COMPREHENSION

Figure 2–1 depicts the primary processes that are involved in spoken language. In language production, senders encode their thoughts into some form of a language code. This code is usually spoken or written, but it can also be signed. In speech, which is the most common means of expressing language, the sounds, words, and sentences that express the speaker's thoughts are formed by sending commands to the muscles responsible for respiration (primarily the diaphragm), phonation (primarily the larynx), and articulation (primarily the tongue, lips, and jaw). Sequences of spoken sounds leave the oral cavity in the form of sound waves.

In listening and comprehension, the sound waves enter the receiver's ear, where they are turned into electrical impulses. These impulses are carried to the brain, where they are recognized as speech and then decoded into words and sentences. Listeners interpret the words and sentences based on their understanding of the meaning of the words in relationship to the other words that were spoken and the speaking context.

THE BUILDING BLOCKS OF SPEECH

Phonemes

Languages have two basic types of sounds, consonants and vowels. Think about the words *bee, key,* and *tea.* Each word ends with the same vowel, the long [ee] sound. They are spelled differently because, in English, sounds in words can be represented by many different letters. But, let's put spelling aside

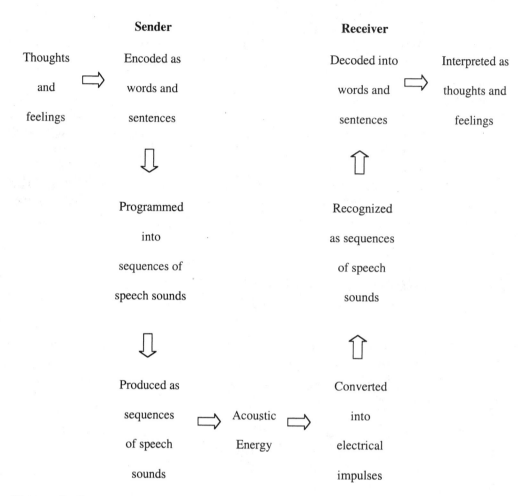

Figure 2–1. A basic model of speech communication processes.

for the moment. In English, these are three words with different meanings because the first consonant in each one differs. The sounds /b/, /k/, and /t/ differ in the way they are produced, and that difference results in a change in meaning. Sounds of a language that cause changes in meaning are called **phonemes.** It is worth noting, however, that not all changes in the way a sound is produced result in a change in meaning. The phoneme /l/ has several variants (e.g., the "light" /l/ produced in a word such as *lip* is a little different than the "dark" /l/ produced in a word like *dull*). These variants of a sound are called **allophones.** Try saying "light" with both a light and a dark /l/. It's still the same word even though the /l/ at the beginning is not produced quite the same way.

Consonants and vowels differ in their basic manner of production. Vowels are produced with no constriction in the vocal tract, whereas consonants are produced with a significant blockage in the vocal tract. The vowels of English, listed in Table 2–1, are classified by jaw height and placement of the tongue in the mouth. The tongue can move in the front back dimension (represented across the top of the table) or in the high to low dimension (listed in the left-hand column of Table 2–1). Lip position is associated with the front back dimension in English. Front vowels are produced with spread lips (i.e., feel how your lips are positioned when you say the word *eat*). Back vowels, such as the *u* sound in *boot,* are produced with the lips rounded. English also makes use of diphthongs, which are two vowels produced in close proximity to one another. The difference is that the tongue is moving in diphthongs. Some diphthongs that are contrastive or phonemic in English are /ɔɪ/ (e.g., boy), /aʊ/ (e.g., cow), and /aɪ/ (e.g., bye).

The consonants of English are listed in Table 2–2. Notice in Tables 2–1 and 2–2 that many of the symbols for sounds correspond to the English alphabet. Some symbols look unfamiliar. These symbols are from the International Phonetic Alphabet; a key for these symbols is provided in Table 2–3. This alphabet is a special set of symbols that we use to represent the sounds of speech in phonetic transcription. This is useful because there are many written letters that correspond to more than one speech sound. For example, the word *garage* begins and ends with two different sounds, even though they are both spelled with the letter *g*. If you look ahead to the CD-ROM Box "Examples of Jargon and Early Words" on page 40, you can see an example of phonetic transcription. We will talk more about the speech samples themselves a little later.

English consonants are produced by altering the manner and place of articulation or by voicing. **Manner of articulation** refers to the different ways that speakers can block airflow through the oral cavity using different types of constrictions. Different manners of blocking airflow lead to qualitatively different sounds. These are defined in Table 2–4. Another way of modifying speech sounds is to produce blockages at different places in the oral cavity. This is referred to as **place of articulation,** and these are described in Table 2–4 as well. Finally, consonants differ in **voicing.** They may be voiced or unvoiced. Voiced sounds are produced with vibration of the vocal folds (e.g., /v/) and voiceless sounds are produced with the vocal folds open (e.g., /f/).

Phonetic transcription of speech is useful when we are studying the speech production of young children or the speech of persons with phonological disorders. In both of these cases, speech patterns do not necessarily correspond directly to those of adult or mature speakers. Using the symbols from the International Phonetic Alphabet (Table 2–3) allows clinicians and researchers to capture in writing precisely how children produce sounds in words. This is helpful for maintaining records of the child's speech development and to compare child production to standard adult production.

Table 2–1. The Vowels of English

	Front	Central	Back
High	i		u
	ɪ		ʊ
Mid	e	ʌ, ə	o
	ɛ	ɝ, ɚ	
Low	æ		
	ɑ		ɔ

Table 2–2. The Consonants of English

		Bilabial	Labiodental	Dental	Alveolar	Palatal	Velar	Glottal
Plosive	Voiceless	p			t		k	
	Voiced	b			d		g	
Fricative	Voiceless		f	θ	s	ʃ		h
	Voiced		v	ð	z	ʒ		
Affricate	Voiceless					tʃ		
	Voiced					dʒ		
Liquid	Central				r			
	Lateral				l			
Glide		w				j		
Nasal		m			n		ŋ	

Syllables

Suppose that you are asked to read aloud an invented nonsense word such as "gigafibber." Try reading this pseudoword aloud to yourself right now. How did you go about deciding how this word is to be pronounced? You probably divided the words into shorter chunks or segments. Most likely, you tried to say the word syllable by syllable. **Syllables** are units of speech that consist of consonants and vowels. Vowels are the central component or the nucleus around which the rest of the syllable is constructed. A syllable may consist of a single vowel (e.g., the *a* in *alone*) although syllables usually contain combinations of consonants and vowels. The most common and easy to produce combination is a consonant and a vowel (e.g., *ba, si*), but syllabic complexity

Table 2–3. Key to International Phonetic Alphabet (IPA) Symbols

Vowels		Consonants			
Symbol	Key Word	Symbol	Key Word	Symbol	Key Word
i	key	p	pan	ʃ	shoe
ɪ	lip	b	big	ʒ	garage rouge
e	made	t	tip	h	house
ɛ	been	d	dog	tʃ	chew
æ	mad	k	cup	dʒ	juice
ʌ	mud	g	gap	l	luck
ɚ	butter	f	fan	r	ran
a	hot	v	van	w	wing
u	loot	θ	thin	j	you
ʊ	look	ð	them	m	milk
o	boat	s	sun	n	nose
ɔ	bought	z	zoo	ŋ	ring

can be increased by adding consonants before the vowel (e.g., *ri, tri, stri*) or after it (i.e., *am, amp*).

Syllables are combined to form words and phrases. In English, monosyllabic words such as *car* and *egg* are extremely common. One difference between monosyllabic words and multisyllabic words or connected speech is that not all syllables are produced with the same level of stress. Listen to yourself say words such as *dinosaur* and *telephone*. Some syllables are produced with greater intensity or loudness (e.g., the initial syllables in the above examples). These are stressed or strong syllables. Other syllables are relatively weak in comparison (e.g., the syllables in the middle of these words). These are called weak syllables. Strong syllables are produced with greater intensity, articulated with greater precision, and are longer in duration than weak syllables.

Change in pitch, stress, intensity, and duration of sounds in connected speech production is called **prosody.** Falling pitch and intensity are associated with statements, whereas rising pitch is associated with question forms. Stress patterns distinguish between the multiple meanings of some words. For example, in the sentence *The contrast is startling,* the word *contrast* is a noun but in the sentence *The red and blue flowers contrast with each other,* it is a verb. The difference in stress pattern helps distinguish the two meanings.

Table 2–4. Consonants Can Be Differentiated on the Basis of Manner, Place, and Voicing Distinctions

Manner of Articulation	
Plosives	Airflow through the oral cavity is completely blocked with the lips or tongue and then it is abruptly released.
Fricatives	Airflow through the oral cavity is constricted so that air is released with a gradual hissing sound.
Affricates	Affricates combine the characteristics of plosives and fricatives. The airflow is completely blocked and then it is gradually released with a hissing or fricative quality.
Liquids	Sounds produced with a gap (rather than contact) between the tongue and the roof of the mouth.
Glides	Consonants produced with a small amount of constriction between the articulators.
Nasals	Consonants produced with the velum open allowing nasal (rather than oral) resonance.
Place of Articulation	
Bilabial	Upper and lower lips in contact
Labiodental	Upper teeth in contact with lower lip
Dental	Tongue tip in contact with (back) of upper teeth
Alveolar	Tongue tip in contact with alveolar ridge
Palatal	Body of tongue in contact with the hard palate
Velar	Body of tongue in contact with soft palate or velum
Glottal	Glottis constricted
Voicing	
Voiced	Voiced consonants are produced with the vocal folds approximated so they vibrate and produce noise or voicing. There are several sound classes in English that only have voiced elements. These include liquids, glides, and nasals.
Voiceless	Voiceless consonants are produced with the vocal folds open so they do not vibrate during the production of a sound.

THE BUILDING BLOCKS OF LANGUAGE

Language is often characterized as having three interrelated components: form, content, and use (Bloom & Lahey, 1978). Form refers to the structure of language, content refers to the meaning of language, and use refers to the way speakers select different forms that best fit the communication context. Any sentence requires an interaction of all three components of language.

Language Form

Language form, or the structure of language, involves three linguistic systems: phonology, morphology, and syntax. We introduced the concept of phonology when we were writing about the basics of speech. **Phonology** is the study of the sounds we use to make words. For example, "b", "r", and "l" are English language sounds. In Spanish, there are different sounds, such as the trilled "r" sound, that do not occur in English. Recall that we said a **phoneme** was the smallest meaningful unit of speech. Take the words /fæn/, /mæn/, and /kæn/ (*fan, man,* and *can*). We know that the sounds /f/, /m/, and /k/ are phonemes in English because putting these different sounds in front of the root /æn/ results in a change in meaning.

Morphology has to do with the internal organization of words. A morpheme is the smallest grammatical unit that has meaning. The word *bird* is a morpheme. It cannot be divided into parts that have any meaning in and of themselves (such as "b" and "ird"). *Bird* is an example of a **free morpheme** because it can stand alone as a word. There are also **bound morphemes,** which are grammatical tags or markers in English. An example of a bound morpheme is the final *-s* in *birds,* which adds grammatical meaning. In this case *-s* marks plurality, meaning that there is more than one bird. Other examples of bound morphemes include *-ed* (which marks past tense as in the sentence, "He jumped over the wall") and *-ing* (which marks the present progressive tense as in the sentence, "He is running"). In English, most bound morphemes are placed on the ends of words. However, some are placed on the beginning of words. An example is *-un,* meaning "not" as in *uninteresting.* Some readers may think information about linguistics is uninteresting. However, professionals who assess and treat individuals with communication disorders need to know this information.

Syntax refers to the linguistic conventions for organizing word order. Basically, syntax is the formal term for grammar. In English we say *blue ball;* in French the proper order is "balon bleu" or "ball blue." The meaning is the same, but the rules governing word order are different for the two languages. Sentences that are ungrammatical may still make sense. Imagine a young child who tells her mother, "Him holded baby doggie." The sentence is ungrammatical because an object pronoun is used in place of the subject (he), the regular past tense marker is applied to the word *hold* that has an irregular form (*held*) for the past tense, and the child omitted an article (*the* or *a*) before the object noun phrase (*a baby doggie*). Even though this sentence is ungrammatical, we know exactly what the child meant.

Language Content

We have just shown how the form of language can add to or detract from the meanings that are conveyed by words and sentences. This leads us into a discussion of **language content,** the component of language that relates to meaning. Speakers express ideas about objects and actions, as well as ideas about relationships such as possession or cause and effect. Sometimes, these meanings can be expressed by a single word. Other times, these meanings are expressed through groups of words. The linguistic representation of objects, ideas, feelings, and events, as well as the relations between these phenomena is called **semantics.**

Children develop a **lexicon,** which is a mental dictionary of words. Word learning is a lifelong process primarily because there are so many words that make up a language, but also because new words are being added all the time (think about all the computer-related vocabulary that has become part of our daily language during the past 10 years). What makes word learning even harder is that most words have multiple meanings. For example, the word *bark,* can refer to something that a dog does or the stuff on the outside of a tree trunk. Imagine how confusing the sentence *That tree has funny bark* might be to a young child who had only heard the word *bark* used with reference to the noise her dog made.

Language Use

Words must be combined into sentences to express complex relationships. **Language use** concerns the goals of language and the means by which we choose between alternative combinations of words and sentences. There are sociolinguistic conventions, called **pragmatics,** that help us decide what to say to whom, how to say it, and when to say it. Imagine that you are telling your friend about a movie you saw recently. You might say, "That had to be the most uninteresting screenplay I've ever seen" or, "That film was so dull I could hardly keep my eyes open" or even, "Talk about a boring movie." We choose different sets of words that we believe will best communicate our meanings to the audience we are addressing.

Effective language requires an interaction of content (semantics), form (phonology, morphology, syntax), and use (pragmatics). Speakers think of something to say and the best words to say it (content) and put those words in sentences (form) that address their goal (use) given the nature of the speaking situation (use). Similarly, listeners will interpret the words (content) and sentences (form) they hear with reference to what they already know about the language being spoken (content and form) and the situation they are in (use).

THE DEVELOPMENT OF SPEECH AND LANGUAGE

By the time most children are 3 or 4 years old, they can integrate language content, form, and use in order to understand and produce basic messages. By the time they reach the age of 9 years, most children are capable of understanding and expressing quite complex messages. Communication ability continues to change into adulthood, where it plateaus around age 50. Late in life, communication skills often decline due to hearing loss and the loss of mental functions. Some of the basic milestones of speech and language development are listed in Table 2–5.

We describe some of the important milestones in communication development from infancy to very old age in the next section of this chapter. Then, we turn our attention to reasons why communication develops the way it does. Knowledge of speech and language development is important to

Table 2–5. Basic Milestones of Speech and Language Development and the Typical Age Range at Which They First Appear

Speech and Language Milestones	Age Range of First Appearance
Understands simple words (mommy, daddy, dog)	6–8 months
Reduplicated babbling (ba-ba)	6–8 months
Variegated babbling (ba-do-ke-ga-do)	6–8 months
First word	10–14 months
Two-word utterances	16–20 months
First grammatical morphemes	1;10–2;2 years
Multiword sentences	2;2–2;6 years
Combinations of sentences that describe events	3;2–3;6 years
Understood by unfamiliar listeners (95% of consonants produced in adult-like manner)	3;10–4;2 years
Identifies beginning sounds in spoken words	5;0–5;8 years
Decodes words	6;0–6;6 years
Tells complex stories	8–10 years
Written stories are more complex than spoken stories	11–13 years
Combines information from multiple sources into research papers	14–15 years
Refines personal speaking and writing styles	15–20 years
Uses vocation-specific vocabulary	21–24 years
Consistent difficulty recalling names and content words	45–47 years

speech-language pathologists, audiologists, and deaf educators. To identify atypical development, one must know what is typical. To assist children and adults with communication disorders, you must determine what their communication abilities are. When planning intervention, it helps to have a clear understanding of the factors that influence typical development.

Individual Differences

It is important for readers to understand there is a fair amount of variation in the *rate* of communication development. That is, some children will develop language faster than others, and some adults' language skills will decline faster than others. There is also some variation in the *way* language develops. Some children are risk-takers; they will try to say words that are difficult for them to produce even if the words are not pronounced correctly. Other children prefer not to produce words that may be difficult for them to say until they are sure they can say them correctly. Some children learn lots of nouns (50 or more) before they start producing two-word utterances; other children learn and use social phrases (e.g., *thank you, see ya later, hi daddy*) some time before they have 50-word vocabularies. Finally, there is variation in communication style. Some children and adults are relatively reticent; they tend not to say a whole lot about anything. Other children and adults are quite gregarious; they tend to say too much about everything!

As a result, it is difficult, if not impossible, to pinpoint what is "normal." Nor can we pinpoint what exactly happens in language development at a particular developmental age. Because there is so much individual variation, we will talk about "typical" development instead of "normal" development, and we will provide age ranges for the first appearance of the speech and language behaviors that we discuss. We celebrate diversity in language development and use, and we recognize that differences between speakers makes communication more interesting. However, we also know that some children have developmental difficulties that place them at significant risk for social, educational, and vocational difficulties later in life. The well-informed speech-language pathologist (SLP) knows how to tell when language development is so far outside the typical range that it can result in negative social, educational, or vocational consequences.

Language Content: Semantics

We begin with language content (semantics) because we believe children learn to talk because they have things they want to say to the people around them. We believe that the desire to understand others and to express one's own thoughts motivates language development. Meaning can be expressed by the words that you say. This is known as lexical semantics. Meaning can also be conveyed by the relationships between words. This is known as relational semantics.

From Crying to Short Phrases (0–24 Months)

Children do not seem to understand different words until they are around 6 months of age. Then, they begin to wave "bye-bye" when they are encouraged to do so by their parents, or they may hold up their arms when their sister says, "How big is baby? Soo big!" By the end of their first year of life, infants usually understand about 20 different words. They start to say words other than "mama" and "dada" between the ages of 10 and 14 months, and their vocabulary can expand to 200 or more words by the time they reach 2 years of age.

Once children have built an adequate **lexicon** (a personal mental dictionary), they begin to combine words into two- and three-word utterances. This happens a little before or a little after they are 18 months of age. The ability to produce two-word utterances marks the child's desire to express relationships between ideas, and it shows that children are learning about word order. For example, children will combine a modifier like "big" or "more" with nouns to create such utterances as "big dog" or "more cookie." Many of their utterances describe relationships between agents (someone or something that causes an action), actions (the activities), objects (things that are acted upon), and locations (places). These combinations of meanings result in utterances like the following:

Frog go	(Agent + Action)
Frog pond	(Agent + Location)
Go back	(Action + Location)
Daddy shoe	(Agent + Object)

 CD-ROM

Two-Word Utterances

CD-ROM segment Ch.02.01 contains children of various ages telling a story. They were shown a wordless picture book called *Frog Where Are You?* (Mayer, 1973). This book contains a series of pictures that tell a story about a frog who escapes. A boy and his dog look for the frog. Their search leads them to have a series of misadventures with animals in the forest. The boy and the dog end up in a small pond, and they see their lost frog with his family. They take one of the baby frogs home. Six children were filmed as they told the story. We spliced

(continued)

sections of their narratives together to create the entire story, starting with Erin (age 2) and ending with her sister Brandi who is an eighth grader. Note that as children get older, the length of children's language increases and their descriptions become more complete and complex.

Watch part 1 of segment Ch.02.01. Brandi and her little sister Erin are looking at a book together. Listen to Erin's two-word utterances. How might we describe the utterances, "going night-night" and "getting out"?

From Early Sentences to Stories (2–5 Years)

Children's vocabulary grows almost exponentially during the preschool years. Children *say* approximately 200 different words at 2 years of age, and this increases to approximately 1,800 different words by age 4, when they probably *understand* as many as 3,000 or 4,000 different words. During this period, children continue to expand their noun and verb vocabularies. They also learn prepositions (over, under, in front of, between), words that express time (before, after, until), words that express physical relationships (hard, soft, large, small), adjectives (blue, red, big, little), and pronouns (me, you, they, our, herself).

Children are also busy learning how to create sentences that express complex relationships between words. For example, children say sentences like, "Billy is riding his red bike in his backyard." This sentence expresses at least five different relationships. The basic relationships are agent (Billy) + action (is riding) + object (bike). The words, *red bike* tell about the state (color) of the bike. By adding the word, *his* in front of *red bike,* the speaker specifies an ownership relationship. The pronoun makes it clear that it is the agent (Billy) who is the owner. The prepositional phrase, *in his backyard,* states two important relationships. We know where the event occurs (in the backyard), and we also know that the backyard belongs to Billy. This example shows how many relationships can be expressed in a relatively simple sentence.

From Oral Language to Written Language: The School-Age Years

Children's vocabularies continue to expand dramatically during the school-age years. It has been estimated that children acquire as many as 3,000 different words annually during the school-age years. At that rate, high school seniors may know as many as 80,000 different words (Miller & Gildea, 1987).

About the time children are in kindergarten, they start to think about the nature of their own language. That is, they begin to analyze language as an entity. This ability is called **metalinguistic awareness.** As children begin to analyze the sound system of language they come to realize that words are comprised of individual sounds. Soon they can identify the sounds that words begin and end with. Children also start to analyze grammar. They can tell when sentences sound "right." For example, school-age children can tell you that the sentence, "They wented to the park" is not correct.

Metalinguistic competence brings about greater understanding of relationships between concepts and increasing subtle knowledge about the meanings of words. As a result, school-age children increase their ability to comprehend and use figurative language such as metaphors and idioms. **Metaphors** are expressions in which words that usually designate one thing are used to designate another. For example, *All the world is a stage.* **Idioms** are expressions that have literal and figurative meanings. For example, the expression *reading between the lines* could mean looking for words in the white space between the lines of this book. However, you probably know that this idiom really means to comprehend meanings or to make inferences about meanings that go beyond the literal meanings of the individual words.

Adulthood

Vocabulary continues to expand throughout the adult years. This is especially true for vocation-specific words. Biologists have different vocabularies than pharmacists, engineers, or speech-language pathologists (SLPs) because members of these professions tend to talk about different things. Shared vocabulary is often used to create social and economic bonds among members of a vocation or people with shared interests.

Late in life, there may be neurological changes that lead to declines in some semantic functions. The ability to comprehend words does not decline much with age. However, the number of different words that are used decreases, as does the speed with which words can be recalled (Benjamin, 1988). There appears to be a "use it or lose it" quality to the mental lexicon. Older adults who have remained mentally active (those who still work, have busy social lives, and read and write frequently) have fewer declines in semantic abilities than older adults who watch more television.

Language Form: Phonology

From Crying to Short Phrases (0–24 Months)

Even before they are born, young children are actively sorting out and grouping the sounds of the language they hear. In experiments, mothers have repeatedly read the same nursery rhyme aloud to their unborn children. At birth, these infants have been found to listen longer to the nursery rhyme read by their mothers than to a rhyme read by another woman (DeCasper, LeCanuet, Busnel, Granier-Deferre, & Maugeais, 1994; DeCasper, & Spence,

1986). Also, newborns listen longer to the sound patterns of their own language than to those of another language (Mehler, Jusczyk, Lambertz, Halsted, Bertoncini, & Amiel-Tison, 1988). Thus, from as early as children are exposed to speech, they are beginning to process information about the speech and language patterns of their native language.

Speech is secondary to biological functions such as respiration and feeding. As infants gain control over these motor functions, speech begins to emerge. The earliest phase of speech development is called **babbling,** in which infants begin to produce a number of types of sounds such as growls, squeals, raspberries, and adult-like vowel sounds. As children gain greater independent control of the muscles that produce speech, they combine different consonants and vowels and string sets of different syllables together in a way that has a speech-like quality. Around age 7 months, infants start to repeat syllables over and over (e.g., bababa), a process called **reduplicated babbling,** and they start to combine different syllables (e.g., bawabedo), a process called **variegated babbling.** Later, their babbling starts to take on adult-like intonation patterns. This type of speech is known as **jargon,** which sounds like statements and questions with the exception that none of the sounds are recognizable words. Children exhibit jargon interspersed with real words until they are 2 years old.

 CD-ROM

Examples of Jargon and Early Words

CD-ROM segments Ch.02.02 and Ch.02.03 show a little boy, Ryan, playing with Meghan, who is a graduate student in speech-language pathology. Listen carefully to what Ryan says in segment Ch.02.02. Can you understand anything Ryan says? He sounds like he is talking, but he is not using any identifiable words in this segment. This is a good example of jargon. Sometimes Ryan uses sentence-ending intonation patterns. Toward the end of the segment, you'll hear Ryan say something that sounds a lot like a question. If you can figure out what the words are, you are a better transcriber than we are.

When you play segment Ch.02.03, you will hear Ryan say the word, "cup" pretty clearly. The rest of his utterances are examples of babbling and jargon. Notice that his babbling sounds a lot like English. One longer utterance contains variegated babbling and ends with the word, "cup."

As children approach their first birthday, they begin to use words. Early words contain the same sounds observed in the later stages of babbling. Common first words, such as *mama, dada,* or *papa,* contain those sounds that the child regularly uses in babbled speech. As their vocabulary increases, children are likely to begin to use **phonetically consistent forms.** These are words that children produce that do not necessarily match the adult target for a word. However, when children consistently produce a form in the same way, those around him can identify the meaning of the word. For example, we know a child who said /wagəbi/ (wagabee) whenever he wanted a particular bear. The sounds did not correspond to the bear's name, which happened to be Paddington. However, if his parents gave him Pooh when he said, "/wagəbi/," the child would adamantly shake his head, "no" and repeat /wagəbi/ louder and more insistently. Soon, his parents learned what this phonetically consistent form meant and did not make any more mistakes.

From Early Sentences to Stories (2–5 Years)

From age 2 years on, children begin to produce speech sounds with increasing accuracy. The earliest set of phonemes acquired by children is /m, b, n, w, d, p, h/; these sounds are often acquired by the time children are 3 years old. The next set of phonemes that children acquire, typically between 3 to 5 years of age, includes /t, ŋ, k, g, f, v, tʃ (ch), dʒ (j)/. The last set of phonemes to be acquired includes /ʃ (sh), θ (voiceless th), s, z, ð (voiced th), l, r, ʒ (ge as in *garage*)/. These sounds are sometimes referred to as the "late 8" sounds. Children may start to acquire these sounds as early as 4 years of age, but these may not be fully acquired until 7 or 8 years of age. It is important to remember that children will use these phonemes inconsistently for a long time before they are mastered. Thus, children might use a phoneme in places where it doesn't belong in a word, as when they substitute /t/ for /k/ resulting in /tæp/ *tap* for /kæp/ *cap* or distort a sound such as /s/ (e.g., young children may produce a "slushy" sound in which the air comes out over the sides of the tongue instead of /s/ in which the air comes out over the tip of the tongue). Speech sound acquisition is a gradual process.

 CD-ROM

Speech Sound Acquisition

If you look at the transcriptions of the speech samples in parts 1, 2, and 3 of the CD-ROM segment Ch.02.01, you can see that each child uses increasingly more of the sounds that are expected for their age. You can also see that individual children differ from the norm. For example, /g/ was in the middle set of sounds acquired for 3 to 5 years, but Erin, who is 2, is already using it in her speech.

Part 1: Erin (Age 2) and Brandi

> B: What is that?
> E: A frog. / ə fag/

(continued)

> **B:** A frog!
> **B:** And what are they in, Erin?
> **B:** Look, what are they in?
> **E:** A room. [ə bum]
> **B:** A room, that's right.
> **B:** And do you know what that is?
> **E:** M-hum. [mhəm]
> **B:** What is that?
> **B:** Is that a window?
> **E:** (nods head yes)
> **B:** Yea. Now what is going on, what are they doing there?
> **E:** Going night-night. [go nɑɪnɑɪ]
> **B:** They're going night-night.
> **B:** What's the frog doing?
> **E:** Get, getting out. [gɛ gɛɪ aʊ]
> **B:** He's getting out!
>
> **Part 2: Older Erin (Age 4)**
>
> There was a little frog. [dɛ wa ð ə lɪdəl fag]
> And then, he, the frog, that frog was mean and that frog was happy. [æn dɛn hi
> də fag dæ fag wʌð min æn dæ fag wʌð hæpi]
> And he would. [æn hi wʊð]
> And there was a possible thing. [æn dɛr wʌð ə pasəbəl fɪŋ]
> And the frog look like. [æn də fag lʊk lɑɪk]
> And he was mean. [æn hi wʌð min]
> And he, and he was sad. [æn hi æn hi wʌð sæd]
> And he was mad. [æn hi wʌð mæd]
> And they were mad. [æn deɪ wʌ mæd]
> And he was mad and he was sad. [æn hi wʌð mæd æn hi wʌð sæd]

Children do not communicate by producing isolated sounds; they need to produce words. Children systematically simplify adult word forms. These simplifications can be described as **phonological processes.** Some processes commonly observed in the speech of children 2 to 3 years of age are weak syllable deletion, final consonant deletion, and velar fronting. Applying the process of weak syllable deletion, we might expect a child to realize the word *telephone* as [tɛpo]. When children delete final consonants they change a word so that it no longer ends with a consonant (e.g., [tɪ] for *tick*). Velar fronting involves substituting the velar stops /t/ and /d/ (front sounds) for back stops /k/ and /g/ (e.g., [tʌp] *tup* for [kʌp] *cup*).

After age 3, processes that children used to simplify word production earlier in development are no longer observed, but other processes emerge that facilitate the production of more complex phonological forms such as consonant clusters (groups of two or more consonants such as /sp/ as in *speak* or

/str/ as in *street*). Processes observed include cluster reduction (e.g., the production of a single consonant instead of a cluster as in the production of [ti] for *tree*), gliding (the substitution of a glide for a liquid such as [twi] for *tree*), and epenthesis (i.e., insertion of a schwa into a cluster as in [təwi] for *tree*).

 CD-ROM

Phonological Processes

Listen carefully to Erin (part 1 of CD-ROM segment Ch.02.01), older Erin (part 2 of segment Ch.02.01), and Trey's (part 3 of segment Ch.02.01) speech samples and look at their transcripts. Which of the phonological processes we discussed in the chapter can you identify in the speech of these children?

From Oral Language to Written Language: The School-Age Years

Beyond the age of 5 years, children's speech continuously becomes more adult-like. As mentioned earlier, some of the latest sounds are not perfected until children are 7 or 8 years old. Children this age also become more adept at producing consonant clusters such as str- and sl-. Most words are produced accurately, but some phonological processes are occasionally observed in the production of complex words or in the production of words containing sounds that are late to be acquired. For example, children may still have difficulty producing multisyllabic words such as *spaghetti* or *pharmacy*.

We wrote earlier about **metalinguistics,** which is the ability to think of language as its own entity. In the late preschool years and early school-age years, children become aware of and start to mentally manipulate the sound structure of the words they say and hear. This ability is known as **phonological awareness,** and it has been shown to be a skill that is critically important for learning to read. For example, children can tell that *fan* and *man* rhyme. Later, they realize that *hot* and *horse* begin with the same sounds. By the time they are in second grade, children should be able to segment words into all their constituent phonemes (*sun* is /s/ -/ʌ/ - /n/) and to delete phonemes (say *school* without the /s/).

Adulthood

As part of the aging process muscles atrophy and cartilage stiffens. These physiological changes lead to some changes in the voice. For example, older male speakers may use a somewhat higher pitch, and their voice may sound hoarse compared to younger male speakers. In addition, respiratory support for speech diminishes so it may be necessary for some speakers to pause more frequently. Specifically in regard to articulation, it has been observed that speakers produce consonants less precisely than do younger speakers. Speaking rate may also slow. Generally speaking, articulatory changes in speech production of older adults are not considered problematic.

Language Form: Morphology and Syntax

From Crying to Short Phrases (0–24 Months)

The ability to sequence actions is one of the critical foundations of language, which involves sequences of sounds to make words and sequences of words to make sentences. Therefore, sequenced organized behaviors such as combinations of symbolic play schemes (pretending to pour tea into a cup and then pretending to put the cup to a doll's mouth) are important prerequisites of morphology (sequences of morphemes) and syntax development (sequences of words that form sentences).

As most children near 2 years of age, they start to use two-word utterances such as *Billy go* or *go there*. These utterances are best characterized by semantic relations such as "agent + action" and "action + location." Utterances of this type are the building blocks of syntax because they usually reflect the word order of language.

From Early Sentences to Stories (2–5 Years)

During this period, children progress from producing primarily one- and two-word utterances to producing sentences that may contain up to 10 words. As children begin to express more precise meanings with multiword utterances, the use of grammatical morphology and syntax becomes important.

Some of the earliest grammatical morphemes to emerge include forms such as the plural -s (*The boys ride*), the possessive -s (*The girl's bike*), and the progressive -ing (*The dog's barking*). Around 3 years of age, children begin to mark verb tense using the third person singular -s (e.g., *My sister swims*) or the past tense -ed (e.g., *The man jumped*). Later, children increase the complexity of their utterances using the copula and auxiliary form of "Be" as in, "Daddy *is* a clown" (a copula form) or "He *is* running" (an auxiliary form).

As children produce longer sentences, they must use appropriate word order (syntax) if they are to be understood. From the time that children use two-word combinations, changes in word order reflect differences in meaning. For example, a child may say, "daddy shoe" to indicate the shoe belongs to daddy, and, "shoe daddy" to ask her daddy to put her shoes on. Ways that young children (between 2 and 3 years of age) add syntactic complexity include using modifiers (e.g., *Want blue ball*) and using new forms such as ques-

CD-ROM

Morphosyntactic Development

Go back to the speech samples in CD-ROM segment Ch.02.01 again and notice how the children's sentences increase in morphosyntactic complexity. For example, when Erin uses a two-word utterance to describe an action, she uses the progressive -ing only (i.e., "going night-night"). The older Erin is able to express past tense forms such as "was" and "were." However, she does not use the past -ed on the end of "look" as might be expected. Even after children have begun to use these forms, they may apply them inconsistently.

tions (e.g., *See ball?* with a rising intonation). By age 3, children start to use prepositions (It's *on* my chair), they use *and* to conjoin elements (I want juice *and* cookie), and they use longer question forms (e.g., *Why you not here?*). By age 4, children are using passive sentences such as, *The girl was bitten by the snake,* and some complex forms like, *I know how to cut with scissors.*

From Oral Language to Written Language: The School-Age Years

Children use a greater variety of complex sentence forms during the school-age years. That is, they become adept at putting multiple clauses (subject-verb combinations) into single sentences. The earliest and most common complex sentences are formed with conjunctions such as *and* (He came to my party *and* brought me a present). Later, children learn to use adverbial clauses that express time (*After we went to the movie,* we got an ice cream cone) or causality (I want you to come over *because* I don't like to play alone). By the time they are 8 years old, children routinely form sentences that have multiple clauses such as, *We wanted Steve to help us study for our science test but he wouldn't because he thought he was so much smarter than everyone else.*

CD-ROM

Complex Sentences

Watch part 6 of CD-ROM segment Ch.02.01 again. Brandi produces three complex sentences in a row. These sentences are complex because they have multiple clauses. We have underlined the main verb in each clause in the sentences below.

(continued)

> Then they <u>climbed</u> over and <u>noticed</u> a whole bunch of little babies were <u>hopping</u> through some grass.
>
> And the little boy <u>said</u>, "There<u>'s</u> our frog!"
>
> So the little boy <u>scooped</u> up their frog, and the dog and him started <u>going</u> back home.
>
> And they said, "Goodbye" to the little frog family saying they would come back to see them soon.

An important part of language development during the school-age years is learning literate (more formal) language structures. As they read and write with greater frequency, childrens' language sometimes takes on a "literate" sound. For example, the sentence, *Readers might be pleased to discover that we will not require memorization of the cranial nerves,* sounds more like written language than, "I'll bet you will be glad to hear this. We are not going to make you memorize the cranial nerves." Near the end of the elementary school years and into the middle school years, children experiment with the kinds of syntactic devices that are required for "literate" language, and they discover when and how to use these structures.

Adulthood

Older speakers demonstrate some changes in their use and understanding of morphology and syntax. Older speakers tend to use a diminishing variety of verb tenses and grammatical forms. Older speakers also may produce grammatical errors somewhat more frequently than younger speakers do. Some changes observed in the area of syntax are more closely related to changes in the lexicon and pragmatics. For example, older speakers may rely more on pronouns than on specific nouns when telling a story. Errors may be observed in the production of complex structures such as passive sentences or embedded structures that place demands on memory. It may also be more difficult for older speakers to understand syntactically complex utterances such as "I saw the lady who had a rose in her hair that the little girl picked from a garden on her way to school." Again, this has to do with memory demands rather than a decline in the comprehension of words.

Language Use: Pragmatics

From Crying to Short Phrases (0–24 Months)

In mainstream American culture, we communicate with our children from the first minute we see them. Mothers and fathers hold their infants, look into their faces, and talk to them. When infants make gurgling noises, their parents are quick to say things like, "Yes, I know. You're all full now, aren't you?" We build conversations with our children by treating everything they say and do *as if* it was true intentional communication. It is important to remember that parents from some cultures do not treat their young children in quite the same way. This cultural aspect is discussed in greater detail in Chapter 3.

Children communicate without words before they communicate with words. For example, when infants want something they cannot reach, they may point to it and vocalize loudly, "uh, uh, uh!" Even though they are not saying words, they are clearly communicating a form of a command, *Get that for me, mom!* Other forms of early intentional communication include looking at a parent, then looking at an object, then looking back to the parent, then back to the object, and so on until the parent gets what they want. This behavior is very important, because it shows children that communication gives them some degree of control over their environment.

Once children start to produce words, they can communicate many different functions with just a few words. In a famous study of his son's early language development, Michael Halliday identified eight communication functions that Nigel used before he was 2 years old. These functions are listed in Table 2–6.

From Early Sentences to Stories (2–5 Years)

Before children can produce short sentences, adults assume most of the responsibility for conversing with them. By age 3, children begin to play a much larger role in conversation. Look at the example of a conversation between Jennifer and her mother. Notice that Jennifer does not have control over all the morphology and syntax necessary to express her ideas grammatically.

Table 2–6. Early Communication Functions Evident During the First Two Years of Life

Label	Function	Words and Gestures
Instrumental	To satisfy needs	"want" + pointing
Regulatory	To control others	"go" (meaning, go away)
Interactional	To establish contact	"hi"
Personal	To express individuality	"mine"
Heuristic	To get information	"What that?"
Imaginative	To pretend	"You batman"
Informative	To explain	"Sara ball" (meaning, that ball belongs to Sara)

Source: Based on Halliday (1975).

Nonetheless, she is assertive as she expresses new ideas and asks a question, and she is responsive when she answers her mother's question.

Jennifer: Sara be at school.
Mother: She'll be home pretty soon.
Jennifer: Can I go school mommy?
Mother: Some day. Right now, you get to go to Mother's Day Out. Don't you like Miss Sally?
Jennifer: Yea, that fun to go there.

One important development during the preschool years is the beginning of narration, the ability to express a chain of events in the form of a story. Children's first stories are personal narratives that consist of one or two sentences. For example, an early personal narrative might go as follows:

Look, I painted a picture. And it got on me. See my shirt? I washed it and it's not go away.

Toward the end of the preschool period, children start to tell stories that contain fictional elements. Many fictional stores follow a similar sequence called a **story grammar.** Stories usually contain **setting** information plus one or more **episodes.** To have a minimally complete episode, the narrator needs to say what motivated the main character to take an action (the **initiating event**), what actions the character took in response to the initiating event (**attempts**), and what the result of the action was (**consequence**). As children develop, they produce more complete and complex episodes that include character thoughts and feelings about the initiating events (**internal responses**), character's ideas about the actions they can take (**plans**), their thoughts or feelings about the consequence of their actions (**reactions**), and the resolution or moral of the story (**ending**).

 CD-ROM

A Fictional Story

CD-ROM segment Ch.02.01 shows six children who were filmed as they told the story, *Frog Where Are You?* (Mayer, 1973). We spliced sections of their narratives together to create the entire story, starting with Erin (age 2) and ending with her sister Brandi, who is an eighth grader. Note that as children get older, the length of children's language increases and their descriptions become more complete and complex. Notice that, beginning at age 8, the children's language sounds more literary. The story propositions are named in parentheses following the children's utterances.

Frog Where Are You?

Part 1: Erin (Age 2) and Brandi

B: What is that?
E: A frog.
B: A frog!
B: And what are they in, Erin?
B: Look, what are they in?
E: A room. **(Setting)**
B: A room, that's right.
B: And do you know what that is?
E: M-hum.
B: What is that?
B: Is that a window?
E: (nods head yes)
B: Yea. Now what is going on, what are they doing there?
E: Going night-night. **(Setting)**
B: They're going night-night.
B: What's the frog doing?
E: Get, getting out. **(Initiating Event)**
B: He's getting out!

Part 2: Older Erin (Age 4)

There was a little frog.

And then, he, the frog, that frog was mean and that frog was happy.

And he would.

And there was a possible thing.

And the frog look like.

And he was mean.

And he, and he was sad.

And he was mad.

And they were mad.

And he was mad and he was sad. **(Setting)**

Segment 3: Trey (Kindergartner)

Trey: Well, he escaped while they were sleeping. **(Initiating Event)**
Trey: And then they woke up. And and it was morning, and he was gone

(continued)

Adult: Oh no.
Trey: He looked in the book and the puppy looked in the jar a little bit more closer. **(Attempt)**
Trey: He stuck his head in there.
Adult: M-hum.
Trey: And then the little boy, and Tom and Spot looked out the window. **(Attempt)**
Adult: Yes they did.
Trey: And Spot fell out.
Adult: And then, then what?
Adult: Well, what's happening here?
Trey: Then the glass broke.
Adult: It sure did.
Trey: And then they were yelling with, and and see if the frog would come out. **(Attempt)**

Segment 4: Ashley (Grade 3)

Jimmy went outside in the woods with Spot calling, "Mr. Frog, Mr. Frog, where are you?" **(Attempt)**

Jimmy looked in a mole hole and called, "Mr. Frog." **(Attempt)**

And the mole shot up, scolding Jimmy. **(Consequence)**

While Spot was near a beehive shaking a tree, and it fell.

Jimmy was looking in an owl hole calling, "Mr. Frog, Mr. Frog." **(Attempt)**

The owl came out and Jimmy fell. **(Consequence)**

Segment 5: Jorge (Grade 6)

The boy was surprised to find the owl in the hole and fell to the ground, **(Reaction)** while the bees were still chasing the dog.

The owl chases the boy around the rock.

When the owl leaves, he climbs the rock.

And the owl said the frog's name. **(Attempt)**

And then, then a deers, a deer lifted his head, and the boy was on top of the deer's head. **(Setting)**

Segment 6: Jennifer (Grade 6)

And the moose took off! **(Initiating Event)**

The dog was barking at the moose. **(Attempt)**

Then the moose stopped at a cliff, and the dog and the boy flew over the cliff into a marshy area.

The boy fell in the water. **(Consequence)**

Then the boy heard a sound. **(Initiating Event)**

The dog crawled on top of the boy's head.

Ribbit, ribbit.

Shhhhh, the boy said to the dog.

Segment 7 Brandi (Grade 8)

The little boy told the dog to be very quiet.

He was going to peek over to see what was there. **(Plan)**

So the boy and the dog looked over the wall. **(Attempt)**

They found two frogs, a mother and a father. **(Consequence)**

Then they climbed over and noticed a whole bunch of little babies were hopping through some grass.

And the little boy said, "There's our frog!" **(Reaction)**

So the little boy scooped up their frog, and the dog and him started going back home. **(Reaction)**

And they said, "Goodbye" to the little frog family, saying they would come back to see them soon. **(Ending)**

The end.

Regardless of the language children learn or the culture they are raised in, most 3-year-olds tend to produce descriptions instead of fictional stories. Between the ages of 4 and 5 years, children tell fictional stories that contain some setting information, and they include a sequence of actions. Children do not routinely tie the actions together into a whole story that makes sense until they are about 5 years old. In addition, children's personal stories tend to be more complex than their fictional stories. If you show a preschool child a picture and ask the child to make up a story about it, he or she is likely to describe the picture rather than create a sequence of events.

From Oral Language to Written Language: The School-Age Years

There are a number of important changes in language use that occur during the school-age years. School-age children engage in longer conversations. They also become more adept at shifting topics and at shifting the style of

CD-ROM

Descriptions

Look at CD-ROM segment Ch.02.01 again. This time, pay attention to the differences between parts 1, 2, and 3. Notice that Erin (age 2) is naming characters in response to her sister's questions.

Erin (age 4) is describing the characters, but she is not incorporating any information about the characters' actions. Trey (age 6) is describing actions. He also provides information about the temporal and causal relationships that underlie the events.

---

their speech to match the nature of the speaking context and their relationship with the person they are talking too. Similarly, their narratives become longer and more complex. School-age children can weave multiple episodes into their stories, and they can tell and write in different **genres** (personal accounts, mysteries, science fiction, horror stories, etc.).

Children also improve at persuasion and negotiation during the school-age years. To be persuasive, speakers need to be able to adjust their language to the characteristics of their listeners and state why the listener should do something that is needed or wanted. Politeness and bargaining are often helpful as well. The first grader's use of persuasion may be limited to getting a friend to share a new toy. However, by high school, students need to use persuasion and negotiation quite well in order to gain privileges such as use of their parent's car for the evening.

Adulthood

Throughout their adult lives, individuals continually refine their discourse to match the needs of the situation. They use persuasion, argument, narration, and explanation in different ways depending on their communication goals, their understanding of the formality of the situation, and assumptions they make about what their listeners already know or think about the topic. Communication style is also related to social and cultural expectations. Manners of expressing oneself are used to create bonds among members of subgroups of society. For example, compare the way newscasters explain a story on National Public Radio's, "All Things Considered," to the way the same story might be reported by the newscaster on your local rock and roll station.

With aging, there are shifts in income levels, employment, social status, and leisure time. Many times, the elderly relocate to settings like retirement communities or nursing homes where there are few younger individuals. A recent study on perceptions of older persons' communication noted changes in discourse style that included dominance of conversations, unwillingness to select topics of interest to listeners, increased verbosity, failure to take the listener's perspective, and more of a rambling style (Shadden, 1988). Discourse changes like the ones just mentioned could be related to memory loss, a desire for prolonged contact, and decreases in opportunities for socialization with a wide range of people. Once again, it is worth mentioning that there are large individual differences in the degree of discourse change and the ages at which these changes occur.

HOW DO SPEECH AND LANGUAGE DEVELOP?

Communication, cognition, language, and speech are interrelated and develop together. As children get older, they practice producing speech sounds, and they think about their environment in more complex ways. Their desire to communicate and their capacity for thinking complex thoughts motivate them to produce increasingly more complex language. At the same time, they are gaining more control over muscles that are used to produce speech, leading to an ability to put different kinds of sounds and syllables together to produce words. Their continuing speech development makes them more intelligible, so people understand what they are trying to say and are more responsive to their needs. Increased socialization facilitates the development of more complex thoughts, and the cycle continues. Thus, we may envision speech, language, cognition, and socialization as having dynamic, reciprocal relationships that drive development in many domains.

Figure 2–2 is a very simple model of the dynamic relationships among factors that are known to influence language development: heredity, social experiences, prior knowledge, learning mechanisms, and language. Most researchers and clinicians believe that both environmental and hereditary factors contribute to development. They do not always agree on the extent of the

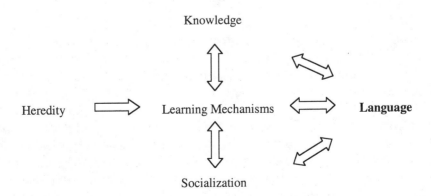

Figure 2–2. The factors that contribute to language development.

contribution that environmental and hereditary factors make to the developmental process. Some scholars believe that heredity plays a larger role than the environment (they might put a larger arrow leading from heredity to learning mechanisms); other scholars hold the opposite opinion (they might put a larger arrow leading from socialization to learning mechanisms).

Learning Mechanisms

We placed learning mechanisms in the center of our model because language learning is a mental activity. However, there are two basic ideas about what that activity consists of. Some believe that the mental activity involved in language development is the same as the mental activity involved in learning anything else (Gardner, 1985; Gathercole & Baddeley, 1993). From this perspective, children must attend to the sounds their parents and teachers say and figure out what the sequences of sounds mean. Once they do that, they need to retain that information so they can use it the next time they hear those same sequences of sounds or the next time they want to express a similar meaning themselves. This requires attention, perception, and memory.

Other scholars argue that these general information-processing mechanisms are not enough to account for the ease and rapidity at which language is learned (Chomsky, 1975; Pinker, 1994). These scholars say language is special and that humans are endowed with innate psychological mechanisms that are specific to language learning. They argue there is a basic design to grammar, regardless of the language being spoken, and human brains have special language-learning mechanisms that enable us to break the grammatical code of the language that surrounds us. Unfortunately, we do not yet know exactly what those innate mechanisms might be or how they work.

Heredity

Children inherit a genetic code from their parents that influences many aspects of mental functioning. Genes are important, whether they affect general sorts of cognitive mechanisms that can be applied to language or specific language-learning mechanisms. The importance of heredity is demonstrated quite clearly by the fact that there is a higher incidence of language impairment in the children of parents who are language impaired. Notice in Figure 2–2 that the arrow leading from heredity to learning mechanisms goes one way. Children are endowed with a particular genetic structure that, presently, cannot be changed. Given the rapid advances that are occurring in genetic engineering, it is entirely possible that we will be able to alter human genetic structure at some point in the future.

Socialization/Education (Experience)

Socialization and education play important roles in language development. Parents are their young children's social partners and educators, and they routinely do a number of things that facilitate language development in their children. First, they often engage their children in routine events (i.e., bathtime, bedtime, meals, routinized play with toys) in which they do and say the same things each time the event takes place. Parents work to establish a shared focus of attention with their children during these routine events and during other instances where they and their children are interacting. That is, parents tend to name the objects and comment on the actions their children are attending to. When they label, parents usually say short phrases (*See baby!*) or sentences (*That's a doggy*). They often produce these words slowly and clearly, with exaggerated intonation, and they may repeat them two or three times. You can imagine how this assists the mental mechanisms that influence language learning. This speech style, sometimes referred to as **motherese,** captures children's attention, holds it, and makes the sounds in words distinct. This clarifies the relationships between meanings and words and makes it likely that children will remember the words, phrases, and sentences in the future.

Parents and teachers engage children in a variety of experiences that contribute to language development. One of the most important experiences involves book reading. The stories and pictures in books expose children to new places, new experiences, new words, and new ways of communicating. Studies have shown there are considerable language-learning benefits to reading to children and, later, to children reading to themselves (see Adams, 1994, and Teale, 1984). At present, we do not know how much social input is necessary or exactly what kinds of input are critically important for language development. Studies of child-rearing practices in differing cultures are necessary to help us resolve answer these questions.

In Figure 2–2, there is a double arrow between socialization and learning mechanisms because there are recursive influences. The more you socialize, the more language demonstrations you encounter, and the more information about language you have to work with. Also, the more advanced your language-learning mechanism is, the more you will contribute to and get out of your socialization experiences.

Knowledge

Prior knowledge affects learning. When you learn something new, you build on what is already known. Some linguistic patterns are more complex than others and require prerequisite knowledge. For example, you would not expect children to produce complex sentences that contain complex auxiliaries like, "Susan *should have been listening* to me more closely," before they create sentences that contain basic auxiliary forms like, "Susan *was* listening." In addition, some concepts are more difficult than others. Prepositions are a good example of this. Children begin learning prepositions at age 2, and they are still learning them at age 4½. Prepositions nearly always take the same form. That is, the preposition comes at the beginning of the prepositional phrase (e.g., *in* the yard, or *on* the front porch). However, some prepositions are learned later than others because they are more complex. For example, children learn *in* and *on* relatively early, but they learn *beside* and *between* later because they are more difficult concepts.

In Figure 2–2, notice that the arrow between knowledge and learning mechanisms is facing both ways. Again, this represents the dynamic relationship between these two factors. The more individuals know, the more language they can process. Similarly, the better people are at information processing, the better they are at using the language they know to learn more. Quite simply, the more one knows, the more one is capable of learning.

Language

Figure 2–2 has three arrows leading to language, suggesting that the language a person comprehends or produces is the outcome of prior knowledge, learning mechanisms, and socialization experiences. The arrows face both ways to indicate the dynamic, reciprocal relationships among knowledge, information processing, socialization/educational experiences, and language. More complex knowledge, mental processes, and social/educational experiences lead to the child's use of more complex language. Similarly, more complex language use contributes to greater complexity of social and educational experiences, language knowledge, and mental mechanisms.

SUMMARY

People communicate by exchanging meanings with one another. This can be done nonverbally, through gestures and facial expression, but meanings are usually exchanged through spoken, signed, or written language. Languages are symbolic systems that require the integration of form (phonology, morphology, and syntax), content (semantics), and use (pragmatics). Nearly all children begin to develop language during the first year of life, but there is a great deal of individual variation in the rate of development.

During infancy, children explore the world around themselves with their sensory and motor systems, begin to communicate a variety of meanings nonverbally, and learn their first words. Children begin to produce two-word utterances around age 18 months, and they create their first short sentences around age 2. Language development literally explodes during the preschool years. By the time children are 5 years old, they know more than 4,000 different words, produce nearly all the sounds of speech correctly, use complex sentences, and tell short stories. The development of reading and writing creates many more opportunities for language development during the school-age years. By the time students graduate from high school, they know as many as 80,000 different words; they can created complex stories with multiple episodes; and they know how to weave sentences together to explain, persuade, and negotiate effectively. Language becomes more specialized during the adult years to match career and social choices. There is a gradual reduction in language skills in the elderly. Just as there was individual variation in the rate of language growth, there is also a great deal of individual variation in language decline. The most common aspects of language decline involve word retrieval difficulties, difficulty comprehending nuances of meaning, and a tendency toward a more rambling verbal style.

There are a number of factors that contribute to language development across the lifespan. Individuals inherit the basic biological mechanisms that support speech and language development. Their cognitive and linguistic learning mechanisms create knowledge out of social experiences. As they communicate more, they are understood better, and they take a more active role in their language interactions. Heightened levels of engagement and sensitivities mix with increased opportunities for language experiences, and this drives the development of even more complex language. In this way, speech, language, cognition, and socialization are involved in dynamic relationships that generate further development in each of these domains.

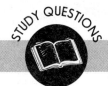

STUDY QUESTIONS

1   What is the difference between language production and comprehension?

2   What is the critical difference among these terms: phonemes, syllables, and morphemes?

3   What linguistic systems are involved in language form, language content, and language use?

4   Why can't we pinpoint the language abilities a child should have at 3 years and 9 months of age?

5   Name one important development that occurs in each area of language (form, content, and use) during each of the four major developmental periods (infancy, the preschool years, the school-age years, and adulthood).

6 What are some examples of sounds that may be difficult for children to produce at the time they enter kindergarten?

7 How would a child who uses the process final consonant deletion pronounce the word *boot?*

8 What are the critical factors that influence language development? How are they related to each other?

REFERENCES

Adams, M. J. (1994). *Beginning to read: Thinking and learning about print.* Cambridge, MA: MIT Press.

Benjamin, B. J. (1988). Changes in speech production and linguistic behaviors with aging. In B. B. Shadden (Ed.), *Communication behavior and aging: A sourcebook for clinicians.* Baltimore, MD: Williams and Wilkins.

Bloom, L., & Lahey, M. (1978). *Language development and language disorders.* New York: John Wiley & Sons.

Chomsky, N. (1975). *Reflections on language.* New York: Pantheon.

DeCasper, A., LeCanuet, J-P., Busnel, M-C., Granier-Deferre, C., & Maugeais, R. (1994). Fetal reactions to recurrent maternal speech. *Infant Behavior and Development, 9,* 133–150.

DeCasper, A., & Spence, M. (1986). Prenatal maternal speech influences newborn's perception of speech sounds, *Infant Behavior and Development, 17,* 133–150.

Gardner, H. (1985). *The mind's new science: A history of the cognitive revolution.* New York: Basic Books.

Gathercole, S., & Baddeley, A. (1993). *Working memory and language processing.* Hove, East Sussex, England: Lawrence Erlbaum.

Halliday, M. A. K. (1975). *Learning how to mean.* London: Arnold.

Mehler, J., Jusczyk, P., Lambertz, Halsted, N., Bertoncini, J., & Amiel-Tison, C. (1988). A precursor of language acquisition in young infants. *Cognition, 29,* 143–178.

Miller, G. A., & Gildea, P. M. (1987). How children learn words. *Scientific American, 257,* 94–99.

Meyer, M. (1973). *Frog where are you?* New York: Dial Press.

Pinker, S. (1994). *The language instinct: How the mind creates language.* New York: William Morrow.

Shadden, B. B. (Ed.). (1988). *Communication behavior and aging: A sourcebook for clinicians.* Baltimore, MD: Williams and Wilkins.

Teale, W. H. (1984). Reading to young children: Its significance for literacy development. In H. Goelman, A. Oberg, & F. Smith (Eds.), *Awakening to literacy* (pp. 110–121). Exeter, NH: Heinemann.

SUGGESTED READINGS

Aitchison, J. (1994). *Words in the mind: An introduction to the mental lexicon.* Cambridge, MA: Blackwell.

Bates, E., Bretherton, I., & Snyder, L. (1988). *From first words to grammar: Individual differences and dissociable mechanisms.* Cambridge, England: Cambridge University Press.

Berman, R. A., & Slobin, D. I. (1994). *Relating events in narrative: A crosslinguistic developmental study.* Hillsdale, NJ: Lawrence Erlbaum.

Brown, R. (1973). *A first language: The early stages.* Cambridge, MA: Harvard University Press.

Hirsh-Pasek, K., & Golinkoff, R. (1966). *The origins of grammar: Evidence from early language comprehension.* Cambridge, MA: MIT Press.

Jusczyk, P. W. (1997). *The discovery of spoken language.* Cambridge, MA: MIT Press.

Nippold, M. A. (1998). *Later language development: The school-age and adolescent years.* Austin, TX: Pro-Ed.

Pinker, S. (1994). *The language instinct: How the mind creates language.* New York: William Morrow.

GLOSSARY

Allophone: A variant of a phoneme that does not change meaning.

American Sign Language (ASL): The language of the Deaf community in the United States. ASL has its own set of phonological, morphological, semantic, syntactic, and pragmatic conventions that differ from those of English.

Attempt: In an episode, information about the actions that the main character takes to achieve his or her goal.

Babbling: Prespeech vocalizations.

Bound morpheme: A morpheme that cannot stand alone as a separate word

Communication: Any exchange of meaning, whether intended or unintended.

Consequence: In an episode, information about the results of the main character's attempts.

Ending: In an episode, the moral of the story, or final statements that bring the episode to a close.

Episode: A part of a story that consists of an initiating event, attempt, and consequence. Episodes may also contain internal responses, plans, and reactions/endings.

Free morpheme: A morpheme that can stand alone as a word.

Genre: A literary style (narration, description, persuasion, mystery, horror, fairy tale, etc.)

Idiom: An expression that can have both a literal and a figurative interpretation (e.g., skating on thin ice).

Initiating event: Background information about the event that propels the main character into action. The initiating event is usually a problem.

Internal response: Information about the main character's thoughts or feelings about the initiating event.

Jargon: Preverbal and early verbal speech pattern in which sequences of syllables sound like statements and questions. Sometimes, children intersperse a few real words into the strings of syllables.

Language: A standardized set of symbols and the conventions for combining those symbols into words, phrases, sentences, and texts for the purpose of communicating thoughts and feelings.

Language content: The meaning of an utterance or word. Content relates to the linguistic system of semantics.

Language form: The structure of language. Form relates to the linguistic systems of phonology, morphology, and syntax.

Language use: Choices that speakers, signers, and writers make about the words and sentence structures that will best express their intended meanings. These choices are made with respect to the formality of the speaking situation. Language use relates to the linguistic system of pragmatics.

Lexicon: A mental dictionary of words.

Manner of articulation: The amount and type (i.e., oral vs. nasal) of constriction during the production of phonemes.

Metalinguistic awareness: Awareness of one's own knowledge about language. For example, the ability to say what sounds comprise a word or the ability to explain why a sentence is not grammatical.

Metaphor: Figurative language in which a word that is normally associated with one thing is associated with something unusual (e.g., That car was a rocket waiting to blast off).

Morphology: The part of grammar that concerns the study of morphemes (the smallest units of meaning).

Motherese: The language and speech style that parents use when they talk to very young children. The sentences are shorter, speech is slower than normal, and the words are pronounced more clearly.

Phoneme: A speech sound that can change meaning.

Phonetically consistent forms: Word-like forms that are always produced in the same way by the child but that do not match the adult target.

Phonological awareness: Knowledge of the sequence of sounds that make up words (*soup* starts with an "s").

Phonological processes: Simplifications of adult-like productions of words. Some of the more common processes are weak syllable deletion, final consonant deletion, and velar fronting (substitution of a /t/ or /d/ for a /k/ or /g/).

Phonology: The study of the organization of sounds.

Place of articulation: The place of constriction during the production of phonemes.

Plan: In an episode, information about what the main character intends to do and why.

Pragmatics: Conventions related to the use of language in various speaking situations.

Prosody: Changes in pitch, stress, intensity, and duration of sounds during connected speech.

Reaction: In an episode, information about the main character's thoughts or feelings about the consequence.

Reduplicated babbling: Babbled sequences in which the same syllable is repeated.

Semantics: The meaning of individual words (lexical semantics) or the meanings that are expressed when words are joined together (relational semantics).

Setting: In a narrative, background information about the characters, the place where the story occurs, or the time of the story.

Story grammar: Conventions for the ways in which meanings are sequenced to form a story (e.g., initiating event, internal response, plan, attempt, consequence, reaction/ending)

Syllable: A basic unit of speech production that must contain a vowel.

Syntax: Conventions related to the way words are ordered to create sentences.

Variegated babbling: Babbled sequences in which the syllable content varies.

Voicing: Vibration of the vocal folds during the production of a phoneme.

3

The Social and Cultural Bases of Communication

Elizabeth D. Peña and Janice E. Jackson

LEARNING OBJECTIVES

1 To learn how individuals learn to use, speak, and understand the language of their community in meaningful ways.

2 To understand how culture is reflected within communication.

3 To compare and contrast the processes of socialization and acculturation.

4 To understand the implications of a mismatch between the culture of the home and the culture of the school.

5 To understand how dialects are formed.

6 To understand the origin and nature of African American English (AAE) and how it is used today.

INTRODUCTION

As social beings, humans learn to use language in a remarkably short span of time. We are able to use language to communicate, problem solve, cooperate, teach, learn, and plan. All of these tasks take place within social contexts, and they follow conventions that are agreed upon by the particular community. Whether we learn English, Spanish, Farsi, Tagalog, or multiple languages depends on the language that is spoken in the home and in the community. Languages are different structurally (e.g., their grammar and phonology). There are also cultural differences and similarities that go beyond linguistic rules. In this chapter, we consider the social and cultural bases of language and their implications for working with people from different cultural and linguistic backgrounds.

 CD-ROM

CD-ROM Summary

The CD-ROM that accompanies this chapter contains eight short video segments of children from diverse cultural and linguistic backgrounds. In addition, there is an audio segment of adults who are from different parts of the United States or who learned English as a second language. The first segment (Ch.03.01) demonstrates how a young child might learn to point in response to an adult request that later leads to school-like activities and testing behavior. The second segment (Ch.03.02) shows a typical, English-as-a-second-language error that may lead to misdiagnosis. The third segment (Ch.03.03) demonstrates different varieties of English. The following four segments (Ch.03.04, Ch.03.05, Ch.03.06, and Ch.03.07) highlight features of African-American English. Finally, the last two segments (Ch.03.08 and Ch.03.09) demonstrate code switching between languages and between dialects.

THE SOCIAL CONTEXT OF COMMUNICATION

Children learn rules of communication through everyday interactions with their family. In addition to learning the specific language that the family speaks, children learn how, when, why, and with whom to use their language.

Different families have different customs, some of which involve ways of talking and interacting. For example, some families may interact in a quiet manner while others use a loud tone of voice. Some families expect children to "show off" and perform certain kinds of communicative behavior for others. They may ask their children things like, "Show me your head" or "Tell Aunt Sally what happened to us yesterday." Other families may expect children to "speak when spoken to" and not perform in front of others. Some families teach and value more indirect ways of communicating while others value more direct styles. We have all heard statements like, "I wish she'd come out and say what she means" or "He is always so blunt." These differing beliefs are related to a number of variables such as ethnic background, religious beliefs, socioeconomic background, familial education, region, family type (nuclear/extended), neighborhood, country of origin, and gender.

Society and culture influence how we view communication. There is no "correct" or "incorrect" belief about when communication begins. However, we need to have an understanding of the variation in these beliefs in order to understand how they can influence parent-child communication. If you are a person who believes that communication begins early, then you might interact with babies in a way that assigns meaning to things that babies do. When your child cries you might say things like, "Oh, you're hungry?" or "Do you want to be held?" On the other hand, if you don't believe that these early signals have intentional meaning, you might try to meet the baby's needs, but you might not say anything to him. You may not think you are communicating with your child. Rather, you may think of yourself as being "in tune" with your baby's needs.

What constitutes "first words" for parents also varies according to what they believe about communication. In mainstream American society, we focus on first words as demonstrating an important early milestone in development. However, other cultures may not view this as an important time. Some cultures think of complete sentences or phrases as an indication of "talking." An example that comes to mind is a referral for a speech-language evaluation where a Spanish-speaking mother had stated that her son had not started talking until age 2. At first, we were concerned that this child spoke so "late." However, in discussion with the mother, we found out that her son began combining words at age 2. For this mother, "talking" meant the use of phrases and sentences, but single words did not count. To understand this mother's concerns with respect to her child's development, we needed to better understand what she was reporting from *her* point of view and what her expectations were.

We have seen that individual families may have different beliefs and customs that relate to communication. Families function within a society and culture that guide and influence their beliefs and customs. However, each individual within the family has slightly different experiences, which in turn influence the greater culture. Culture is constantly changing and adapting. Consequently, **culture** can be defined as a set of beliefs and assumptions shared by a group of people that guide how individuals in that group think, act, and interact on a daily basis. The members of the cultural group implicitly understand these beliefs. The way language is used can be a reflection of the cultural group to which that person belongs.

SOCIALIZATION: LEARNING THE RULES OF FAMILY AND SOCIETY

Socialization and **acculturation** are two terms that are used to describe how people learn about their culture. In our discussion, we will refer to socialization as the process by which one learns one's own culture, and we will refer to acculturation as the process by which one learns or adapts to another culture.

The process of socialization includes learning how to interact with others. This interaction is reflected in how we use language to communicate. Language learning is an important step in becoming a fully integrated member of a cultural group. When we learn a mutual language, and the syntactic and pragmatic rules that govern that language, we can communicate. In learning English for example, we learn that word-order dictates meaning. For example, "She kissed him," tells who did what and who received what, on the other hand, "He kissed her" has the opposite meaning. In addition, we learn the social or pragmatic rules for using the language that we've learned. For example, when he was President, Lyndon B. Johnson should have been addressed as "Mr. President" instead of "Hey Lindy!" even though both are linguistically accurate.

There are specific customs and conventions that govern how language is used. Anyone who has tried to learn another language knows that the grammar is different. For example, in some languages, such as Spanish and French, nouns have gender, and the article is used to mark gender and number. This is different from the English articles "a" and "the" that are neutral to gender. English speakers can use "a" and "the" in front of masculine or feminine nouns as in "a girl" or "a boy."

There are also different conventions that govern language use (pragmatics). How close should you stand when talking to someone? How much time is given to order in a restaurant? How long must a customer wait before receiving a bill? There is a whole ritual of behavior and communication in restaurants. For example, in many U.S. restaurants it is not unusual to receive the bill toward the end of the meal, even while eating dessert. However, in other countries, the customer must ask for the bill, because the bill signals that the customer is getting ready to leave. Bringing the bill before the customer finishes a meal might be interpreted as hurrying them along, which would be rude.

There are regional differences within countries as well. For example, in the United States, the amount of information that is given when asking questions is indicative of different social interaction rules. On the East Coast, it has been our experience that you get an answer to the question you ask, and nothing more. The respondent may not want to assume lack of knowledge and thus will not give additional information. On the other hand, West Coast respondents may give additional information "just to be friendly." When visiting the East Coast, someone from the West Coast may ask a general question expecting information beyond that which was specifically requested and be disappointed that his or her "real" question was not answered.

The rules of your community may determine whether you "get right to the point" or "beat around the bush." In Appalachia, it is considered appropriate for people to carry on a conversation for a while, asking about family and friends, discussing the weather, and then sitting a spell before they even begin to broach the "true" nature of their visit (e.g., to ask for someone's assistance or to negotiate the price of a car). If a teacher who was an outsider introduced him- or herself and then began to ask a series of straightforward questions, he or she might be considered rude and highly suspect.

Variation in Socialization Practices

We tend to interpret behavior based on our own expectations and experiences. Someone who has a different set of expectations may misinterpret a behavior that seems perfectly reasonable for someone else. This is especially true for communicating across cultures. It is important for speech-language pathologists (SLPs) and audiologists to remember that parents may teach ways of interacting that reflect their own culture and their own values. Parents teach children both directly and indirectly by providing them with examples and models of appropriate communication. Through these interactions, children learn to be active participants in their own culture. Parents universally want their children to be contributing adult members of the society. What differs is the path that learning takes. Parents, based on their own culture and experiences, teach the behaviors that are important to them (Rogoff, 1991).

Potential for Home and School Mismatch

Because parents do not universally socialize children in the same way, there is a potential for **mismatch** when two cultures come into contact with each other. This is seen particularly when children from nonmainstream cultures enter the public school system. In most mainstream public schools, educators have selected the curriculum content, the way that it is delivered, how children are taught, and the language in which children are taught (English). Educators in the public schools have a shared knowledge of child development and the skills that children have when they begin school. However, this shared knowledge is based on mainstream culture and experiences that influence and reinforce each other. When children who are not from the mainstream culture enter the school system, their experiences may not match educators' expectations about what it is they should know. Furthermore, children may enter the mainstream school system with little knowledge of the language that is spoken in the school. When families know and value educators' expectations, they will likely socialize their children in ways that will help them to be successful in academic settings. However, children socialized in homes with different interaction styles may not match school expectations.

 CD-ROM

"Show Me"

CD-ROM segment Ch.03.01 shows an 18-month-old child pointing to body parts in response to the parent's request. Because the parent is an educator, she knows the types of question demands that will occur later in school and uses questioning that matches that of schools. By the time this child begins school, he will have had many opportunities to practice this type of question-answer routine.

WHAT SHOULD WE DO IF THERE IS A MISMATCH?

There is a potential for speech-language pathologists, audiologists, and other educators to reach inappropriate conclusions about the abilities of children from diverse backgrounds if they do not understand issues related to normal cultural and linguistic variation. We need to have an understanding of how first and second languages are learned, how languages and dialects vary, and how past experiences might impact school performance. It is important that those who work with individuals from different cultural and

 CD-ROM

Learning English as a Second Language

CD-ROM segment Ch.03.02 shows a 4-year-old Spanish-speaking girl speaking in English. In response to a statement by the English-speaking adult, "She's a boy," Magali says, "No, her a girl." This grammatical error is typical for a child in the process of learning English, but could be mistaken for an indication of language impairment. Additionally, notice that this young language learner is relatively fluent in English even though she has been speaking it for less than a year. Because of her limited exposure and experience with English, it would not be appropriate to assess her only in English.

linguistic backgrounds keep these issues in mind so as not to interpret a mismatch as a disorder.

Learning a Second Language

Second language learners take from 1 to 3 years to learn face-to-face communication—what Cummins (1984) calls **"basic interpersonal communication skills" (BICS).** These children may take as long as 5 to 7 years to learn higher-level, **decontextualized language,** which Cummins termed **"cognitive academic language proficiency" (CALP).** Sometimes, children who are assessed in their second language may appear to be fluent in English because they have good BICS. However, they may score poorly on educational tests because they have yet to master the nuances of CALP. Thus, it is important that educators take both languages into account when making educational decisions about children who are second language learners and those who are from bilingual environments.

Differences in Language Form and Acquisition

A second issue with respect to children from different cultural and linguistic backgrounds has to do with the ways that languages are structured and the order of acquisition of these structures. For example, earlier in this chapter we said that gender agreement was important in Spanish and French. Gender agreement is not learned in English because it does not exist in English. Examining performance in only one language of a bilingual child may exclude important information that is not specific to that language.

There may be differences in the order of acquisition across languages. We have the expectation that children learn certain things at a given age, and generally easier things are learned early and harder things are learned later in development. Children's performance is often judged either informally or formally by comparison to what is known about this developmental progression. However, some language tasks may be more complex in one language in comparison to another language. One example is the acquisition of prepositions that convey directionality or location. In English, these occur relatively early in development (about age 1–2). In Spanish, directionality is often expressed in a verb phrase and is learned relatively later in comparison to English. So, we have to have an understanding of the development of both languages in order to make appropriate judgments about development.

The Effect of Experience on School Performance

The school situation has communicative demands and unwritten rules about how children and adults interact. In American mainstream schools, children are expected to be able to tell stories, relate known events, ask and respond to direct questions, respond to "known-answer" questions (names of objects, attributes), and respond behaviorally to indirect requests. A typical question format that is seen in classrooms is responding to "known-answer" questions. Here, we may see teachers asking children questions that adults know the answer to. The purpose of this type of question is to elicit a display of knowledge. This allows the teacher to assess whether children know a certain concept, whether they understood a lesson, or whether they have certain background knowledge.

Children who have had experience with adult-child interaction in which the adult asks the child to respond to known-answer questions are likely to respond in a way that is consistent with an adult's expectations. We see a lot of this kind of questioning in American mainstream parent-child interaction. Mother and father may ask known-answer questions that require pointing (such as looking at books and responding to, "Where's the cat, dog, shoe, ball?") or choices ("Do you want up or down?"), or naming ("What's this?"). However, some children may have little experience with this style of questioning. They may be more familiar with responding to questions that require them to provide information that is not known to the adult, so they may see this type of question as a request for relating an event or story. Thus, care must be taken to ensure that children's classroom interaction differences are not misinterpreted as low performance or low ability.

These three issues (the nature of second language learning, differences in language form, and different experiences) together may lead to mismatch between communication expectations and experiences. This mismatch potentially leads to miscommunication, lowered expectations, stereotypes, and inappropriate referrals and classification. Understanding how culture and language can affect these decisions can help to lessen the negative impact that mismatches may have.

DIALECTS AND BILINGUALISM

There are different languages and different dialects in the world. What makes a dialect a dialect and what makes a language a language? A **dialect** is typically defined as a variation of a language that is understood by all speakers of the language. One language may have several different variations. Everyone speaks a dialect— some variety of the "mother" language that we learned as a child. Often it is the "sound" of a particular dialect that we notice first. In the United States, we notice that people in New York sound different from people in the South, yet they are both understandable to a speaker of English. On the other hand, different languages have different phonology, lexicon, and syntax (sound system, vocabulary, grammar) and are not understood by people who don't speak those languages.

At what point does a dialect become a language? According to Pinker (1994) the linguist Max Weinrich maintained that, "A language is a dialect with an army and a navy." That is to say, the primary determination of what is called a dialect and what is called a language is one of power—not of linguistics. Dialects are as linguistically legitimate as any language, but without the power to "promote" themselves to the level of "language." Therefore, you can be sure that whatever the "standard" language is in any given community, it belongs to those with the most power in that community.

How Are Dialects Formed?

Historically, dialects have evolved as the result of social transitions such as large scale geographical patterns of movement by people, the development of transportation routes, or the establishment of education systems and government. Languages change over time. When a group of people are separated by geographical barriers such as oceans, rivers, or mountain ridges, the language that was once spoken in similar ways by everyone will change within each of the two groups. The two resulting varieties are usually understandable to both groups. A perfect example is the English spoken in the United States and the English spoken in England. When the first settlers arrived in the Americas they sounded the same as their fellow countrymen left behind in England. Over time, the lack of contact between those in the Colonies and those in England resulted in two distinctly different forms of English. In this way American English and British English are both dialects of the language of English. Within the United States there are even more dialect varieties of English. Most of these varieties are related to geographical regions.

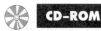 **CD-ROM**

"Mary Had a Little Lamb"

Watch CD-ROM segment Ch.03.03, "Accents." You will hear people with different accents and dialects recite this familiar poem. Listen to the rhythm and intonation patterns of each of the different samples. Listen to how they produce the vowels and consonants. Speech patterns typically affect rhythm, intonation, and individual sounds. Can you guess where each person is from? Are there patterns that you really notice? Typically, one notices a speech pattern that is different from one's own or from what one has heard often. Are there some that sound more pleasing to you than others? Know that both positive and negative attributes can be assigned to the same speech pattern. It is important to note that these attributes are assigned based on individual experiences and not on some "objective" value of the language.

There are Northern dialects, Southern dialects, and Mid-Western dialects. A dialect may be spoken by as many as several thousand people or as little as a few hundred people. A hallmark of dialect variation is intonation, prosody, and phonology. We often refer to these sound differences as **"accents."**

Because language is dynamic, dialects change and evolve as communities change and evolve. The more isolated a speech community is, the more preserved the speech style will be. For example, there are small coastal islands (like Tangier Island off the coast of Virginia or the Gullah Islands off the coast of southern Georgia) in which speech patterns have remained relatively unchanged for generations. To outsiders, groups of people like these might have speech that sounds quite old fashioned or unusual.

The Social Context of Dialects and Languages

Although language scientists have no difficulty in defining dialect in a neutral manner, society seems to have much more difficulty with this. Because language occurs in a social context, it is subject to certain societal judgments. Individuals attribute, often unfairly, certain characteristics to people with certain dialects. Certain dialects may be seen as exotic or romantic, whereas others may be viewed as problematic and "difficult to understand." To know more than one language can be seen as a positive or a negative depending on which languages the individual speaks. In any given society the ways of a "favored" group become favored as well. The customs themselves have no inherent value, but become valued or favored simply as a result of their use by a favored group. Most people would not consider cucumber sandwiches or snails inherently desirable. Yet, because they are consumed in favored "upper-class" circles, they become desirable to many. In much the same way, the dialect of any favored group will become the favored dialect in a community. It is crucial to understand that this "favored" status has no basis in linguistic reality, just as cucumbers and snails are not in any real sense better than any other food. Because a particular dialect is considered to be the standard to be achieved, the language itself is not necessarily better or more sophisticated than the other varieties of the language. Conversely, the speech patterns of a stigmatized group will often become as stigmatized as the group themselves. In truth, the dialect of a socially stigmatized group may not be linguistically impoverished or more unsophisticated than the standard variety.

Historically, the dialects of American English evolved as immigrants came to the United States. Immigrants from different parts of England had different varieties of English, as was the case with immigrants coming from Poland, Ireland, and Italy. In the areas of the northeast United States where these people immigrated, the different varieties of English are quite distinct—New Yorkers sound different from Bostonians who sound different from those living in Maine and so on. As settlers moved West, the different varieties of

English began to blend more as groups interacted more. That is why dialect differences in the western United States are not quite as distinct.

Dialects can also be indicative of close contact with other languages. As we noted before, the languages that many immigrants spoke when they initially came to this country had an impact on English. This phenomenon is seen today with our newest immigrant populations. Again, in individuals learning a second language, the home language and the language of the larger community influence each other. These issues are seen in both AAE and in bilingualism. In the next two sections we will examine issues regarding AAE and bilingualism within this social context.

The Case of African-American English

The speech variety used by the African-American population in the United States illustrates most of the dialect issues discussed so far, as well as the bilingual issues discussed in the next section. Linguists and language specialists most often refer to this variety of speech as African-American English or AAE. In the past, it has also been called Black English, Negro dialect, Non-Standard Negro dialect, and Ebonics. African-American English (AAE) may be viewed as a dialect of English because English words are used and there is much overlap with English grammar. However, when viewed from historical and political perspectives, African-American English can be viewed as a unique language form.

African-American English (AAE) has been the subject of great debate over the past several decades. Early debates centered on the legitimacy of AAE as a language form and the true linguistic competence of those who spoke AAE. Recent debates in the late 1990s have centered on the legitimacy of using AAE as an educational tool to improve classroom performance in schools where children speak primarily AAE. While the latter is too in-depth a topic for this discussion, we can provide some insight on what linguists and other language specialists do know about AAE.

When groups are socially stigmatized, their language will likely be stigmatized as well. This is certainly true of AAE, which is used by a large segment of the African-American community. Frequent misconceptions and myths have long surrounded the use of AAE. Consequently, it is pertinent to first briefly discuss what AAE is not. AAE is not "bad English," "broken English," or slang. AAE is not an impoverished form of Standard American English (SAE), and it is not spoken solely by African-Americans. That is to say, some features of AAE are used by members of other ethnic groups who are familiar with AAE features and who find value in their usage. Moreover, AAE is not what some refer to as "hip-hop" or "jive"; that is to say, AAE is not synonymous with "yo baby, yo baby," "she's dope," "she's all that," or "what's up." These types of sayings and word usages are simply part of a small vernacular used by a particular social group that is most typically young and urban.

Recently, it has also been adopted by some young people in suburban settings. This type of speech (e.g., "What up?" "She's all that") is no different than other types of rapidly changing vernaculars such as "Valley Girl" and "Surfer Dude" talk. But, it is not AAE. So what then is AAE?

AAE is a speech form used by a large segment of the African-American population that has ties to the West African linguistic roots of the community's slave ancestors. AAE's unique evolutionary history is directly linked to the trans-Atlantic slave trade. Most of the Africans-turned-slaves were taken from the West Coast of Africa. Linguists understand that the languages spoken in this part of Africa are a part of the Niger-Congo family of languages, which consists of some 500–600 different languages. These languages, although not mutually intelligible, have similar grammars. For example, members of the West African family of languages tend to follow the same sound rules (e.g., no consonants clustered at the ends of words); conjugate verbs by requiring that the verb remain constant for person and number; and have similar tense and aspect patterns such as habitual aspect, and past, present, future, near past, and remote past tense). In other words, Niger-Congo languages exhibit a grammar different from the Northern European or Germanic family of languages of which English is a member.

Upon their arrival in America, Africans initially retained their African linguistic patterns. The majority of slaves working as field laborers had limited direct contact with English, which reinforced the retention of the African-turned-slave's primary linguistic patterns. Conversely, those slaves working in plantation homes or on small plantations had more direct contact and interaction with English. It is hypothesized that the slave did what all learners of second languages do—first, they learned the names of things (nouns); then, verbs; and later, adjectives and other forms. As with all learners of second languages, what remained most constant were the grammatical patterns that were initially learned by the speaker in his first language; for example, word forms like nouns and verbs were frequently organized according to the slave's African linguistic patterns. This is akin to the way English speakers initially say *blanca casa* (*white house*) when learning Spanish, instead of using Spanish grammar where the adjective follows the noun (e.g., *casa blanca*).

It is crucial to the understanding of evolution of AAE that one realizes that slaves were never taught English. The common penalty for literacy during slavery was death. This is an important distinction in understanding how the African-American is unlike the immigrant who had access to programs designed to teach English to encourage assimilation. The African-American was not welcome to assimilate into society. Indeed, it is this unacceptance that served to retain the speech patterns of the African-turned-slave.

Once slavery formally ended in 1865, **"Jim Crow" segregation** immediately followed. Blacks were legally denied access to social and political interactions with mainstream society, which dictated that blacks could not live where whites lived, go to school where whites went to school, eat where whites ate, attend church where whites worshipped, swim where whites swam, or even drink from a fountain where whites drank. Linguistically, this social stratification preserved the speech patterns of the African-American community. The dismantling of "Jim Crow" segregation did not begin until the mid 1960s—a mere 30 years ago. Despite the official desegregation of the African-American community, many sociologists contend that the socioeconomic stratification that continues has sustained the isolation of a large segment of the African-American population from the mainstream population. Harvard sociologist Orlando Patterson (1998) notes that the African-American community today still remains highly isolated from the rest of America. Table 3–1 highlights some of the features found in AAE, many of which are known to be reflective of West African language rules, especially the tense and aspect patterns which are notably different from SAE. An example is the use of the aspectual marker "be," which does not exist in SAE (e.g., She "<u>be</u>" running). Although this "be" appears to be used like an SAE auxiliary (e.g., She <u>is</u> running), it is an aspect marker that denotes an activity or state of being (mad,

Table 3–1. African-American English Grammatical Features

Grammatical Feature	Examples
Copula/Auxiliary Deletion	He running to the store He a doctor
Verb Regularization (same verb form for all subject cases)	"I play, you play, he play, we play, they play."
Zero Possessive Marker	That my brother car I go to my auntie house
Zero Past Tense -ed Marker	Yesterday we play ball
Zero Plural Marker	Fifty cent Four chair
Reflexive Pronouns	He did it hisself She gonna hurt herself, itself, theirselves
Expletive "it" (it used for "there's")	It's a girl in my class named Amber It's a dog in your yard (vs. there's a dog . . .)
Tense and Aspect Features	
Habitual "be"	She be sewing (She sews habitually on specific occasions over time)
Completive past tense	He done gone (He already left)
Remote past tense	He been gone (He left a long time ago)
AAE Sound Rules	**Example**
No consonant pairs on word endings	"jus" (for just) "men" (for mend)
/th/ sound substitution: /d/ or /f/ used in its place	"dis" (for this) "birfday" (for birthday)

sad, happy, etc.) that occurs habitually over time, but may or may not be happening now.

In the social quest to achieve the mainstream English, the truly interesting part of AAE has been overlooked. Within the speech of many African-Americans today remain some of the last true vestiges of the motherland left behind by the community's ancestors. The fact that AAE utilizes different tense patterns than SAE is not a reflection of an "error" of SAE, but rather of the encompassing of not only the three tenses of SAE but the five tenses found in many West African languages. The collapsing of groups of consonants at the ends of English words (e.g., *tesses* instead of *tests*) is not an "error" of SAE pronunciation rules, but an adherence to pronunciation patterns found in some West African languages (see Table 3–1 for commonly used features).

 CD-ROM

AAE Features

CD-ROM segments Ch.03.04, Ch.03.05, and Ch.03.06 show children using specific features of African-American English. Segment Ch.03.04 is an example of non-use of past tense -ed marker. Notice here that the past tense context is indicated by the use of the irregular past tense verb *went*, which precedes the nonmarked *graduate*, "When she, um *graduate*, everyone was there for her party."

Segment Ch.03.05 shows 3rd person /s/ regularization in the form of using *eat* instead of *eats*, copula deletion in the form of substituting *they* for *they're*, and the phonological pattern of using /d/ for /th/ in the sentence, "But the real principal *eat* lunch with *dem*, because *they* bad."

Another example of 3rd person regularization is seen in segment Ch.03.06. In this clip, the feature is not as easily identified because of the phonetic context. Listen and see what you hear. Is Danny saying *"He teach us college stuff like . . ."* or *"He teaches college stuff like . . ."*?

Today AAE is used on a continuum by its speakers, some of whom use many features frequently while others use a few features infrequently. Some speakers move up and down the continuum depending on the particular communicative context. In formal work settings some speakers may use only SAE patterns. Then, in a casual home and family environment, these same individuals may use more AAE features. This ability to use AAE in some settings and not in others, or to vary its usage throughout one event, is known as **code switching.** For many in the African-American community, the use of AAE features has become a social identity marker that they embrace. That is, some speakers willingly move between SAE and AAE and have no desire to abandon AAE in favor of SAE. They feel this way because AAE is part of their cultural identity and their connection to the African-American community. Still others wish to use only the socially esteemed variety of SAE that is more accepted in mainstream American society.

 CD–ROM

Code Switching: AAE and SAE

CD-ROM segment Ch.03.07 shows Danny performing intonational code switching when imitating SAE-speaking classmate. He uses intonation and pitch indicative of SAE that differ from his typical use of pitch and intonation, "Stop, stop, get off, I'm telling Mr. Naughlin."

Segment Ch.03.08 shows Danny performing grammatical code switching to SAE in the presence of a non-AAE-speaking visitor. He starts to use aspectual "be," which has no SAE equivalent word, and then changes to an SAE translation, "He *be putting* big words *he puts* big words." Note that, although *he puts big words* is similar in meaning to *he be putting big words,* it does not highlight the same habitual aspect that "be" refers to in AAE. He also switches from a regularized 3rd person /s/ production to the SAE irregular 3rd person /s/, "He *don't* He *doesn't* need to . . ." These types of switches were not observed in Danny's speech before the visitor arrived and appeared to be a result of accommodating a non-AAE speaker.

We have discussed the difference between languages and dialects as relating primarily to power and influence as opposed to any linguistic reality. The major difference between AAE and other dialects of English is the base language. Typically, dialects emerge as the speakers of one language diverge and experience differences in that language. AAE differs from this model in that, at its core, there appear to be at least two languages: English plus the grammatical core of a group of West African languages. Despite this difference, though, most linguists typically consider AAE to be a dialect of English since it uses all English words and has more similarities than differences to SAE. But its differences have been significant enough, historically, to cause debate about its legitimacy as well as misdiagnosis of children's linguistic competence. Similar issues of misdiagnosis also occur with children who are bilingual, as will be seen in the next section.

Bilingualism

Most of us would probably agree that a **bilingual** individual is someone who uses and understands two languages. However, when we start to look at the nature of bilingualism and at people who are bilingual we see enormous variation. How do we define bilingualism and what are the implications for the practice of speech, language, and hearing sciences?

It used to be that bilingualism was defined as a "balanced" use of two languages by a person. However, studies of these so-called "balanced" bilinguals demonstrated that they had different strengths in each of their languages and that the two languages did not, in fact, mirror each other. Grosjean (1989) points out that the way we define bilingualism influences how we interpret bilingual behavior. He suggests that the "balanced" definition of bilingualism (meaning, two monolinguals in one) reflects the idea that a bilingual individual must have equal fluency in both languages, and that anything short of that is therefore inadequate. However, even bilinguals who are highly fluent in two languages have different strengths depending on the situations in which they use each of the languages. Over time, bilinguals move in and out of relative fluency in the two languages based on the social and educational demands that affect their lives.

At any given point in time, it is much more likely that a bilingual individual will present an "unbalanced" profile. This is why Grosjean (1989) suggests that we think of bilinguals as bilinguals, and not as two monolinguals. Because there are different types of bilinguals, it is important to take into account the dynamic nature of language and how two languages might be learned.

It is important to understand how an individual becomes bilingual. There are people who have studied a foreign language in school who then may travel, live, or work in a country where that language is spoken. This type of bilingual is usually referred to as an **elective bilingual.** There are also people who learned a second language because they immigrated to another country, very likely because of economic reasons, and must learn a second language in order to interact in the community. This person is likely to not have formal education learning the second language. This person would be referred to as a **circumstantial bilingual.**

The nature of bilingualism also relates to when the person learned the first and second languages. Some individuals are exposed to two languages from birth. Perhaps their families know and use two languages at home. These bilinguals are considered to be **simultaneous bilinguals.** There are individuals who learn a second language when they go to school (often kindergarten or preschool) or who learn a second language as an adult. These individuals are considered **sequential bilinguals.** It's important to examine the status of each language and understand that different types of bilinguals will have different profiles. A kindergarten child who was exposed to two languages from birth will perform differently from a child whose first exposure to English is in kindergarten, even though both of these children may be classified as bilingual.

Young children present a special case as they are still learning language. They may still be learning their primary language when they begin to learn a second language, or they may be learning two languages at once. Thus, their bilingualism is not fully established.

We consider bilingualism to be a continuum of relative proficiency in a speaker's first language (L1) and their second language (L2). Proficiency in any language is task dependent. So, individuals who are bilingual may be highly proficient in their first language (L1) for certain tasks, while they may be more proficient in their second language (L2) for a completely different set of tasks. For example, it is not uncommon for young children to know "home" vocabulary (e.g., functions, body parts, names of relatives, social routines) in the home language and "school" vocabulary (e.g., colors & numbers) in English. Finally, bilinguals in interaction with other bilinguals may mix, switch, or borrow words across languages in a rule-governed way. Additionally, they may code switch in response to the situation or to their listeners.

 CD-ROM

Codeswitching: Spanish and English

Watch CD-ROM segment Ch.03.09. At first, Magali interacts with an adult who only speaks Spanish to her, and that is her stronger language. Together, Magali and the adult make up a story about a frog's birthday party. They also draw a frog, adding water, a table, and a birthday cake. Magali turns to the other adult once the drawing is complete and says to her, "There we go," while picking up the puppet. The Spanish speaker continues to address Magali in Spanish only, telling her to explain to the other adult what is happening in the picture. Once again, Magali turns to the second adult and explains in English, "That is the happy birthday." You can see that Magali is aware of her audience and switches between the two languages appropriately and effortlessly.

Why are these descriptions important? When working with bilinguals it is important to understand how and when they came to know two languages. Understanding of their language learning circumstances and timing may help us make more appropriate clinical judgments about their language learning abilities and may help us to respond to their needs in a culturally sensitive manner. Also, it is important to assess in both (or all) the languages of an individual to gain a complete understanding of their speech and language functioning. Finally, because bilingual status is constantly changing due to social and academic interactions, language testing should be viewed as having only short-term stability.

When two languages come into contact with each other, there are typically mutual influences between them. One common occurrence is that the grammar of the home language may influence word order in the second language. For example in Spanish, articles and nouns must agree on number and gender (masculine/feminine), but in English gender is not marked, and the article "a" is singular, while "the" can be singular or plural, with plurality marked on the noun. An English speaker learning Spanish may make article-noun agreement errors, "el casa" *the* (masculine, singular) *house* (feminine, singular) instead of the correct "las casas." There is also evidence that the second language may influence the first language. In several studies of bilinguals across several languages, Bates and her colleagues (Bates, Devescovi, & D'Amico, 1999; Hernandez, Bates, & Avila, 1994; Liu, Bates, & Li, 1992) have found that, in comparison to monolinguals, bilinguals employ the grammatical cues of both their languages at the same time. For example, Spanish speakers rely heavily on noun-verb agreement as an important grammatical cue, whereas English speakers rely on word order as a primary cue. Spanish-English bilinguals were seen to utilize both word order and noun-verb agreement in Spanish and English.

A final issue that is important to consider when working with individuals who come from a different language background is that of culture. In the earlier part of this chapter we discussed the process of socialization—or coming to know one's own culture and language. We also need to consider the process of acculturation. We'd said that this was the process by which a second culture was acquired. It is important to realize that there are several processes in action in the acculturation process. Just as with learning a second language, the reasons for acculturation may vary. On one hand, an individual or family may want to maintain the home culture but may have to make some adaptations in order to succeed in school or work. On the other hand, some families feel that their culture may be stigmatizing, and they may want to adapt to the new culture as fast as possible. Still other families may blend aspects of the home and host culture.

SUMMARY

This chapter introduced you to some of the issues related to examination of culture and language. We have seen that culture and language change over time, and that culture is reflected in the language that we use every day. It is important to understand the process of learning a first and second language and of learning a first and (possibly) second culture. We know that lack of understanding of cultural and linguistic diversity can lead to erroneous assumptions about someone's ability. Furthermore, this lack of understanding can lead to misdiagnosis in speech-language pathology and audiology. Ultimately, we need to have an understanding of culture and language to better assess and treat individuals from diverse backgrounds.

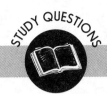

STUDY QUESTIONS

1 Compare and contrast the processes of socialization and acculturation.

    a. How might differences in socialization practices affect school performance?

    b. What are reasons for acculturation?

---

2 Define and describe BICS and CALP.

---

3 How can language and culture affect test taking?

    a. Explain some potential problems with translating tests from one language to another.

    b. How might differences in test-taking experiences impact test performance?

---

4 Describe how dialects are formed.

---

5 List both positive and negative assumptions that might be made about dialects. What are some potential impacts of these assumptions?

---

6 What are some examples of different types of bilinguals?

---

7 Why would understanding how individuals become bilingual matter to a speech-language pathologist (SLP) or audiologist?

---

8 Describe the origins of African-American English (AAE).

    a. Explain how AAE might be considered a language.

    b. Explain how AAE might be considered a dialect.

REFERENCES

Cummins, J. (1984). *Bilingualism and special education: Issues in assessment and pedagogy.* Austin, TX: Pro-Ed.

Bates, E., Devescovi, A., & D'Amico, S. (1999). Processing complex sentences: A cross-linguistic study. *Language & Cognitive Processes, 14*(1), 69–123.

Grosjean, F. (1989). Neurolinguists, beware! The bilingual is not two monolinguals in one. *Brain and Language, 36,* 3–16.

Hernandez, A., Bates, E., & Avila, L. (1994). On-line sentence interpretation in Spanish-English bilinguals:

What does it mean to be "in between"? *Applied Psycholinguistics, 15,* 417–446.

Liu, H., Bates, E., & Li, P. (1992). Sentence interpretation in bilingual speakers of English and Chinese. *Applied Psycholingustics, 13,* 451–484.

Patterson, O. (1998). *Rituals of blood: Consequences of slavery in two American centuries.* Washington, DC: Civitas/ Counterpoint.

Pinker, S. (1994). *The language instinct: How the mind creates language.* New York: William Morrow.

Rogoff, B. (1991). *Apprenticeship in thinking: Cognitive development in social context.* New York: Oxford University Press.

SUGGESTED READINGS

Baker, C. (1993). *Foundations of bilingual education and bilingualism.* Bristol, PA: Multilingual Matters, Ltd.

Gumperz, J. (1982). *Discourse strategies.* New York: Cambridge University Press.

Heath, S. B. (1983). *Ways with words: Language, life, and work in communities and classrooms.* Cambridge, England: Cambridge University Press.

Iglesias, A. (1985). Cultural conflict in the classroom: The communicatively different child. In D. N. Ripich & F. M. Spinelli (Eds.), *School discourse problems* (pp. 79–96). San Diego: College-Hill Press.

Kayser, H. (1995). *Bilingual speech-language pathology: An Hispanic perspective.* San Diego: Singular Publishing Group.

Valdes, G., & Figueroa, R. (1993). *Bilingualism and testing: A special case of bias.* New York: Ablex.

GLOSSARY

Accent: A particular nonnative stress on syllables in words, which connotes the influence of a second language.

Acculturation: The process of learning a second culture.

Basic interpersonal communication skills (BICS): Language proficiency at a level that requires low cognitive load in situations that are highly contextualized.

Bilingual: Use and comprehension of two languages. Level of proficiency in each language may be different across situations, communicative demands, and over time.

Circumstantial bilingual: Someone who becomes bilingual as a result of living in a bilingual environment. May come about due to forced migration or for economic reasons such as traveling to another country to find work.

Code switching: The alternating use of two languages at the word, phrase, and sentence level with a complete break between languages in phonology. In AAE, code switching refers to alternations in intonation, prosody, and specific grammatical features determined by the situational context. More formal settings typically result in "switches" toward Standard American English, and more informal situations typically yield switches toward AAE grammatical and intonational patterns.

Cognitive academic language proficiency (CALP): Language proficiency at a level that requires high cognitive load in situations that are decontextualized.

Communicative demand: The expectations of a specific language interaction.

Culture: The set of beliefs and assumptions shared by a group of people that guide how individuals in that group think, act, and interact on a daily basis.

Decontextualized language: Refers to a language learning environment devoid of significant nonverbal or contextual cues to assist meaning.

Dialect: Variation of a language that is understood by all speakers of the "mother" language. May include sound, vocabulary, and grammatical variations.

Elective bilingual: Refers to someone who learns a second language by choice.

Grammatical patterns: Rule-governed organization of words in sentences.

"Jim Crow" segregation: The legalized segregation (about 1900 through the 1960s) barring African-Americans from public and social interaction with whites.

Language context: The situation in which language is used, including the immediate environment of the speaker and listener and past experiences that each brings to the situation.

Mismatch: Refers to a discrepancy between child socialization and expectations for home language interactions and school language interactions.

Sequential bilingual: A second language is introduced after the primary language is established.

Simultaneous bilingual: Two languages are acquired early in a person's development.

Socialization: The degree to which one is able to interact with others following appropriate social norms.

Socioeconomic status: A family's socioeconomic status is based on family income, parental education level, parental occupation, and social status in the community.

4

An Overview of Communication Disorders

Ronald B. Gillam, Thomas P. Marquardt, and Frederick N. Martin

LEARNING OBJECTIVES

1 To understand how disorders of hearing, speech, and language adversely affect communication.

2 To compare and contrast the meaning of the following terms: impairment, disability, handicap, disorder, and difference.

3 To learn about the major types of speech, language, and hearing disorders.

4 To learn about the incidence and prevalence of communication disorders.

LANGUAGE, SPEECH, AND HEARING IN A SYSTEM OF COMMUNICATION

As noted in Chapter 2, communication is an exchange of meaning between a sender and a receiver. Most of the time, meanings are exchanged via a code, called language, that can be written or signed but is most often spoken. Figure 4–1 depicts speech, hearing, and language as three important interrelated processes that link individuals to each other and to the society that surrounds them. With respect to spoken language, speakers use a series of programmed structural movements to form sequences of sounds that represent words, phrases, and sentences, and then listeners interpret the message by converting acoustic energy that reaches their ears into mental representations of words and sentences. The large shaded arrows at the top and bottom of the figure are meant to represent the reciprocal relationships between individuals and the societies in which they function. Through communication, the individual can influence society at large. At the same time, social and cultural experiences play an important role in shaping the way individuals think and communicate.

Most people communicate effectively by the time they are 3 or 4 years old, and most individuals are experts at this process by the time they are 9 years old. Unfortunately, there are many ways that the processes involved in communication can break down. When they do, people routinely turn to speech-language pathologists and audiologists for help.

This chapter presents a typology of communication differences and disorders and the kinds of communicative disruptions individuals experience when they have difficulties with one or more of the processes that contribute to speech, language, and hearing. It is important to realize that communication is a system with many reciprocal relationships. A problem with one aspect of the communication process often impacts many of the other processes that are related to it. For example, children who have a hearing loss receive limited acoustic input, which adversely affects the development of their language and speech. Language and speech disorders often have an adverse impact on social, academic, and vocational aspects of people's lives.

TERMINOLOGY

Some people have unusual difficulties with communication. What are the best ways to refer to these problems? According to the World Health Organization (Wood, 1980), the word **impairment** should be used to refer to any loss or abnormality of psychological, physiological, or anatomical structure or function. This is a relatively neutral term with respect to the ability to function in society. For example, a hearing impairment means only that there is unusually poor hearing. It doesn't mean that individuals cannot

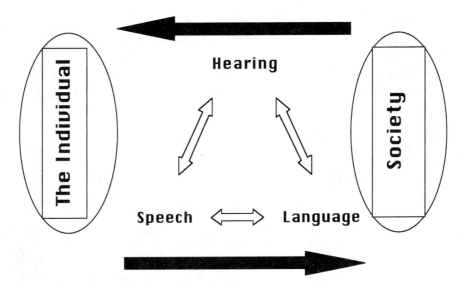

Figure 4–1. Hearing, speech, and language as links between the individual and society.

function well in daily living and working situations. With hearing aids, they might live their lives as completely and fully as people who hear well. The concept of impairment leads us to ask, What is wrong with the person, and can it be fixed? What does this person do well? What skills and abilities can be used to compensate for this person's impairment?

The word **disability** refers to a reduced competence in meeting daily living needs. The person with a disability might not be able to perform a particular life activity in a particular context. For example, people with hearing impairment might not be able to communicate well on the telephone, even when they are wearing a hearing aid. In this case, the hearing impairment led to a disability. The concept of a disability leads us to ask, What are the communication requirements of the environments that the individual functions in every day, and to what extent can the person access important daily living activities if some sort of compensation (like a hearing aid) is provided?

The word **handicap** refers to a social, educational, or occupational disadvantage that results from an impairment or disability. This disadvantage is often affected by the nature of the person's impairment and by the attitudes and biases that may be present in the person's environment. For example, a child with a hearing loss may have a hearing aid that allows her to hear most speech sounds without difficulties. However, she might not be able to hear as well in a noisy classroom environment. Unless the classroom teacher undertakes measures to lessen the extent of classroom noise, the child might not hear important classroom instructions, resulting in an educational handicap. The concept of a handicap leads us to ask, Does this person experience social, educational, and vocational penalties? To what extent can we lessen these penalties by compensating for the person's impairment and by educating important people in the environment about ways they can modify the environment? The term handicap is considered pejorative by many people.

The term **communication disorder** is sometimes used as a synonym for impairment and other times as a synonym for disability. In this text, we use the term *communication disorder* to refer to any communication structure or function that is diminished to a significant degree. In essence, a communication disorder interferes with the exchange of meaning and is apparent to the communication partners. Unless specifically stated, we will not imply any cultural, educational, or vocational disadvantage. Unfortunately, many people with communication disorders experience communication disabilities and handicaps, although this is not necessarily so.

Some people communicate in ways that differ from that of the mainstream culture. Unfortunately, these people may be at risk for social, educational, and/or vocational penalties even though they do not have an impairment. We use the term **communication difference** to mean communication abilities that differ from those usually encountered in the mainstream culture even though there is no evidence of impairment. For example, when they begin school, children who have spoken Spanish for most of their lives will not communicate like their monolingual English-speaking classmates. If these children learned Spanish without any difficulty, they obviously do not have a communication disorder. Unfortunately, these children's communication differences may contribute to periodic social and educational disadvantages within the school environment. These children certainly need extra assistance in learning English as a second language. However, unless children have communication impairments (characterized by loss or decline in communicative structures or functions that adversely affects their communication in all the languages they speak), they should not be diagnosed with a communication disorder, and they should not be treated by speech-language pathologists (SLPs) or audiologists. Table 4–1 presents a list of concepts that speech-language pathologists (SLPs) and audiologists should consider when they assess children from linguistically and culturally diverse backgrounds.

Person-First Language

It is important to recognize that the problems individuals experience do not define who they are. For example, a person who stutters is not just a stutterer. That person may be a caring parent, a good friend, a successful business owner, or even a good communicator. For this reason, most researchers and clinicians use **person-first language** to refer to individuals with communication disorders. By "person-first," we mean the communication disorder is a

Table 4–1. Critical Concepts To Consider When Conducting Assessments with Children From Linguistically and Culturally Diverse (LCD) Backgrounds

- Lack of proficiency and skill in Standard English does not necessarily indicate a communication disorder.
- Children and adults who speak two or more languages sometimes have difficulty discriminating differences between English words due to differences between the sound patterns in their first and second language.
- Children do not need to forget their first language in order to learn a second language.
- All tests are culturally biased because they represent the cultural values and expectations of the test authors.
- Some learning styles are culturally determined.
- Speech-language pathologists and audiologists should not assume that the learning needs and learning styles of all children from LCD backgrounds are similar.
- Individuals from culturally and linguistically diverse backgrounds may not have the same perceptions or attitudes about "disability" or "impairment" as individuals from mainstream American culture.
- Individuals from culturally and linguistically diverse backgrounds and their family members have valuable information about communication expectations that must be taken into consideration when determining how to best address their communication needs.

Source: Adapted from Leadholm and Miller (1992).

single descriptor of the individual and not their primary attribute. We will follow that convention as much as possible in this book by using such phrases as, "children with language disorders" instead of "language-disordered children." When we refer to groups of individuals who present a particular disorder, we might sometimes use the name of the disorder alone (i.e., "aphasics") instead of always having to write the somewhat more convoluted phrase, "individuals with aphasia." When we use the name of a communication disorder to refer to the group of individuals who present that disorder, readers should know that we do not mean to imply that the disorder is the sole defining characteristic of persons who happen to present that kind of problem. As a matter of fact, our patients tell us that they do not like to be defined by their disabilities.

A classification of the various types of communication disorders is presented to demonstrate the wide diversity of disorders that professionals in communication sciences and disorders (CSD) must be prepared to work with. Each of these disorders is considered in more detail in later chapters. We present a broad overview here so you will have a concept of the breadth of the field of communication sciences and disorders (CSD) before you start learning about the specifics. Common types of communication disorders are listed under the headings of hearing, speech, and language.

TYPES OF COMMUNICATION DISORDERS

Communication disorders typically are classified into hearing, speech, and language categories, but as we noted, this is an artificial separation because these processes are not functionally isolated within the system of communication. Additional parameters of classification include the etiological basis (cause) of the disorder and the point during the maturation of the individual that the disorder occurred. **Organic** disorders have a physical cause. For example, an adult with difficulty retrieving words after a stroke and a child who has problems producing speech sounds due to inadequate closure between the nose and mouth after the repair of a cleft palate have physical problems that account for their communication problems. In contrast, there are communication disorders termed **functional** for which a physical cause cannot be found. For example, a man may continue to speak at the same pitch as a child even though the vocal folds are normal. In this case there is no physical basis for the problem. For some communication disorders, it is difficult to determine whether the cause of the disorder would best be described as organic or functional. A young child may have difficulty producing speech sounds in comparison to his peers, but it is not known with surety whether the disorder is organic in nature (e.g., a result of delayed maturation of the nervous system) or functional (e.g., a result of poor speech models or lack of environmental opportunity for speaking).

When the disorder occurs is also an important consideration. Developmental disorders, such as delays in speech and language development, occur early in the maturation of the individual but may continue into adulthood. Acquired disorders, such as speech and language disorders due to brain trauma following an accident, occur after communication skills have been fully developed.

With these distinctions in mind, we will provide a brief overview of hearing, speech, and language disorders. Some reference is made to the **incidence** (percentage of the population that experienced a disorder during their lifetime) and **prevalence** (number of individuals with a disorder at some point in time). More detailed statistics about specific disorders are provided in individual chapters of the text.

Hearing Disorders

The size and mobility of the U.S. population make it difficult to find precise incidence figures for any medical condition. However, according to the American Speech-Language-Hearing Association (ASHA, 2000), of the estimated 46 million citizens with a communication disorder, more than 28 million have some kind of hearing disorder.

People with hearing disorders have a deficiency in their ability to detect sounds. This deficiency can vary in terms of how loud sounds need to be presented before they can be heard. Hearing can also vary with respect to the pitch level of sounds that are heard. Some individuals can hear low-frequency sounds like the notes from a bass guitar better than they can hear high-frequency sounds like a small bell. Other individuals do not hear sounds at any frequency very well.

Hearing loss can have a large or small effect on communication depending on the degree of loss and the type of sounds that are affected (see Table 4–2). People with mild degrees of hearing loss that affect only their ability to hear high-pitched sounds will miss out on final sounds of words like "bath," but they will hear most other sounds well enough so they can usually fill in the missing pieces. For example, you can probably read the following sentence even though the letters representing the final sounds are missing, "Joh_ wen_ upstair_ to ta_ a ba_." However, people with a hearing loss that affects their ability to hear high- and low-pitched sounds produced at conversational speech levels will be at a significant disadvantage in communication.

If you could not hear conversations, it would be difficult for you to interact with your friends, to take notes in your classes, or to perform the duties

Table 4–2. The Impact of Hearing Loss on Communication

Degree of Loss	Severity	Impact on Communication
15-30 dB	Mild	Can hear all vowels and most consonants spoken at conversational loudness levels. Children with this degree of loss typically experience some difficulties with communication development until they receive appropriate amplification. Adults with this degree of loss will have some difficulty understanding women and children with high-pitched voices, and they may struggle with conversation in noisy environments like restaurants.
30-50 dB	Moderate	Can hear most vowels and some consonants spoken at conversational loudness levels. It is difficult to hear unstressed words and word endings. Children with this degree of loss experience significant delays in communication development. Adults with this degree of loss have some difficulties understanding others during conversations.
50-70 dB	Severe	Can hear most loud noises in the environment (car horns) but not speech unless it is spoken very loudly. Children usually have marked communication difficulties and delays. Adults miss a significant amount of information spoken in conversations.
70 dB+	Profound	Can hear extremely loud noises (jet planes landing) but cannot hear language spoken at conversational levels. Without suitable amplification, individuals with this degree of hearing loss are not able to communicate through speech.

associated with most jobs. Thus, there can be serious social, educational, and vocational consequences of moderate-to-severe hearing losses. Other important factors that influence the degree of the impact that a hearing loss has on communication include whether the hearing loss is unilateral (one ear) or bilateral (two ears), the kind of amplification that is provided, the length of time the individual has had amplification, and the attitudes of family members.

The age of the person with a hearing loss also plays an important role in the degree of impact that a hearing loss has on communication. A moderate hearing loss that is present from birth is much more problematic than a moderate hearing loss that is contracted when an individual is 40 years old. That is because good hearing is critical for communicative development. Children who do not hear well have considerable difficulties understanding language that is spoken to them, learning to produce speech sounds clearly, and developing the words and sentence structures necessary for expressing complex ideas. Early detection of hearing loss is absolutely critical so that children can receive intervention as soon as possible. Some children can profit a great deal from being fitted with a hearing aid. The sooner they receive appropriate amplification, the better it is for speech and language development. Other children do not hear much even with amplification. These children need to be exposed to sign language or specialized speech training in order to develop language.

Many people believe that people who have a hearing loss simply cannot hear sounds as loud as others hear them. If this were the case, the obvious solution to any hearing loss would be to simply make sounds louder in order to make them audible. While this conception of hearing loss is sometimes accurate, more often the ability to hear speech is more complicated. Not only do people with hearing impairments perceive sounds as being less loud, they also perceive sounds as less clear. So, even when speech is amplified so that it is louder, individuals with some kinds of hearing losses may still have difficulty **discriminating** (hearing differences) between sounds due to a loss of the clarity of sounds. For example, they may confuse the word *ball* for the word *doll*. In effect, they hear but do not understand because the auditory information is distorted. The degree of deterioration of the auditory image is often directly related to the degree of the hearing loss. The result is that it can be difficult to find the kind of hearing aid that will assist some people with hearing loss. Fortunately, in its short life (about 50 years), audiology has advanced to the point where diagnosis and rehabilitation measures can assist the majority of children and adults who have hearing impairments.

Speech Disorders

Speech disorders result from interruption in the process of speech production. This process starts with the programming of movements and ends with the acoustic signal that carries the meaning of the message. In some cases, speech disorders result from impairment in a single structure, such as the larynx or tongue. In other cases, the disorder may involve almost the entirety of the process. By historical convention, speech disorders are categorized on the basis of the aspect of speech production (articulation, fluency, voice, etc.) that is affected. There are implicit assumptions that speech disorders may be observed at any time across the lifespan (during the developmental period or later in life). Some speech disorders result from **congenital** or **acquired** conditions (see Table 4–3). Others are considered to be functional or developmental (the cause is not known). Speech disorders can only be assessed adequately when the characteristics of a person's speech are considered as one part of the entire communication process.

Articulation and Phonological Disorders

Individuals with **articulation disorders** have problems with the production of speech sounds. Such problems result from deviations in anatomical structures, physiological functions, and learning. When the problem is thought to be related to the way sounds are represented in the brain, it is commonly referred to as a phonological disorder. The problem may be minimal (interfering with the way one or two speech sounds are produced) or severe (rendering speech unintelligible). Included in this category are developmental speech disorders, neuromuscular speech disorders in adults and children, and articulation disorders resulting from orofacial anomalies like cleft palate. Approximately 10% of preschool and school-age children have articulatory or phonological disorders (ASHA, 2000).

Table 4–3. Speech Disorders Associated With Congenital or Acquired Conditions

Disorder	Characteristics
Cleft Palate	Nasal loss of air during consonant production; abnormal resonance, speech sound production errors.
Cerebral Palsy	Articulation and voice disorders associated with abnormal muscle function in children.
Laryngeal Pathology	Changes in voice quality due to injury, vocal nodules, tumors of the vocal tract, or other diseases.
Laryngectomy	Surgical removal of larynx necessitates an alternative form of communication.
Dysarthria	Disorders of respiration, phonation, and articulation due to abnormal muscle function in children and adults.
Apraxia	Neuromuscular speech disorders and deficits in programming speech movements.
Brain Trauma	Injury to the brain that results in a variety of communication disorders.

Fluency Disorders

A **fluency disorder** is an unusual interruption in the flow of speaking. Individuals with fluency disorders have an atypical rhythm and rate and an unusual number of sound and syllable repetitions. Their disruptions in fluency are often accompanied by excessive tension, and they may struggle visibly to produce the words they want to say. Approximately 1% of the general population stutters, but as many as 5% of all adults report they stuttered at some point in their lives.

Voice Disorders

This category is usually divided into two parts: phonation and resonation. **Phonatory disorders** result from abnormalities in vocal fold vibration that yield changes in loudness, pitch, or quality (e.g., breathiness, harshness, or hoarseness). Problems closing the opening between the nose and the mouth during production of speech sounds result in excessive or insufficient nasality. These problems are termed **resonance disorders.** It is estimated that 3 to 9% of the U.S. population has some type of a voice disorder (ASHA, 2000).

Language Disorders

Language refers to the words and sentences that are used to represent objects, thoughts, and feelings. A language disorder is a significant deficiency in understanding or in creating messages. There are three main types of language disorders: developmental (or functional) language disorders that occur during childhood, acquired language disorders that can occur during childhood but most often occur in older adults, and dementia, which nearly always occurs in older adults. It has been estimated that between 6 and 8 million individuals in the United States have some form of language disorder (ASHA, 2000).

Language Delay

During the preschool years, some children have delayed language development. These children have smaller vocabularies, shorter sentences, and they may not say as much as most other children their age. Approximately half of the children who have significant early language delays (i.e., vocabularies less than 50 words) at 2 years of age will have language growth spurts that enable them to catch up to their same age peers by the time they are 5 years old (Paul, Hernandez, Taylor, & Johnson, 1996). Unfortunately, we do not yet know how to predict which children with early language delays will outgrow them and which children will not.

Developmental Language Disorder

Some children have impaired language comprehension and/or production that significantly interferes with socialization and educational success. These children might have a variety of problems including difficulty formulating sentences that express what they want to say, an unusual number of grammatical errors, difficulties thinking of words they know at the moment they need them, and/or difficulties with the social use of language (they tend to say the wrong thing at the wrong time). Until children are in the late preschool and early school-age years, it is difficult to distinguish a language delay from a language disorder. Between 6 and 8% of all children have language disorders. The primary types of childhood language disorders are presented in Table 4–4.

Acquired Language Disorders

These disorders are caused by brain lesions (specific areas of damage to the brain). The most common type of an acquired language disorder is aphasia, which typically occurs in elderly adults after they have suffered a cerebrovascular accident or stroke. Individuals with aphasia frequently have trouble remembering words they once knew or using sentence structures they once

Table 4–4. Common Developmental Language Disorders

Disorder	Characteristics
Mental Retardation	Significantly subaverage mental function with associated difficulties in communication, self-help skills, independence, and motor development.
Specific Language Impairment	Significant deficits in language abilities that cannot be attributed to deficits in hearing, intelligence, or motor functioning.
Autism Spectrum Disorders	Unusual disturbances in social interaction, communication, behaviors, interests, and activities that affect the capacity to relate appropriately to people, events, and objects.
Central Auditory Processing Disorder	Difficulty identifying, interpreting, or organizing auditory information despite normal auditory acuity.
Learning Disability	Difficulties in the acquisition and use of listening, speaking, reading, writing, reasoning, or mathematical abilities.
Dyslexia	A specific reading disorder that results from difficulties with representing and analyzing sounds in words.

used without any problems. It has been estimated that about 1 million Americans have aphasia, and approximately 80,000 individuals acquire aphasia each year (ASHA, 2000).

Traumatic injury to the brain results in a syndrome of cognitive and language disturbances. The communication deficits associated with the injury are primarily a consequence of impaired cognitive processes related to memory, orientation, and organization and include problems more apparent in communication than in speech and language functioning. Most cases of brain trauma are due to motor vehicle accidents with an incidence of approximately 7 million new cases each year.

Dementia

Dementia is a general loss of mental functions due to pathological deterioration of the brain. Dementia is characterized by disorientation; impaired memory, judgment, and intellect; and shallow affect. It is most often seen in individuals who have Alzheimer's disease. Many of the estimated 2 million Americans with dementing diseases such as Alzheimer's disease and Parkinson's disease also have significant language impairments.

SUMMARY

This chapter has introduced some of the differences and disorders that interfere with communication abilities. These disorders are discussed in greater detail in the sections that follow this chapter. We wanted readers to have a general sense of the breadth of the field of communication sciences and disorders before they reviewed specific types of disorders in greater detail. Some communication disorders relate to the way individuals receive information. These disorders involve various degrees and kinds of hearing abnormalities. Other communication disorders involve the way information is processed after it is received. These disorders involve various degrees and kinds of language difficulties. Finally, there are communication disorders that affect output, including difficulties related to speech articulation, voice, and fluency.

As you read the rest of this book, we hope you will remember there are recursive relationships between input, processing, and output systems. A disorder in hearing, speech, or language will have negative consequences for the other two. The specific consequences vary somewhat from person to person. This is why speech-language pathologists and audiologists need to work closely with individuals with communication disorders, their families, and with other professionals. This is also why any type of a communication disorder requires careful analysis and description before therapy begins.

REFERENCES

American Speech-Language-Hearing Association. (2000). *Communication facts.* Rockville, MD: Author.

Leadholm, B., & Miller, J. (1992). *Language sample analysis: The Wisconsin guide.* Madison, WI: Wisconsin Department of Public Instruction.

Paul, R., Hernandez, R., Taylor, L., & Johnson, K. (1996). Narrative development in late talkers: Early school age. *Journal of Speech and Hearing Research, 39,* 1295–1303.

Wood, P. (1980). Appreciating the consequences of disease: The classification of impairments, disabilities, and handicaps. *The World Health Organization Chronicle, 34,* 376–380.

SUGGESTED READINGS

Martin, F. N., & Clark, J. G. (2000). *Introduction to audiology* (7th ed.). Needham Heights, MA: Allyn and Bacon

Nelson, N. W. (1993). *Childhood language disorders in context: Infancy through adolescence* (2nd ed.). Needham Heights, MA: Allyn and Bacon.

Paul, R. (1995). *Language disorders: From infancy through adolescence.* St. Louis, MO: Mosby.

GLOSSARY

Acquired: Disorder that occurs after speech and language skills have been developed.

Articulation and phonological disorders: Problems producing speech sounds correctly due to differences in anatomical structures, physiological functions, or learning.

Communication differences: Communicative abilities that differ from those of other individuals in the same environment in the absence of an impairment.

Communication disorder: Sometimes used as a synonym for impairment, and other times as a synonym for disability.

Congenital: Disorder that occurs at birth or early in the developmental period.

Disability: A reduced ability to meet daily living needs.

Discrimination: The ability to hear differences between sounds.

Fluency disorder: Unusual disruptions in the rhythm and rate of speech. These disruptions are often characterized by repetitions or prolongations of sounds or syllables plus excessive tension.

Functional: Disorder with no known physical cause.

Handicap: A social, educational, or occupational disadvantage that is related to an impairment or disability. This disadvantage is often affected by the nature of the person's impairment and by the attitudes and biases that may be present in the person's environment.

Impairment: Any loss or abnormality of psychological, physiological, or anatomical structure or function

Incidence: Number of individuals who experience a disorder during their lifetime.

Organic: Disorder with a known physical cause.

Person-first language: When describing a person with a communication disorder, professionals should refer to the individual first, then the disorder that they present. For example, it is better to say, "children with autism" than "autistic children." Similarly, "He has aphasia" is preferred over, "He is an aphasic."

Phonatory disorders: Abnormalities in the pitch, loudness, or quality of the voice.

Prevalence: Percentage of a population that demonstrates a disorder at a given point in time.

Resonance disorders: Abnormalities in the use of the nasal cavity during speaking. Individuals can be hypernasal (excessive nasality) or denasal (insufficient nasality).

II

HEARING AND HEARING DISORDERS

5

Hearing Science

Craig A. Champlin

LEARNING OBJECTIVES

1 To learn how sound is generated.

2 To understand how sound travels through a medium.

3 To learn the names of important structures in the auditory system.

4 To understand how different parts of the auditory system work.

INTRODUCTION

Simply defined, hearing is the sense of perceiving sound. Closer examination reveals that hearing is the result of a complicated series of events. First, an object or sound source must be set into motion. A back-and-forth movement called vibration is then transferred from the source to the surrounding medium, which is usually air. When the air particles closest to the source begin to vibrate, the sound travels away from the source in all directions via a domino-like effect. Eventually, the sound reaches the listener who is equipped with an exquisite apparatus, the ear, for catching sounds as they fly through the air. Ear structures channel the sounds deeper inside your head, where the vibrations are converted to neural impulses. The impulses travel to the brain, and sound is perceived.

This chapter discusses the generation and propagation of sound. It will also name important structures of the ear and auditory nervous system and describe their function. The information that is provided in this chapter is necessary for understanding much of the rest of the book. Dr. Martin considers the measurement of hearing in Chapter 6. Chapter 7 (Audiologic Rehabilitation) and Chapter 8 (The Habilitation of Children With Severe to Profound Hearing Loss) concern ways we can assist individuals who do not hear well. We will return to issues related to hearing and the hearing mechanism in Chapter 9 (Speech Science) and Chapter 16 (Language Science).

FUNDAMENTALS OF SOUND

Generating Sound

As mentioned previously, sound needs to be generated before it can be heard. To be a sound source, an object must have mass and elasticity. **Mass** is defined as the amount of matter present in a given object. All objects have mass. **Elasticity** refers to an object's ability to return to its original shape after being deformed (e.g., compressed or stretched). The more elastic the object, the more likely it will be a good sound source.

Perhaps a practical example will help to illustrate the process of **sound generation.** In Figure 5–1, a guitar string has been tightly stretched between two posts. The string is at rest. This position is indicated by the solid line labeled A. The string can be deformed by pulling it upward, away from its resting position. This is position B in the figure and is shown by the long dashed line. When the string is released from position B, it is drawn downward, toward its resting position. The elastic force attempts to restore the string to its original shape. However, the string does not suddenly stop once it reaches its resting position. Because the moving string has mass and thus inertia, momentum drives it, causing it to overshoot the target. As the string continues to move away from its resting position, the elastic force steadily builds. At some point, the elastic force exceeds the opposing force of momentum and the string stops, albeit briefly. This position is indicated in the figure by the short dashed line, which is labeled C. Elasticity pulls the string toward its resting position, but again it fails to stop as momentum pushes the string past its mark. As before, the elastic force increases in strength until it overcomes the force of momentum. Again, the string reverses its direction of travel and moves back the other way. This up-and-down motion continues until the

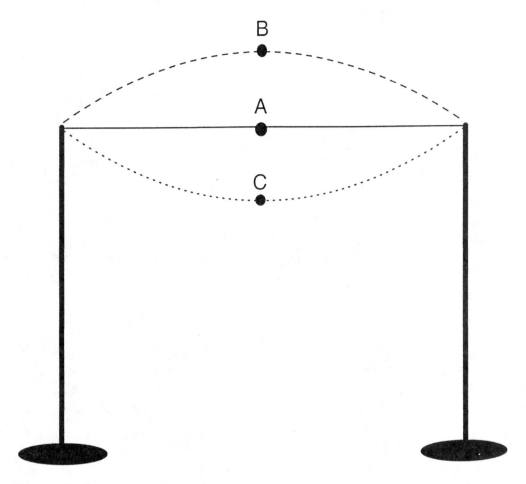

Figure 5–1. Drawing of a guitar string at three different positions during vibration. Position A indicates the resting position. Position B corresponds to the maximum, positive amplitude. Position C indicates the maximum, negative amplitude.

force of friction eventually overpowers the forces of elasticity and momentum to halt the vibration.

Measuring Sound

In the previous example, the string generated vibrations, which created sound. To understand sound better, it may be instructive to consider what properties of vibration can be quantified or measured. When the string vibrates, it moves up and down. If you were to make a drawing of the string's movement over time, it would look like Figure 5–2. This graph is known as a **waveform.** The x-axis (horizontal line) of the graph represents the passage of time (in seconds). It shows when the vibration starts (where time equals

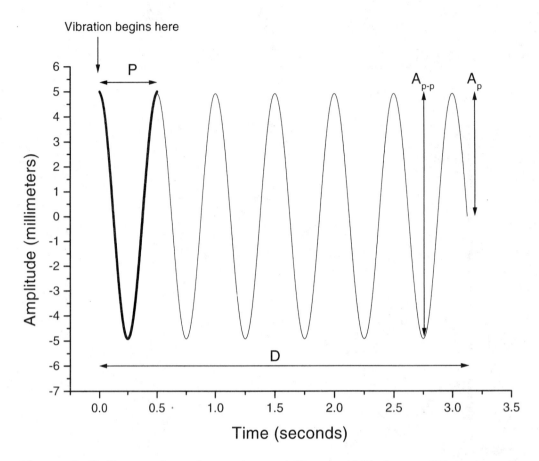

Figure 5-2. The waveform of a simple sound. The period (P), duration (D), peak amplitude (A$_p$) and peak-to-peak amplitude (A$_{p-p}$) are marked. The bold line shows one cycle of vibration.

zero) and when the vibrations stops, 3.25 seconds later in this case. The y-axis (vertical line) shows the distance from the resting position (in millimeters). A positive number indicates upward displacement, and a negative number indicates downward displacement. The position where displacement equals zero denotes the resting position.

Recall that plucking the guitar string generated sound. The string was pulled away from its resting position and then quickly released. For this purpose, the sound began immediately following the release of the string. On the waveform graph, this point corresponds to time of zero seconds and a displacement of +5 millimeters. The string moves downward initially, shooting past the resting position. At a displacement of −5 millimeters, the string stops briefly before reversing its direction. The string now moves upward, zipping past the resting position, but then it slows and finally stops again when it reaches a displacement of +5 millimeters. The process begins to repeat itself—the string moves down, then up, then down again, then up again, and so on.

When describing something, particularly in science, one strives to be as specific as possible. Making quantitative measurements is one way to provide accurate descriptions. The waveform is useful because it allows you to quantify all the characteristics of a simple sound, for example, the vibration of the guitar string. The four quantities that will be considered are frequency, amplitude, duration, and starting phase.

Frequency refers to the number of cycles of vibration that occur in 1 second. The unit of measurement is Hertz, abbreviated Hz. The frequency of a sound is not directly available from the waveform; it must be derived from another measurement called the **period.** However, before discussing the period, you must understand what a cycle of vibration is. Examining the waveform reveals that vibration is repetitive or cyclical. A cycle of vibration is the series of unique movements an object makes. In our working example, the guitar string moved downward, then upward. This sequence of movements corresponds to one cycle of vibration. The bold line segment in Figure 5–2 indicates a cycle. The period, abbreviated P, is the amount of time needed for one cycle of vibration. As shown in Figure 5–2, P equals 0.5 seconds (500 milliseconds) because that is how long it takes the string to complete one cycle of vibration.

Once you know the period, the frequency of vibration can be calculated using the formula $f = 1/P$, where f represents the frequency and P represents the period. From the example waveform, you know that P equals 0.5 seconds. Dividing this number into 1 yields a frequency of 2 Hz. This number means the guitar string vibrates at the rate of 2 cycles per second. It is worth noting that the frequency and period are inversely related—as P increases, f decreases and vice versa. You can prove this to yourself by inserting different values for P into the formula. In practical terms if a sound source vibrates slowly (i.e., the period is long), it will produce a low-frequency sound. Conversely, if the source vibrates rapidly (i.e., the period is short), it will generate a high-frequency sound. Remember that because the x-axis of the waveform

 CD-ROM

Demonstration of Sound Frequency

CD-ROM Segment Ch.05.01 contains three waveforms that are displayed successively on the screen. The sounds can be heard if the computer is equipped with headphones or a speaker. Use the Pause button on the player to freeze the image. The first wave has a frequency of 200 Hz (period = 0.005 seconds), the second wave has a frequency of 400 Hz (period = 0.0025 seconds), and the third wave has a frequency of 800 Hz (period = 0.00125 seconds). Note that as the frequency increases, the number of cycles visible on the screen increases, too. Conversely, as the frequency increases, the period (e.g., the distance between successive peaks in the waveform) decreases or gets shorter.

is time, it does not tell about frequency directly; you must derive this information by measuring the period, which is a time-based quantity.

Returning to the waveform graph in Figure 5–2, note the y-axis reveals how far away the string is from its resting position. Acoustically speaking, this measure of distance is known as the **amplitude** of vibration, or simply amplitude. The maximum displacement in the positive or negative direction is called the peak amplitude. In Figure 5–2, the peak amplitude is indicated by A_p. Sometimes, the peak amplitude can be difficult to gauge, especially if the resting position cannot be determined precisely. A solution to this problem is to measure the distance from the maximum positive peak to the maximum negative peak. This measurement is called the peak-to-peak amplitude and is shown in Figure 5–2 as A_{p-p}.

CD-ROM

Demonstration of Sound Amplitude

CD-ROM Segment Ch.05.02 presents three waveforms are displayed successively on the screen. The sounds can be heard if the computer is equipped with headphones or a speaker. Use the Pause button on the player to freeze the image. Each waveform has a frequency of 400 Hz. The first wave has peak-to-peak amplitude of 6 centimeters, the second wave has peak-to-peak amplitude of 3 centimeters, and the third wave has peak-to-peak amplitude of 1.5 centimeters.

One feature of everyday sounds is the tremendous variability in amplitude. By comparison, the amplitude of a loud sound may be 10,000,000,000 times greater than that of a soft sound. Writing numbers like this is cumbersome and may lead to inaccuracy. Consequently, the decibel, abbreviated dB, was invented. The decibel is based on a logarithmic scale, rather than a linear one. Without getting into the details, a logarithmic scale is useful when working with very large (or very small) numbers. The decibel then, provides an efficient way of expressing amplitude. To get a better feel for the decibel, the softest sound you can hear is about 0 dB, while the loudest sound you can tolerate is around 120 dB. Conversational speech presented at a comfortable loudness level is between 65–75 dB.

The duration of vibration means how long the sound lasts. In other words, the duration corresponds to the span of time marked when the source starts moving and when it stops. The duration is abbreviated D, and, as shown in Figure 5–2, D equals 3.25 seconds.

The **starting phase** of vibration describes the position of the sound source when the vibration begins. For example, you could pull the guitar string up and then release it or you could pull the string down and then let it go. These two positions are not the same. The starting phase, as measured in degrees (0–360), quantifies the position of the sound source just before it begins to vibrate.

Simple and Complex Sounds

The four quantities just discussed—period (the inverse of frequency), amplitude, duration, and starting phase—characterize **simple sounds.** A sound is considered simple if it vibrates at a single frequency. A pure tone is an example of a simple sound. Simple sounds rarely occur in the everyday world. In fact, virtually all sounds you hear are complex sounds.

Complex sounds are vibrations that contain two or more frequencies. In a way, simple sounds are building blocks. By adding simple sounds together, extremely complex sounds such as speech or music can be created. A music synthesizer is an electronic device capable of generating *any* sound by combining simple tones.

 CD-ROM

Demonstration of Simple and Complex Sounds

CD-ROM Segment Ch.05.03 presents two waveforms that are displayed successively on the screen. Use the Pause button on the player to freeze the image. The first wave is a simple sound, a 200-Hz tone. The second wave is a complex sound, which was synthesized by adding together three, equal-amplitude tones (200, 400, and 600 Hz).

You have seen that the waveform provides a useful way of depicting simple sounds. However, the waveform of a complex sound is not particularly revealing because the specific details (e.g., the period) are obscured. An alternative method for representing complex sounds is to plot the **spectrum.** The graph has as its coordinates frequency on the x-axis and either peak amplitude or starting phase on the y-axis. The amplitude spectrum is used more often in sound applications, so the focus will be on it rather than the phase spectrum.

The top two panels in Figure 5–3 show the waveform (left) and amplitude spectrum (right) of a simple sound. The single vertical line indicates only one frequency is present. The height of the line corresponds to the peak amplitude. For comparison purposes, the waveform and amplitude spectrum of the spoken word *big* are shown in the bottom left and right panels, respectively.

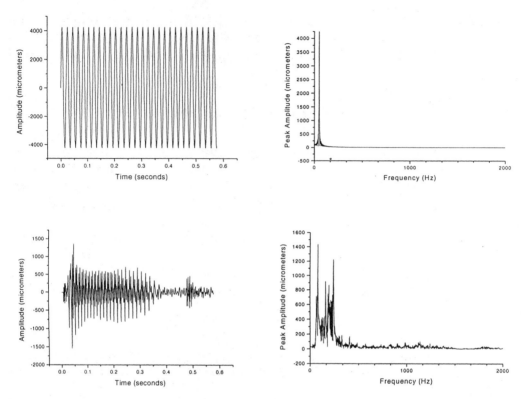

Figure 5–3. Waveforms and amplitude spectra of simple and complex sounds. The upper, left panel shows the waveform of a 50-Hz tone, while the upper, right panel is the amplitude spectrum of the tone. The lower-left panel shows the waveform of the spoken word *big*; the lower, right panel is the amplitude spectrum of the word.

It is difficult to identify the period(s) in the waveform; thus, the frequency composition of this complex sound cannot be determined using this graph. In contrast, the amplitude spectrum reveals the frequency and peak amplitude of each component. Because complex sounds are so common, the amplitude spectrum is widely used for the purpose of visualization.

Sound Propagation

Returning to the guitar string example, recall that plucking the string caused it to vibrate. If this were done in a vacuum like outer space, the string would eventually stop moving, and nothing more would happen. On Earth, however, air surrounds the string. When the string vibrates in this environment, it bumps into the small particles called molecules that make up air. The string pushes and pulls on the neighboring air molecules, which causes them to vibrate, too. Air molecules closest to the sound source are affected first. Then, via a chain reaction, sound energy rapidly moves away from the source in all directions. This process is known as **sound propagation.** Although the speed of sound in air is influenced by several factors including temperature and humidity, 350 meters per second is a reasonable estimate of how fast sound travels. All sounds travel at the same speed.

As you move away from the sound source, the amplitude of the vibrating air molecules decreases progressively. Sound energy is lost due to friction produced by the molecules crashing into one another. By traveling a sufficient distance from the source, the sound's impact on air molecules at that location is minimal, if any. This is why you are not able to eavesdrop on a conversation occurring on the other side of the room.

In this first half of the chapter, you learned how sound is generated and how it is propagated through the medium. As a listener, you strive to perceive sound. In the next section, you will learn about the structures of the ear that enable hearing.

THE AUDITORY SYSTEM: STRUCTURE AND FUNCTION

Vertebrates, such as mammals (including humans), are the only animals that have an auditory system per se. One anatomical characteristic shared by all vertebrates is bilateral symmetry, which means having similar structures on both sides of the body. The auditory system of vertebrates, then, includes a pair of ears. A diagram of the ear is shown in Figure 5–4, which shows the structures of the outer, middle, and inner ears. This cross-sectional view is of the right ear.

The auditory system consists of two parts. The ear (the outer, middle, and inner ear), and the auditory nervous system (neural pathways, associated nuclei, and the brain). The second half of the chapter will name the significant structures of the auditory system and then briefly describe the function of each one. Because sound arrives first at the outer ear, the discussion will begin there.

The Outer Ear

The outer ear consists of the **pinna** and **external auditory meatus (EAM).** The pinna is the visible flap of skin attached of the head. Because the pinna is made of cartilage, it is quite pliable. The primary function of the pinna is to funnel sounds into the EAM. This process is facilitated by the pinna's shape (i.e., the various ridges and hollows) and its slightly forward-facing orientation. The EAM is essentially a tube that is closed at one end. In the male adult, the EAM is about 2.5 centimeters (cm) in length and 1.0 cm in diameter. The skin that lines the EAM contains oil glands that secrete a sticky, yellow or brown substance known as **cerumen** (earwax). The cerumen

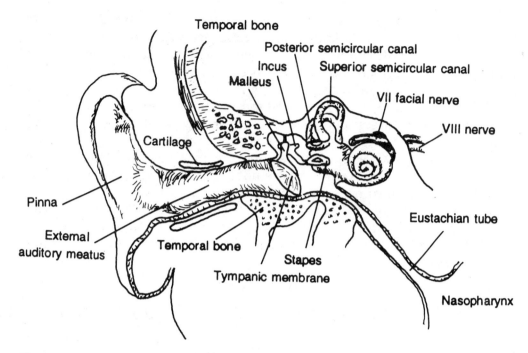

Figure 5–4. Coronal section of the ear, including the outer, middle, and inner ears. (From *Audiology Supplement to Anatomy and Physiology for Speech and Language* [p. 2], by J. A. Seikel, D. W. King, & D. G. Drumright, 1997, San Diego, CA: Singular Publishing Group.)

and the tiny hairs that are also present in the EAM help protect the delicate middle ear by trapping the small debris that may enter the canal. The outer one-third of the EAM is surrounded by cartilage. The inner two-thirds of the canal are supported by the **temporal bone,** which is one of the bones of the skull. The skin becomes more sensitive as one moves inward along the EAM. In fact, tactile stimulation in this area may trigger a cough reflex. The potential for evoking this reflex, with its rapid head movement and accompanying risk of injury, is one reason to avoid using small objects to clean the EAM.

 CD-ROM

Anatomy of the Pinna

CD-ROM segment Ch.05.04 is a photograph of the right pinna of an adult male. The important structures are labeled.

Besides their protective function, the pinna and EAM have the capacity to selectively boost or amplify some sounds. Conceptually, each of these structures partially encloses a small volume of air, as an empty soda bottle would. You have seen that air can vibrate; however, it tends to vibrate at some frequencies better than others depending on the amount (volume) of air that is present. This acoustical phenomenon is known as **resonance.** To demonstrate resonance, blow across empty bottles of different sizes, and listen to the pitch of the sound that is produced. The pockets of air trapped in the pinna and EAM resonate. In the human adult, the resonant frequencies associated with these structures range from 2000 to 5000 Hz. Although the boost provided by resonance is not large (maximum effect = 10–15 dB), sounds passing through the outer ear are influenced by its resonance characteristics.

THE MIDDLE EAR

Opposite the pinna, at the other end of the EAM, the **tympanic membrane (TM)** forms the boundary between the outer and middle ear. Sound traveling down the EAM strikes the TM and causes it to vibrate just like the head of a drum, hence the common name "eardrum." The circular TM is stretched across the EAM, forming an airtight seal between the outside world and the middle-ear cavity. The area of the TM is approximately 80 mm². However, the surface of the TM is not uniformly taut. A small region (about 25% of the total) at the top of the TM is relatively loose, which may help reduce risk of rupture of this membrane. Attached to the center of the TM is the malleus. The **malleus** is one of three bones that make up the **ossicular chain.** The ossicles are the smallest bones in the human body. The other ossicles are the **incus,** which is connected to the malleus, and the **stapes,** which is attached to the incus. The TM in children is nearly transparent, so it is possible to see the ossicles by illuminating the EAM with a special ear light called an otoscope. The TM appears cone-shaped because the ossicular chain tends to pull it inward. Therefore, shining an otoscope on the TM produces the characteristic "cone of light" on the lower, back portion of the TM's surface.

 CD-ROM

Anatomy of the Tympanic Membrane

The left panel of CD-ROM segment Ch.05.05 shows a photograph of the right tympanic membrane of an adult male. The head of the malleus can be seen on the other side of the tympanic membrane. The right panel shows the same view, except the malleus is outlined.

CD-ROM

Anatomy of the Tympanic Membrane and the Ossicles

The left panel of CD-ROM segment Ch.05.06 presents a model of the tympanic membrane and the three ossicles. The key structures are labeled. In the right panel, the model can be rotated, which permits viewing from various orientations. *Note:* There is no sound associated with this image.

Located on the floor of the middle-ear cavity is a passageway, called the **Eustachian tube (ET).** The ET connects the middle ear to the back of the throat. Normally, the ET is closed. When the air pressure in the middle ear is less than the air pressure surrounding the body (e.g., going up in an airplane), the ET rapidly opens, allowing air from the mouth to pass into the middle ear. This action equalizes the air pressure in the middle ear. You know your ET is working properly when you feel your ears "pop." Yawning, swallowing, and chewing are normal activities that help the ET to pop open.

The ossicles are suspended in the middle-ear cavity via a set of ligaments. Additionally, the **tensor tympani** and **stapedius muscles** are attached to the malleus and stapes, respectively. The function of these muscles will be considered shortly. The ossicles provide a pathway for sound to travel from the outer to the inner ear. The vibration's journey, however, is not an easy one as the inner ear is filled with water. Sound energy does not transfer easily from one medium to another. When air-born sound waves encounter water, nearly all (approximately 99.9%) of the energy is reflected; very little (0.1%) energy is transmitted. This opposition to energy transfer is known as impedance. The ossicles exist to help overcome the effect of impedance, thus permitting more sound energy to be transmitted from the outer into the inner ear. The difference in the area of the TM compared to the stapes footplate is the primary method for **impedance matching.** The area of the TM is about 18 times larger than that of the footplate. This means that vibrations striking the TM are increased 18 times by the time they reach the much smaller footplate. The ossicles act as tiny levers, which also boost the sound amplitude. This effect is small relative to the area difference. Without impedance matching, the sound level reaching the inner ear would be reduced and our hearing capacity greatly diminished.

An important role of the middle ear is overcoming the impedance mismatch between air and fluid. There are certain circumstances, however, where high impedance (i.e., low energy transfer) is desirable. Intense sounds are capable of producing excessive motion in the ear. Such movement is potentially harmful to the fragile sensory cells in the inner ear. To help reduce the risk of damage, a reactive mechanism has developed in mammals. The so-called **acoustic reflex** involves the tiny tensor tympani and stapedius muscles that were mentioned previously. Recall that the tensor tympani and stapedius muscles are attached to the ossicles. These muscles, especially the stapedius, contract reflexively when the ear is stimulated with sounds exceeding 80 dB or so. The contraction results in an overall stiffening of the ossicular chain, which increases the acoustic impedance of the ear. By increasing the acoustic impedance, the delicate structures of the inner ear are afforded some protection against intense sounds.

The Inner Ear

Like the middle ear, the inner ear resides in a hollowed out portion of the temporal bone. Actually, the inner ear consists of a series of interconnected cavities known as the bony or **osseous labyrinth.** The osseous labyrinth is filled with fluid called **perilymph,** which is essentially saline or salt water. Floating in the perilymph is a sack known as the **membranous labyrinth.** The flexibility of the membranous labyrinth enables it to conform to the tortuous shape of the osseous labyrinth. The fluid inside the membranous labyrinth is **endolymph.** The chemical content of endolymph makes it somewhat different from perilymph.

The inner ear houses structures used for hearing and balance. The osseous and membranous labyrinths are divided into three distinct areas—the cochlea, vestibule, and semicircular canals. The cochlea contains the hearing organ, while the vestibule and semicircular canals hold the organs of balance. Because this chapter is devoted to sound and hearing, the focus will be on the structures in the cochlea.

The **cochlea** is a coiled tube. There are approximately 2.5 turns in the coil of the human cochlea. The membranous labyrinth actually partitions the cochlea into three smaller tubes. The upper and lower tubes are called scala vestibuli (SV) and scala tympani (ST), respectively. They both contain perilymph. The middle tube is called scala media (SM); it is filled with endolymph. The entrance into the inner ear from the middle ear is provided by the

 CD-ROM

Inside the Cochlea

CD-ROM segment Ch.05.07 shows the cochlea as if it were cut in half. In this view, the cochlea is coiled such that the apical end is at the top of the picture. (From *Neuroscience of Communication* [p. 235], by D. B. Webster, 1995, San Diego, CA: Singular Publishing Group.)

oval window. The stapes footplate is positioned in the oval window, which opens into scala vestibuli. There is another opening into the cochlea called the **round window.** Located on the wall of the middle-ear cavity just below the oval window, the round window leads to scala tympani. The round window is covered with a thin membrane to prevent perilymph from leaking into the middle-ear cavity. A cross-sectional view of the cochlea is shown in Figure 5–5.

When viewed in cross-section, scala media is not round, but triangular. A thin layer of cells known as **Reissner's membrane** forms the top (hypotenuse) of the triangle. Reissner's membrane separates scala vestibuli from scala media. The side of the triangle consists of a collection of vessels called the **stria vascularis,** which supplies blood to the cochlea. The bottom (base)

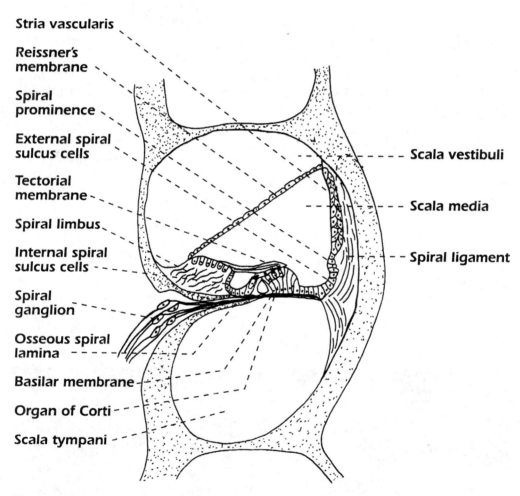

Figure 5–5. Cross-sectional view of the cochlea. (From *Neuroscience of Communication* [p. 182], by D. B. Webster, 1995, San Diego, CA: Singular Publishing Group.)

of the triangle is formed by the basilar membrane. This membrane divides scala tympani from scala media.

The **basilar membrane** is a thin ribbon of tissue. One edge is attached to a lip of bone called the osseous spiral lamina, and the other edge is supported by the spiral ligament. The basilar membrane differs from an actual ribbon in that the width and thickness are not uniform throughout its length. The end closest to oval window, referred to as the base, is narrow and thin, which gives the basilar membrane a stiff consistency. The opposite end of the basilar membrane, called the apex, is wide and thick. The basilar membrane here is relatively flaccid. Moreover, the stiffness of the basilar membrane changes progressively from one end of the cochlea to the other. This stiffness gradient turns out to play an important role in the process of hearing.

Sound waves impinging on the TM cause it to vibrate. These vibrations are conducted to the cochlea via the ossicular chain. The stapes moves in (or out of) the oval window. The footplate pushes (or pulls) on the perilymph in the scala vestibuli, which, in turn, pushes (or pulls) the membranous labyrinth downward (or upward). The motion of the membranous labyrinth affects the perilymph in the scala tympani. The round-window membrane bulges outward (or inward) to counteract the pressure changes generated at the oval window by the stapes. The main point is that many structures in the cochlea, including the basilar membrane, are set into motion when the ear is stimulated by sound.

Recall that the basilar membrane is stiff at one end and loose at the other. One consequence of this mechanical variation is that the entire basilar membrane does not move in unison. Rather, the basal end (the one near the oval window) begins moving first, and the up-down action is transmitted down the basilar membrane toward the apex. This pattern of vibration is called the **traveling wave.** The amplitude of the traveling wave changes as it moves from base to apex. That is, the amplitude increases, reaches a maximum at a particular location on the basilar membrane, and then decreases. The place of maximal displacement is determined by the frequency of the sound. Because the basilar membrane is stiffest at the base, it vibrates best (i.e., greatest amplitude) when stimulated by a high-frequency sound. The apex is less stiff, and thus the greatest amplitude of vibration is brought about by a low-frequency sound. Like a piano, the basilar membrane is laid systematically according to frequency, with the high-frequency "notes" at the basal end and the low-frequency "notes" at the apical end. The arrangement where each frequency is related to a particular place along the basilar membrane is known as **tonotopic organization.**

The intensity of the sound also affects the amplitude of the traveling wave. Low-intensity sounds produce a small traveling wave. Conversely, high-intensity sounds generate a traveling wave of greater amplitude. You have seen that frequency and intensity are primary characteristics of sound. The cochlea, specifically the traveling wave, provides a mechanism for sensing these two properties. Frequency content is conveyed by the location of the peak(s) in the traveling wave, while the amplitude of the peak(s) provides information about the sound's intensity.

The cochlea performs another function that is essential to hearing. For the brain to perceive sound, the vibrations must be converted from mechanical (or movement-based) energy to electrical energy. The general process of converting energy from one form to another is known as **transduction.** In the ear, transduction is accomplished by the hair cells. The **hair cells** rest on top of the basilar membrane, arranged in four rows that extend from the base of the cochlea to its apex. There actually are two types of hair cells. The three rows of outer hair cells lie closer to the stria vascularis than does the single row of inner hair cells. Several small cilia (hair-like structures) project from the top of each hair cell, hence the name. A gelatinous substance called the **tectorial membrane** arches over the tops of the inner hair cells and rests on the cilia of the outer hair cells. The tectorial membrane runs parallel to the basilar membrane. One edge is attached to the spiral limbus, which is on the opposite side of the scala media from the stria vascularis. The structures named in this paragraph are collectively known as the **organ of Corti.**

The organ of Corti moves up and down when stimulated. The basilar membrane is securely attached to the osseous spiral lamina, but less securely to the spiral ligament. Further, the tectorial membrane is only anchored on one side, to the spiral ligament. Because of this arrangement, as the organ of Corti moves it tends to pivot much like a hinge. Recall that the bottoms of the hair cells are rooted in the basilar membrane, while their tips are embedded in the tectorial membrane. Consequently, when the organ of Corti begins to move in response to sound, the cilia are forced to bend. The up-down motion of the organ of Corti is translated directly into back-and-forth movement of the cilia. This form of movement by the hair cells is called "shearing" and is crucial to the transduction process.

 CD-ROM

Organ of Corti

CD-ROM segment Ch.05.08 is a radial section through the organ of Corti. The entire organ of Corti moves up and down in response to sound stimulation. In conjunction with this motion, the tiny cilia located on the top of each hair are bent back and forth. (From *Neuroscience of Communication* [p. 239], by D. B. Webster, 1995, San Diego, CA: Singular Publishing Group.)

As stated previously hair cells perform transduction. More specifically, the mechanical energy of vibration is converted to electrical energy. To understand how the hair cell accomplishes this, a brief discussion of electricity is necessary. An ion is a small (subatomic) particle that carries an electrical charge. Certain kinds of ions are positively charged while others are negatively charged. As the saying goes, "opposites attract," so positive and negative ions are drawn to one another. Electricity is the manifestation of this attraction.

There is electricity in the cochlea. The inside of the hair cell has an overabundance of negative ions. Endolymph, which baths the cilia at the tops of the hair cells, has an excess amount of positive ions. The two groups of ions are kept apart by the insulating membrane that surrounds the cell. Remember that the cilia bend back-and-forth during sound stimulation. This motion opens and closes miniscule "trap doors" that are thought to exist at the tips of the cilia. When the doors are open, the positive ions rush into the hair cells. You may wonder why the negative ions do not flow out of the cell. The current thinking is that the trap doors are too small to allow the larger negative ions to pass through. The influx of positive ions causes the inside of the cell to become depolarized (less negatively charged). The depolarization triggers a reaction at the bottom of the hair cell. Small packets of a chemical substance called **neurotransmitter** are expelled into fluid-filled space outside the cell. The neurotransmitter makes the short trip across the space where it encounters nerve cells adjacent to the hair cell. The transduction process is complete. The hair cell has converted mechanical (cilia bending) to electrical (neurotransmitter release) energy.

The Auditory Nervous System

Sound is now in an electrochemical form that can be interpreted by the brain. Before this can happen, however, the information must be transmitted from the cochlea to the auditory nerve, through the brainstem, then the midbrain, and finally to the auditory cortex. Let us begin our discussion of the auditory nervous system by examining the eighth nerve.

The **eighth nerve** derives its name from the fact that it is cranial nerve VIII. The eighth nerve consists of approximately 30,000 individual cells called **neurons.** Neurons are simple in the sense that they can only conduct information in one direction. Because of this constraint, the eighth nerve contains two neural subsystems. The *afferent* subsystem transmits messages from the cochlea to the brain, while the *efferent* subsystem carries messages from the brain back to the cochlea. Approximately 95% of the afferent cells originate at the inner hair cells; the remaining 5% are connected to the outer hair cells. The fact that most of the afferent neurons are connected to the inner hair cells suggests these cells are the primary ones for carrying information about sound to the brain. If this is the case, then what is the function of the outer hair cells? We will return to this question after a short discussion of the efferent subsystem.

The efferent neurons carry messages from structures in the brain, which have not yet been described, back to the cochlea. Unlike the afferent subsystem, the neurons in the efferent subsystem mostly make connections with the outer hair cells. Remember that outer hair cells are attached to both the basilar membrane and tectorial membrane. Recent evidence indicates that the outer hair cells are capable of rapidly alerting their length. These minute movements may affect the traveling wave by either increasing or decreasing its amplitude. A boost in amplitude may enhance our hearing, while a reduction may serve a protective function. In either case, more work needs to be done to define the specific role of the outer hair cells.

Besides conducting information in only one direction, neurons are simple in their response properties. Neurons communicate with one another via a simple language based on action potentials. An **action potential** is a brief electrical pulse. A neuron produces a series of action potentials in response to stimulation. All action potentials are identical in duration and amplitude; thus, the rate (i.e., number of action potentials per second) provides a convenient means of quantifying the neural response. It turns out that intensity is the dimension of sound coded by rate. The relation is a direct one—as sound intensity increases, neural rate increases. The neuron, however, is limited in that its rate can only vary over a 30–40 dB range. The problem is that human hearing spans a range of at least 120 dB. To provide adequate coverage, the activation level of individual neurons is staggered. To see how this might work, consider three neurons. Neuron #1 responds from 0–40 dB, neuron #2 responds from 40–80 dB, and neuron #3 responds from 80–120 dB. By staggering the activation level, the full 120-dB range can be realized. Moreover, rate and activation level are important mechanisms used by the auditory nerve to code sound intensity.

Two mechanisms exist for coding sound frequency. The first one is based on the idea that the neural site of origin and the frequency are related. Conceptualize the eighth nerve as a rope made up of many individual fibers (the neurons). The neurons coming from the apex form the rope's inner core, while those cells coming from the base make up the outer layer. Because the tonotopic organization in the cochlea is maintained in the nerve, it is possible to predict the frequency information carried by a particular neuron. The location-frequency relation is better known as the place mechanism.

A second mechanism for conveying frequency information to the brain relates to a neuron's predisposition for responding at a specific point in the vibratory cycle. For example, an action potential may be generated only when a sound wave reaches its maximum amplitude. If this were to happen repeatedly, an equal time interval or period would occur between each subsequent action potential. You know from an earlier discussion that frequency and period are inversely related ($f = 1/P$). It is possible that the brain too, understands this association and uses neural periodicity to gain information about frequency. Therefore, both place and periodicity are important mechanisms used by the auditory nerve to code sound frequency.

Information about sound is not transmitted directly to the brain by the eighth nerve. Instead, there are parallel neural pathways running on both sides of the head. This complicated network consists of many individual neurons that begin and end at specific centers called nuclei. Nuclei are situated at various locations throughout the auditory nervous system. For the sake of brevity, the primary nuclei will be listed in the order found in the afferent auditory pathway. Keep in mind that a parallel efferent pathway also exists. A schematic diagram of the afferent pathways is shown in Figure 5–6.

The eighth nerve carries messages from the cochlea to the **cochlear nucleus,** which is located in the lower brainstem. Like many areas in the auditory nervous system, the cochlear nucleus is divided into smaller regions. Providing the names of these nuclei, however, is beyond the scope of this introductory chapter. All afferent neurons coming from the hair cells terminate in the cochlear nucleus.

A second group of neurons leaves the cochlear nucleus and extends to the next cluster of nuclei collectively known as the **superior olivary complex.** Actually, a portion of the neurons leaving the cochlear nucleus travels to the superior olivary complex on the same (ipsilateral) side of the head. The other neurons exit the cochlear nucleus, cross the midline, and connect to the superior olivary complex on the opposite (contralateral) side. One reason you have two ears is to help locate the source of sound. The superior olivary complex likely plays an important role in sound localization because this is the first place in the afferent pathway where information from the right and left ears is integrated or combined.

A third set of neurons goes from the superior olivary complex to the **lateral lemniscus nucleus.** The lateral lemniscus is large in mammals that live underground, but relatively small in primates. This suggests that the role of the lateral lemniscus in human hearing may be a minor one.

A fourth group of neurons extends from the lateral lemniscus to the **inferior colliculus nucleus.** A neural pathway connects the inferior colliculus on the right side to the inferior colliculus on the left side. Such interconnecting tracts or **commissures** are found at several levels in the auditory nervous system.

Extending from the inferior colliculus to the midbrain is a fifth set of neurons. These cells terminate in the **medial geniculate body.** The sixth and final set of neurons leaves the medial geniculate body on its way to the **auditory cortex.** Unlike the medial geniculate body, which lies deep within the head, the auditory cortex is found on the surface of the brain. The brain you can see, once the skull is removed, consists of two cerebral hemispheres. A hemisphere is divided into four sections called lobes. The auditory cortex is located in the temporal lobe, which is the thumb-like region on the side of each hemisphere. The auditory cortex marks the end of the afferent auditory

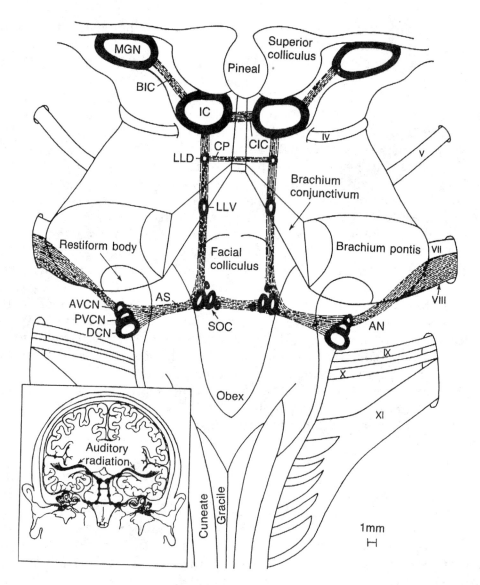

Figure 5–6. Ventral view of the subcortical pathways of the central auditory nervous system. The abbreviations are as follows: VII = cranial nerve 7; VIII = cranial nerve 8; AVCN = anterior ventral cochlear nucleus; PVCN = posterior ventral cochlear nucleus; DCN = dorsal cochlear nucleus; IC = inferior colliculus; LLV = ventral lateral lemniscus; LLD = dorsal lateral lemniscus; MGN = medial geniculate nucleus; SOC = superior olivary complex. (From *Audiologists' Desk Reference, Volume 1, Diagnostic Audiology, Principles, Procedures, and Practices* [p. 36], by J. W. Hall III & H. G. Mueller III, 1997, San Diego, CA: Singular Publishing Group.)

pathway. From there connections are made with other areas of the brain that are responsible for important functions such as language, memory, movement, and so on.

SUMMARY

Sound moves from its source through the medium to the listener. The outer ear of the listener gathers the sound present in the air and directs it to the middle ear. The middle ear is a mechanical system that boosts sound amplitude so the vibration is transmitted more effectively into the inner ear. The inner ear separates complex sounds into simple ones according to frequency. Additionally, the inner ear converts vibration to electrical impulses. The eighth nerve and the auditory neural pathways carry the impulses to the brain, which attempts to assign meaning to sound.

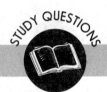

STUDY QUESTIONS

1 Describe the interplay between the forces of momentum and elasticity during vibration.

2 What four measurable quantities characterize all simple sounds?

3 Sketch the waveform of a simple sound.

4 Name five structures of the middle ear.

5 What are the two functions of the cochlea?

6 Contrast the afferent and efferent pathways of the auditory nervous system.

7 Proceeding from cochlea to brain, list the main structures in the auditory pathway.

8 How are changes in the amplitude and frequency of sound communicated to the brain by the auditory nervous system?

SUGGESTED READINGS

Davis, H., & Silverman, S. R. (1970). *Hearing and deafness.* New York: Holt, Rinehart and Winston.

Durrant, J. D., & Lovrinic, J. H. (1995). *Bases of hearing science.* Baltimore: Williams & Wilkins.

Gelfand, S. A. (1998). *Hearing: An introduction to psychological and physiological acoustics.* New York: Marcel Dekker.

Green, D. M. (1976). *Introduction to hearing.* New York: Lawrence Erlbaum Associates.

Hirsh, I. J. (1972). *The measurement of hearing.* New York: McGraw-Hill.

Speaks, C. E. (1997). *Introduction to sound: Acoustics for the hearing and speech sciences.* San Diego, CA: Singular Publishing Group.

Yost, W. A. (1994). *Fundamentals of hearing: An introduction.* San Diego, CA: Academic Press.

Zemlin, W. R. (1968). *Speech and hearing science.* Englewood Cliffs, NJ: Prentice-Hall.

GLOSSARY

Acoustic reflex: The contraction of the middle ear muscles in response to an intense sound. The contraction limits the amount of sound energy passing through the middle ear, thus protecting the delicate structures in the inner ear.

Action potential: A brief electrical voltage generated by a neuron, typically following stimulation.

Afferent: Nerve impulses carried from the periphery to the brain.

Amplitude: The distance an object moves from its resting position during vibration.

Auditory cortex: An area in the temporal lobe of the brain that is responsible for hearing.

Basilar membrane: A ribbon-like tissue in the cochlea that separates scala media (above) from scale tympani (below). It provides the foundation on which rests the organ of Corti.

Cerumen: A tacky yellow or brown substance secreted by oil glands in the external auditory meatus. This substance is commonly known as earwax.

Cochlea: The coiled tube in the inner ear that houses the sensory cells for hearing.

Cochlear nucleus: A way station in the lower brainstem that communicates with the cochlea via the eighth nerve.

Commissure: A group of neurons that cross the midline, from one side of the brain to the other.

Complex sound: A sound composed of at least two, but usually many more, frequency components.

Efferent: Nerve impulses carried from the brain to the periphery.

Eighth nerve: The cranial nerve (VIII) devoted to carrying information about hearing and balance to and from the auditory nervous system. The eighth nerve in humans is made up of about 30,000 individual neurons.

Elasticity: The property that enables an object to return to its original shape after being deformed.

Endolymph: The fluid found within the membranous labyrinth.

Eustachian tube (ET): The canal that connects the middle-ear cavity to the back of the throat. The Eustachian tube opens briefly to equalize pressure in the middle ear.

External auditory meatus (EAM): The canal that directs sound from the pinna to the tympanic membrane.

Frequency: The number of cycles of vibration completed in 1 second, measured in Hertz (Hz).

Hair cells: The sensory cells of hearing and balance that convert sound energy from one form to another.

Impedance matching: A technique that helps energy move from one medium to another with minimal loss. The ossicles in the middle ear perform this function.

Incus: Middle bone in the ossicular chain, attached at either end to the malleus and stapes, respectively.

Inferior colliculus nucleus: A way station in the midbrain that lies between the lateral lemniscus nucleus and the medial geniculate body.

Labyrinth: A system of canals connecting portions of the inner ear. The larger osseous labyrinth contains perilymph and the smaller membranous labyrinth which contains endolymph.

Lateral lemniscus nucleus: A way station in the brainstem that lies between the superior olivary complex and the inferior colliculus nuclei.

Malleus: The outermost bone in the ossicular chain. One end is attached to the tympanic membrane; the other end is connected to the incus.

Mass: The amount of matter an object has.

Medial geniculate body: A way station in the brainstem that lies between the superior olivary complex and the inferior colliculus nuclei.

Membranous labyrinth: A flexible sac found within the osseous labyrinth that houses the structures of the inner ear.

Neuron: A specialized cell that conducts bioelectrical messages in the nervous system.

Neurotransmitter: A substance released by hair cells or neurons that affects neighboring neurons.

Organ of Corti: A collection of sensory and supporting cells that extends from the base of the cochlea to its apex.

Osseous labyrinth: A hollowed out portion of the temporal bone that encases the inner ear.

Ossicular chain: The three interconnected bones in the middle ear that conduct vibration from the tympanic membrane to the cochlea.

Oval window: The opening between the middle ear and scala vestibuli of the cochlea. The stapes footplate seals the opening.

Perilymph: The fluid found within the bony labyrinth.

Period: The amount of time needed to complete one cycle of vibration.

Pinna: The cartilaginous flap of skin attached to the side of the head around the opening to the external auditory meatus.

Reissner's membrane: The thin layer of tissue that separates scala vestibuli from scala media.

Resonance: The frequency at which an object vibrates best.

Round window: The opening between the middle ear and scala tympani of the cochlea. The round window membrane covers the opening.

Simple sound: A sound composed of a single frequency component.

Sound generation: The process where an object is set into motion through the application of an external force.

Sound propagation: The movement of vibration through a medium brought about by collisions between neighboring particles.

Spectrum: A graph that shows the amplitude or phase as a function of frequency.

Stapedius muscle: A middle-ear muscle that is attached to the stapes. This muscle contracts in response to intense sound.

Stapes: The innermost bone in the ossicular chain. One end is attached to the incus; the other end, or footplate, occupies the oval window.

Starting phase: The position occupied by an object at a particular time within one cycle of vibration. Starting phase may be measured in degrees or radians.

Stria vascularis: A collection of blood vessels that is found within the scala media. The stria vascularis delivers nutrients and removes waste from cells in the organ of Corti.

Superior olivary complex: A way station in the brainstem that lies between the cochlear nuclei and the lateral lemniscus nucleus.

Tectorial membrane: A gelatinous substance that is attached at one edge to the spiral limbus. The bottom of the tectorial membrane is connected with the cilia of the hair cells.

Temporal bone: One of the seven bones that form the skull. The temporal bone contains the middle and inner ear.

Tensor tympani muscle: A middle-ear muscle that is attached to the malleus. This muscle contracts in response to intense sound and to tactile stimulation of the face.

Tonotopic organization: An arrangement where one of a structure's dimensions is systematically laid out according to frequency.

Transduction: The process where energy is converted from one form to another. The hair cells change mechanical energy to electrical energy.

Traveling wave: The displacement pattern of the basilar membrane brought about by stimulation with sound.

Tympanic membrane (TM): The cone-shape layer of tissue that separates the external auditory meatus from the middle ear cavity. The malleus is connected to the inner surface of the tympanic membrane.

Waveform: A graph that shows the amplitude as a function of time.

6

Hearing Disorders

Frederick N. Martin

1 To understand what the profession of audiology is designed to accomplish.

2 To determine what a hearing loss is.

3 To differentiate among different kinds of hearing losses.

4 To understand the causes of hearing loss.

5 To grasp the kinds of difficulties in understanding speech encountered by people with different kinds of hearing loss.

6 To understand the basics of hearing testing.

7 To understand the kinds of instrumentation required for adequate hearing testing.

8 To grasp the concepts of tuning fork tests and their relationships to modern audiometry.

9 To be able to interpret basic hearing test results.

INTRODUCTION

The previous chapter described the anatomy and physiology of the auditory system, that is, how it is constructed and how it works. This chapter introduces the kinds of hearing disorders encountered by audiologists and speech-language pathologists, the diagnostic procedures available for making the appropriate appraisals of these disorders, and their effects on the communication process. Although audiological test procedures are discussed, it is important for the reader to realize that the practice of audiology goes far beyond the performance of tests and their interpretation. These tests help to determine the kinds of intervention that are necessary to improve the communication of those with hearing impairment and others with whom they interact. At the conclusion of this chapter the reader should be able to interpret the basic tests described, including the audiograms and related tests using speech stimuli. This chapter assumes a basic knowledge of the anatomy and physiology of the auditory system as described in Chapter 5. An understanding of the principles of this chapter is essential for understanding Chapter 7 on auditory (re)habilitation.

HEARING TESTS

The evolution of hearing tests has been ongoing for centuries. I have no doubt that as long as humans have relied on their hearing for receptive communication, there have been individuals whose hearing has been impaired. Just when informal testing began and how it was carried out is unknown, although a little educated guessing may give us some insights.

Informal Tests

The early hearing tests, some of which have carried over to modern times, probably included the production of gross sounds and the search for some kind of acknowledgment by cooperative individuals and overt responses from those who could not cooperate. Noncooperative individuals include small children, the elderly, the infirm, and those who feel they can benefit by having people believe they have a hearing loss that does not exist. These stimuli could be produced by the human voice, by hand clapping, or by hitting two objects together. Perhaps the clicking of two coins was used to see if a person reported hearing this predominantly high-frequency sound or the spinning of a coin on a tabletop that produced a ringing sound. Whispered and soft speech are still used by some physicians as gross estimates of hearing sensitivity, although no quantitative information can be gleaned from such tests.

Sound Pathways

Sound travels through the air as a series of waves, with their respective compressions and rarefactions. The **air-conduction** pathway is the natural way by which most land-living animals hear. Those sounds reaching the head are gathered by the pinna of the outer ear, carried down the external auditory canal, and directed to the tympanic membrane (eardrum). Vibration of the tympanic membrane sets the chain of middle-ear ossicles into motion, which, in turn, disturbs the fluids of the cochlea of the inner ear. The cochlea, acting as a sort of microphone that converts mechanical energy into an electrochemical code, sends information to the brain via the auditory (VIIIth cranial) nerve. It has been said many times, and it bears repeating here, that we do not hear with our ears but rather with our brains. The ear is a necessary, but not totally efficient means of enabling "hearing."

Sound energy may also reach the inner ear by vibrating the bones of the skull, thereby setting the bony labyrinth into sympathetic vibration and eliciting the same response from the cochlea as is produced by air conduction. This process of bypassing the conductive mechanism (the outer ear and middle ear) and going directly to the sensorineural mechanism (the inner ear, and then the auditory nerve) has been given the obvious name of **bone conduction.**

Tuning-Fork Tests

During the 19th century, several creative German physicians borrowed the use of a device from tuners of musical instruments (Johnson, 1970). This was the *tuning fork,* a metal tool capable of vibrating at specific frequencies. Several tuning forks can be used, with their frequencies determined by the size of the forks, that is, the larger the tuning fork the slower it vibrates because of its mass and the lower the frequency emitted. Since Western music utilizes the octave scale, most tuning forks, which continue to be used today by many otolaryngologists (physicians specializing in the treatment of disorders of the ear, nose, and throat), are designed to produce sounds on the musical C scale. A tuning fork vibrating at 128 Hz is close to Low C, 256 Hz is Middle C, 512 Hz is High C, and so on. Tuning forks can be used as gross tests of hearing by comparing the audibility of a tone between the examiner and the patient or by comparing patients' hearing by air conduction to their hearing by bone conduction.

The way tuning-fork tests measure the integrity of the air-conduction pathway is to hold the stem of the fork in one hand with the vibrating tines next to the patient's external ear. In this way the sound travels in all directions, including down the external auditory canal. Bone-conduction tests can be carried out by pressing the stem of the tuning fork against the patient's skull, usually on the bony protuberance behind the pinna of the external ear called the **mastoid process.** The tuning fork can be moved from the patient's head to that of the examiner as the amplitude of vibration diminishes over time to see whether the patient stops hearing the tone before, after, or at the same time as the examiner. In such tests it is assumed that the examiner has normal hearing. The loudness of the vibrating tines of a tuning fork held next to the ear (air conduction) can also be compared to the loudness of the sound produced by the stem of the tuning fork held against the skull (bone conduction).

No single tuning-fork test is particularly useful on its own, but the use of several different tuning-fork tests can help determine the general type of hearing loss that a patient has at specified frequencies. Because tuning forks cannot reveal the extent of any hearing loss, they have given way to more quantitative procedures.

Pure-Tone Audiometry

Among the many notable inventions of the 20th century was the pure-tone **audiometer** (see Martin & Clark, 2000, and Figure 6–1). Although improvements in technology have resulted in vastly different circuitry from the early instruments, all pure-tone audiometers have certain things in common. They produce a series of pure tones, which are signals with only one frequency and no harmonics. These tones can be delivered via earphones to a patient's ears or via a bone-conduction oscillator affixed to the skull. Frequencies are generated that are close to the C scale and are usually available at octave intervals over a fairly wide frequency range. The usual frequencies found on pure-tone audiometers include 125, 250, 500, 1000, 2000, 4000, and 8000 Hz (note the correspondence to the musical C scale). Some mid-octave frequencies are typically included such as 750, 1500, 3000, and 6000 Hz.

Pure-tone tests are designed to determine a patient's **threshold of audibility** at a number of different frequencies for each ear. Air conduction is tested by using a pair of earphones held firmly to the head by a headband (Figure 6–2) or, preferably, inserted into the ears (Figure 6–3). Bone-conduction testing is accomplished with a specially designed steel band holding an oscillator against the skull. Many audiologists measure bone conduction on each mastoid process independently to obtain threshold information for both cochleas (Figure 6–4). However, the reality is that it is often impossible to

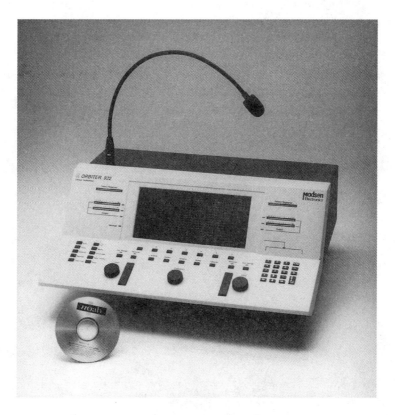

Figure 6–1. An example of a diagnostic audiometer. (Photo courtesy of Madsen Electronics)

know which cochlea is responding, since vibrating the skull from any spot usually results in both cochleas being stimulated equally. For this and other reasons the forehead is the preferred testing site (Studebaker, 1962).

As stated, the frequencies produced by audiometers are measured in cycles per second (cps) or hertz (Hz). Intensity changes are measured in decibels (dB). Chapter 5 discussed the decibel as a unit of sound pressure that is expressed as a logarithmic unit because of the large range of intensities that can be heard by normal-hearing persons. The reference described was specified as sound-pressure level (SPL). The audiometer uses the decibel in a different way, which brings us to the concept of **hearing level (HL).**

While sound-pressure level (SPL) has a specific intensity reference (20 micropascals), hearing level refers to the intensity necessary to evoke a threshold response from persons with normal hearing. Since the human ear is not equally sensitive at all frequencies, the audiometer produces different SPLs at different frequencies to reach 0 dB HL (hearing level). Theoretically, a person with normal hearing would show threshold responses at about 0 dB HL at all frequencies tested, even though the sound-pressure level required to produce 0 dB HL is different at each frequency. Therefore, persons using pure-tone

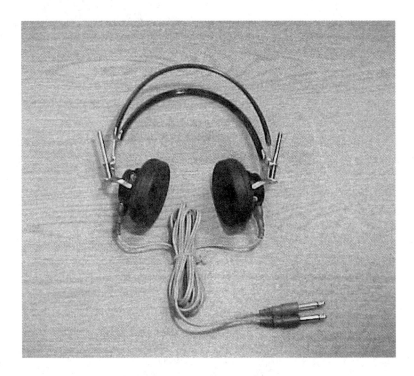

Figure 6–2. Photograph of a pair of supra-aural earphones. (Photo courtesy of Madsen Electronics)

audiometers need to compare the thresholds of their patients to 0 dB HL at each frequency to determine how much hearing loss is present. Although there is some disagreement about this, normal hearing, as described in this book, is said to encompass a range from −10 to 15 dB HL. Any threshold found to be greater than 15 dB HL is considered to demonstrate a hearing loss by air conduction, bone conduction, or both.

Another reference for the decibel is **sensation level (SL),** which is simply the difference (in decibels) between the level of a signal presented and the threshold of the individual receiving that signal. For example, a tone of 50 dB SL (sensation level) is 50 dB above a listener's threshold, regardless of what that threshold might be. For example, a person with a threshold of 20 dB HL would hear a signal of 50 dB HL at 30 dB SL. It is essential whenever discussing the intensity of a sound that the reference for the decibel be specified.

Hearing sensitivity is normally displayed on a graph called an **audiogram.** Unlike most graphs, which show the larger numbers near the top and the smaller numbers near the bottom, audiograms are inverted. The lowest number of decibels is shown near the top of the graph. The number of decibels (hearing level) is shown to increase going down the page. The different test frequencies are displayed on the horizontal axis of the audiogram, with the lowest test frequency (usually 125 Hz) on the left side and the highest

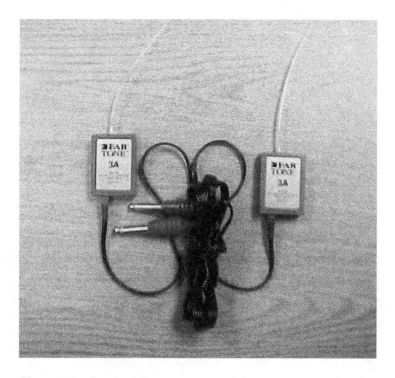

Figure 6–3. Photograph of a pair of insert earphones. (Photo courtesy of Madsen Electronics)

frequency tested (usually 8000 Hz) on the right side of the graph. A grid is thereby created (e.g., see Figures 6–6 through 6–9). As the patient's hearing is tested, each test signal is raised and lowered in intensity until the sound is so soft that it can only be detected about 50% of the time. This level is called the **threshold of audibility** and is expressed in decibels with a hearing level (HL) reference. By placing symbols where the horizontal and vertical axes of the audiogram intersect, the audiologist plots the patient's threshold for each frequency for each ear by air conduction and bone conduction. The right ear air-conduction thresholds are usually shown in red using a circle, and the left ear air-conduction thresholds are shown in blue using an X. When bone-conduction thresholds are measured from the mastoid, they are also plotted in red (for the right ear) and blue (for the left ear) using the symbol < for the right and the symbol > for the left.

Speech Audiometry

Pure-tone tests have remained the mainstay of diagnostic audiology for many years. They supply information about hearing sensitivity over a range of frequencies and are helpful in determining the type and degree of hearing

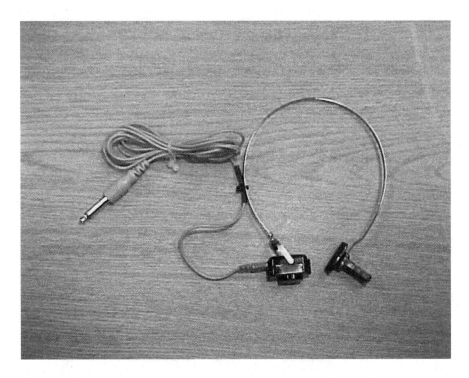

Figure 6–4. Photograph of a bone-conduction oscillator. (Photo courtesy of Madsen Electronics)

loss so that appropriate remediation can be instituted. However, since pure tones do not exist in nature, they are abstract stimuli. People who seek help for their hearing difficulties, or for the hearing problems of significant other persons, generally do so because of difficulties in hearing speech.

In consideration of that statement, it was only natural that testing devices would be developed to measure different aspects of speech. These include how intense speech must be to be barely audible (the **speech-recognition threshold [SRT]**), and how well speech can be discriminated when it is loud enough to be heard (the **word-recognition score [WRS]**). The degree of hearing loss expressed as an SRT is described in hearing level, and it usually approximates the degree of hearing loss by air conduction at the average of the thresholds obtained at 500, 1000, and 2000 Hz. In this way, the SRT (speech-recognition threshold), in addition to expressing how much hearing loss a patient has for speech, also lends verification to the pure-tone audiogram. If the two measures disagree by more than about 5 dB, an explanation should be sought, for the accuracy of one or both of these tests is in question.

Speech-recognition thresholds (SRTs) are customarily measured using two-syllable words called **spondees,** where both syllables are uttered with the same stress. Examples of spondaic words are *hotdog, baseball, toothbrush,* and *sidewalk.* Although spondaic stress is not used in English discourse, spondaic words are clinically useful in that they are fairly easy to discriminate, even close to threshold.

The word recognition score (WRS) of patients is of clinical interest in that it helps both in determining the cause and possible treatment of their hearing loss. WRS is a useful predictor of the outcome of audiological rehabilitation. Most clinicians measure WRS using lists of 50 one-syllable **phonetically balanced (PB)** words, so called since they are said to contain all the phonemes of the language with their approximate frequencies in connected discourse. While this is not necessarily the case, these word lists have been popular for more than half a century. Unlike the tests described earlier, WRSs are measured in percent, rather than in decibels. When a list of 50 words is presented, the patient is asked to repeat each word. The number of words correctly repeated is multiplied by 2%, and the result is the WRS.

People with normal hearing usually have very high WRSs (90 to 100%), as do people with conductive hearing losses, regardless of the degree of impairment. This is because there is little distortion in their auditory systems. In the case of a significant sensorineural hearing loss, there is almost always some measurable distortion. Therefore, as a general rule, there is a relationship between the degree of sensorineural hearing loss and the drop in WRS. For example, patients with mild sensorineural hearing loss (15 to 30 dB HL) may show WRSs of 80 to 90%, those with moderate losses (30 to 60 dB HL) may show WRSs of 60 to 80%, and those with severe losses (65 to 85 dB HL) may show WRSs of 40 to 60%. Patients with profound hearing losses sometimes have such great difficulties in discriminating speech that the scores are extremely low or not even measurable. It goes without saying that the preceding statement is intended only as a set of examples. Usually, the greater the sensorineural hearing loss the greater the distortion and the poorer the WRS, but there are many exceptions to these assumptions.

Electrophysiological Tests

The tests just described all require some measure of cooperation from the patient and have been called *subjective tests*. It has long been thought desirable to have tests that can be carried out without direct patient response to a signal. The evolution of these procedures has been most pronounced in the last few decades and is described briefly in the following sections.

Acoustic Immittance

The term **immittance** was coined by the American National Standards Institute (ANSI, 1987) as a combination of *impedance* (the sound energy that is reflected from the tympanic membrane) and *admittance* (the energy that is admitted via the tympanic membrane to the middle ear). Since no system, including the human ear, is totally efficient in sound transmission, there is always some impedance, and thus admittance is never total. The development of immittance meters has introduced a number of procedures that have become standard in clinical audiology. An example of a modern acoustic immittance meter can be seen in Figure 6–5.

The measurement of the mobility of the tympanic membrane and middle-ear system is called **tympanometry.** The mobility of the middle-ear system is measured by varying the amount of positive and negative air pressure imposed against it. Air pressure changes are applied by a probe placed in the external auditory canal. As the air pressure is varied up and down from normal atmospheric pressure, the tympanic membrane becomes stiffer by being gently pushed into the middle ear (with positive pressure) and pulled out into the external auditory canal (with negative pressure). A test sound is introduced into the canal, and the amount of sound energy bouncing back is monitored as the pressure is varied. This procedure is called tympanometry and can reveal such conditions as tympanic membrane perforation, interrupted ossicular chain, fluid in the middle ear, and stiffness of the ossicles.

In addition to tympanometry, it is possible to measure the **acoustic reflex,** which is the contraction of the middle-ear muscles in response to the

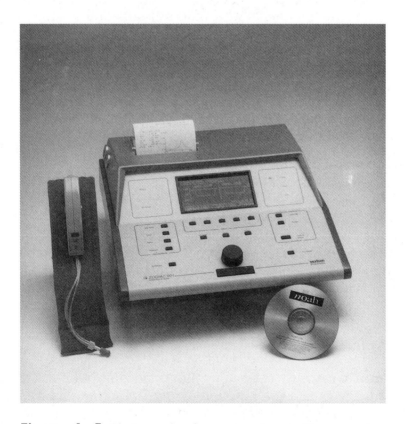

Figure 6–5. Photograph of an acoustic immittance meter. (Photo courtesy of Madsen Electronics)

introduction of intense auditory signals (about 85 dB SL for normal hearers). A great deal of insight can be gleaned from acoustic reflex thresholds that can be obtained at normal sensation levels, high sensation levels (greater than 100 dB), low sensation levels (less than 65 dB), or reflexes that cannot be obtained at all.

Performance of a basic hearing evaluation is demonstrated on the accompanying CD-ROM.

 CD-ROM

A Hearing Evaluation

CD-ROM segment Ch.06.01 is a movie that shows portions of a hearing evaluation. The procedures that are demonstrated include pure-tone air- and bone-conduction audiometry, speech-recognition thresholds, and word-recognition scores.

Auditory Evoked Potentials

Whenever a sound is heard, it is recognized as changes in electrical activity by a number of relay sites along the auditory path in the brain. These responses are small in comparison to the ongoing electrical activity that is present in any living brain. As such, they are difficult to observe, but the development of computers has allowed for averaging the signals in such a way as to make the responses recognizable. Within 300 milliseconds after the introduction of a sound (called the *latency period*), the signal has reached the higher centers of the brain. The earlier the response occurs (the shorter the latency), the lower in the auditory system the response is generated. Probably the most widely used diagnostic results are those that are obtained within the first 10-millisecond latency. These early responses are called the **auditory brainstem response (ABR).**

The ABR (auditory brainstem response) is presently used for a number of purposes, including testing newborn infants for hearing loss, determination of the site of lesion in the auditory pathway, and measuring hearing in non-cooperative individuals such as small children, the elderly, and individuals willfully or unconsciously attempting to make their hearing appear worse than it is.

Otoacoustic Emissions (OAE)

The scientific community was rocked a little over two decades ago with the realization that the inner ear actually produces some very faint sounds

(Kemp, 1978). These sounds have been called spontaneous **otoacoustic emissions (OAE)** and are present in about half of all individuals with normal hearing. For some reasons yet to be explained, spontaneous otoacoustic emissions (OAEs) are found more often in females than in males and are more often seen in right ears than in left ears. It was then learned that an emission could be produced as a kind of "echo," by introducing a signal to the ear and then monitoring the sound that is returned from the tympanic membrane. The sound is mechanically generated by the outer hair cells of the cochlea of the inner ear. These have been called evoked otoacoustic emissions.

OAEs have leapt into clinical prominence since their development, and there are now devices used for this purpose that are so small they can be held in one hand. OAEs have taken their rightful place beside acoustic immittance and auditory evoked potentials in the battery of tests available to clinical audiologists.

TYPES OF HEARING LOSS

Hearing status is generally classified as being normal or showing one of three types of hearing loss: conductive, sensorineural, or mixed, as described in the following sections.

Normal Hearing

People with normal hearing sensitivity show auditory thresholds below (less than) 15 dB HL at all frequencies, as can be seen in Figure 6–6. The patient shown here would be expected to have little or no difficulty hearing under most circumstances.

Conductive Hearing Losses

Individuals with **conductive hearing losses** show impairment by air conduction (which measures the total amount of loss they experience), but they have normal hearing by bone conduction. This is because the air-conducted signal must pass through both the outer and middle ears, where the conductive problem presumably resides, and where the sound, coming from the earphone of the audiometer via air conduction, is attenuated (made weaker). When the test is carried out by bone conduction, which bypasses the conductive system, hearing appears to be normal since the sensorineural system is undamaged in conductive hearing losses. Figure 6–7 shows a moderate conductive hearing loss. Note that there is a loss by air conduction in both ears at each frequency, but that bone conduction is normal throughout. The de-

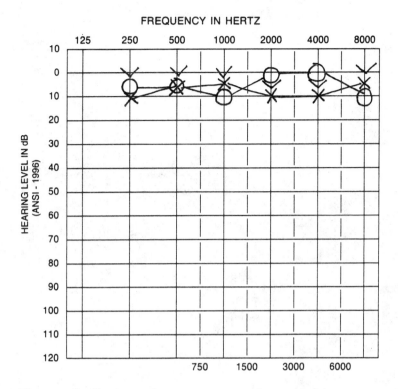

Figure 6-6. An audiogram representing normal hearing in both ears.

gree of hearing loss will vary for air conduction based on the cause and extent of the problem, but bone conduction will always remain within the normal range. The configuration of the audiogram is fairly flat, that is, there is approximately the same degree of loss at each frequency. This is fairly typical of conductive hearing losses, although there is naturally some variation.

Causes of Conductive Hearing Losses

Conductive hearing losses are caused by damage to the outer ear or middle ear.

Outer-Ear Hearing Losses

There is disagreement among experts on whether the tympanic membrane should be considered a part of the outer ear or a part of the middle ear, since it is the boundary that separates these two cavities. This argument is like asking whether a closed door between the living room and dining room is in one room or the other. It is really a part of both. So it is with the tympanic

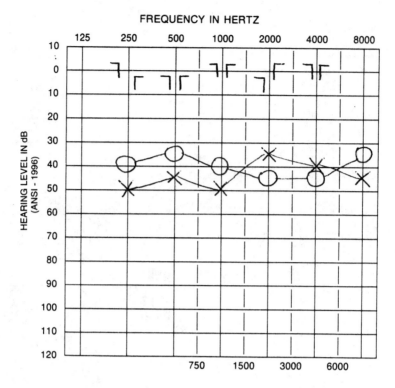

Figure 6-7. An audiogram representing a conductive hearing loss in both ears.

membrane, but for purposes of this chapter, we will consider the tympanic membrane to be a part of the middle ear.

Outer-ear conditions produce hearing losses when the external auditory canal becomes occluded. While loss of or damage to the pinna is known to effect changes in the acoustics of the external auditory canal, pinna abnormalities do not produce measurable hearing loss when hearing is tested using earphones. Nevertheless they should be considered when working with people who have pinna abnormalities.

The lumen of the external auditory canal can be partially or completely blocked by such things as foreign objects (like pencil erasers), ear wax, the buildup or debris from infection, or swelling of the canal walls because of infection or irritation. There are also conditions that occlude the canal like tumors, or burns (which cause the canal to collapse), or congenital partial or complete closure of the canal. All of these conditions require careful scrutiny by an ear specialist before otological or audiological rehabilitation should begin.

When hearing losses occur because of external auditory canal disorders, the hearing loss is of the conductive type, and word recognition scores are generally excellent. The value afforded by immittance measures is denied to the audiologist, because the fact that the external auditory canal is closed makes inserting the immittance probe tip impossible.

Middle-Ear Hearing Losses

The primary cause of hearing loss in the middle ear is infection called **otitis media.** In fact, otitis media is the largest single cause of hearing loss in general. Most people have at least one bout of otitis media in childhood, and while it is most common in children, it can occur at any age. Otitis media causes hearing loss in several ways: the fluid that forms in the middle-ear space secondary to the infection can act as a sound barrier, or the infection may cause thickening or destruction of the tympanic membrane or ossicular chain. Otitis media should be viewed primarily as a medical condition, and treatment should be sought as soon as symptoms appear. Audiological intervention is indicated if there is any indication that the treatment for hearing loss secondary to otitis media will be prolonged.

While the term *otitis media* literally means infection of the middle ear, many of these cases do not involve infection per se, but rather the accumulation of sterile fluid because of the negative middle-ear pressure that results from eustachian tubes that do not function properly. Children and adults who suffer from chronic eustachian tube dysfunction may have a simple operation called **myringotomy.** A small plastic tube is placed through an incision made in the tympanic membrane, allowing the middle ear to ventilate by the passage of air through the tube from the external auditory canal to the middle ear. These tubes are often worn for periods up to a year or so, at which time they often extrude spontaneously.

Other causes of conductive hearing loss in the middle ear include a variety of congenital disorders. Some occur in isolation and some as one symptom of a syndrome that includes other abnormalities (as of the bones of the cranium and face). Other causes include tumors, trauma, or fixation of the ossicular chain by a condition called **otosclerosis** (most commonly seen in adult white females).

It is now commonly agreed that even very mild conductive hearing losses in young children may interfere with normal language development, and hearing aids are often prescribed at very young ages in these cases. A condition called **minimal auditory deprivation syndrome (MADS)** may result from the lack of sensory input to the auditory centers of the brain, resulting in what has been referred to as **central auditory processing disorder (CAPD).**

Sensorineural Hearing Losses

Chapter 5 discussed the functions of the inner ear as being responsible for the body's balance and equilibrium, as well as for its role in hearing. The balance portion, called the **vestibular mechanism** (the utricle, saccule, and semi-circular canals), can go awry for a number of reasons, resulting in the disturbing symptom of vertigo, the sensation of whirling or violent turning. Damage to the **cochlea** produces what is called a **sensorineural hearing loss.** Sensorineural hearing losses may range from very mild, sometimes showing virtually normal hearing for low frequencies and depressed hearing for higher frequencies, to profound or even total hearing loss.

The term *sensorineural* suggests that the lesion causing the hearing loss is either sensory (in the cochlea) or neural (either in the neural structures of the cochlea or the **auditory [VIIIth cranial] nerve**). As can be seen in Figure 6–8, cochlear hearing losses evince an absence of an air-bone gap, which is the hallmark of the conductive hearing loss. That is, in sensorineural hearing loss the thresholds for air-conducted tones are about the same, in decibels, as the thresholds for bone-conducted tones. The word-recognition scores are almost always poorer than those seen in patients with normal hearing or those with conductive hearing losses (caused by either outer-ear or middle-ear disorders), and the degree of speech discrimination difficulty is often linked directly to the degree of hearing loss.

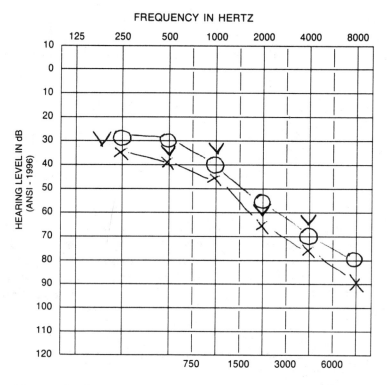

Figure 6–8. An audiogram representing a sensorineural hearing loss in both ears.

The degree of loss illustrated in Figure 6–8 is moderate. Notice that the audiogram tilts downward, suggesting greater hearing difficulty in the higher frequencies than in the lower frequencies. Although this configuration is typical of sensorineural hearing loss, there is great variation in the type and severity of these losses. In addition to high-frequency losses, it is common to see flat audiograms, low-frequency losses, and a variety of shapes. The degree of loss may be quite different at different frequencies and may range from mild to profound.

Causes of Sensorineural Hearing Losses

Sensorineural hearing losses usually involve damage to the cochlea or the auditory nerve. Like conductive losses, sensorineural hearing losses may occur prenatally (before birth), perinatally (during the birth process), or postnatally (after birth).

Cochlear Hearing Losses

Prenatal cochlear hearing losses may be inherited, either in isolation or as a part of a syndrome. They may be caused by anoxia (oxygen deprivation) of the fetus, trauma, viral infections that cross the placental barrier, fetal alcohol syndrome, or variance between the blood of the mother and the fetus, such as in Rh incompatibility.

Perinatal cochlear hearing losses are usually caused by some disruption in the normal birth process. Complications like umbilical strangulation or other trauma may affect the cochlea by causing anoxia. Such conditions often affect not only the auditory structures but the brain as well, resulting in conditions like cerebral palsy and mental retardation.

Postnatal cochlear hearing losses often result secondary to prolonged otitis media, occurring first as conductive, then as mixed, and finally as pure sensorineural losses. Postnatal causes include a variety of viral and bacterial infections such as meningitis, a number of sexually transmitted diseases, high fevers, exposure to loud noise, and the aging process.

Auditory Nerve Hearing Losses

Hearing losses that result from damage to or irritation of the auditory nerve are usually unilateral (occur in only one ear). The most common cause is **acoustic neuroma,** a tumor that forms on the vestibular branch of the auditory (VIIIth cranial) nerve. It eventually presses on the cochlear branch, usually causing **tinnitus** (ringing or roaring sounds in the ear[s]), then difficulty in discriminating speech, then hearing loss, which progresses either rapidly or slowly from very mild to total. The decision to surgically or radiologically remove acoustic neuromas, or to inhibit their growth is based on a number of factors, including the patient's age, general health, and symptoms. There are other causes of VIIIth nerve hearing losses, but acoustic neuroma and acoustic neuritis (inflammation) are the most common.

Mixed Hearing Loss

As shown in Figure 6–9, a mixed hearing loss is a combination of both the conductive and sensorineural varieties. The amount of sensorineural impairment is expressed as the difference, in decibels, between 0 dB HL and the bone-conduction threshold at each frequency. The amount of conductive hearing loss is the difference, in decibels, between the bone-conduction threshold and the air-conduction threshold at each frequency (this is called the **air-bone gap [ABG]**). As the sensorineural component increases, the bone-conduction threshold gets higher (lower on the audiogram), and as the conductive component gets greater, the air-bone gap increases. The air-conduction threshold reveals the total amount of hearing loss at each frequency.

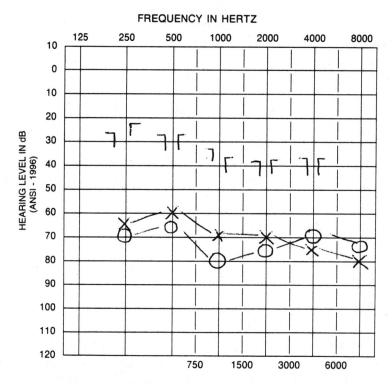

Figure 6–9. An audiogram representing a mixed hearing loss in both ears.

Central Auditory Processing Disorders

Central auditory processing disorder (CAPD) was mentioned earlier as occurring among children suffering from sensory deprivation in the auditory path. Both children and adults may appear in the audiology clinic with complaints of difficulty in hearing that do not relate to how loud particular sounds are. The difficulty appears to be in processing or discriminating speech, and the problem is exacerbated in noisy or otherwise untoward listening situations.

For a time, in the history of diagnostic audiology, the emphasis was on the diagnosis of central disorders and pinpointing the site of lesion (i.e., brainstem vs. cortex). Since the emergence of modern imaging techniques like positron emission tomography (PET), magnetic resonance imaging (MRI), and computed tomography (CT) scanning, the contribution of audiology to these diagnoses has been lessened, although some of the recent breakthroughs in evoked-potential testing show great promise. What appears to be more important than diagnosis is to understand the individual's specific difficulty and, after the possibility of a health or life-threatening lesion has been eliminated, to focus on improving the skills these patients need to cope with their difficulties. Solutions to this type of problem are addressed in Chapter 7.

SUMMARY

Audiology has evolved over a little more than 50 years from a profession dedicated to the development and performance of accurate diagnostic hearing tests to one that is involved in every aspect of auditory rehabilitation. The diagnostic audiologist must determine the need for medical and nonmedical (rehabilitative or psychological) intervention to improve the quality of life of people with hearing loss. Modern techniques now permit early diagnosis of hearing loss in children so that appropriate education and training may begin. Chapter 7 delves further into audiological (re)habilitation, which is one of the primary justifications for diagnostic audiology.

STUDY QUESTIONS

1 List causes for conductive hearing loss caused by damage to the outer ear.

2 List causes for conductive hearing loss caused by damage to the middle ear.

3 List causes for sensorineural hearing loss caused by damage to the inner ear.

4 List causes for sensorineural hearing loss caused by damage to the auditory nerve.

5 What are the principal features of conductive hearing loss in terms of the relationships between air conduction and bone conduction? What is typical in the way of word-recognition scores?

6 Answer question #5 in terms of sensorineural hearing loss.

7 What is a mixed hearing loss?

8 What is otitis media?

REFERENCES

American National Standards Institute (ANSI). (1987). *American national standard specifications for instruments to measure aural acoustic impedance and admittance (aural acoustic immittance).* ANSI S3.39-1987. New York: Author.

Johnson, E. W. (1970). Tuning forks to audiometers and back again. *Laryngoscope, 80,* 49–68.

Kemp, D. T. (1978). Simulated acoustic emissions from within the human auditory system. *Journal of the Acoustical Society of America, 64,* 1386–1391.

Martin, F. N., & Clark, J. G. (2000). *Introduction to audiology* (7th ed.). Boston: Allyn & Bacon.

Studebaker, G. A. (1962). Placement of vibrator in bone conduction testing. *Journal of Speech and Hearing Research, 5,* 321–331.

SUGGESTED READINGS

Clark, J. G., & Martin, F. N. (Eds.). (1994). *Effective counseling in audiology.* Englewood Cliffs, NJ: Prentice-Hall.

Katz, J. (Ed.). *Handbook of clinical audiology* (4th ed.). Baltimore: Williams & Wilkins.

Martin, F. N., & Clark, J. G. (1996). *Hearing care for children.* Boston: Allyn & Bacon.

Martin, F. N., & Clark, J. G. (2000). *Introduction to audiology* (7th ed.). Boston: Allyn & Bacon.

Stach, B. A. (1998). *Clinical audiology: An introduction.* San Diego: Singular Publishing Group.

GLOSSARY
G

Acoustic neuroma: A tumor arising on the auditory (VIIIth cranial) nerve.

Acoustic reflex: The measurable contraction of the muscles of the middle ear in response to an intense sound.

Air conduction: The pathway of sounds that includes the outer ear, middle ear, inner ear, and the structures beyond.

Air-bone gap (ABG): The difference, in decibels, between the air-conduction threshold and the bone-conduction threshold.

Audiogram: A graph depicting the threshold of audibility (in decibels) as a function of different frequencies.

Audiometer: A device used for the measurement of hearing.

Auditory brainstem response (ABR): Measurable responses in the brainstem to a series of acoustic stimuli.

Auditory nerve: The VIIIth cranial nerve that carries information from the inner ear to the brain about hearing and balance.

Bone conduction: The pathway of sound that bypasses the conductive mechanisms of the outer and middle ear by vibrating the skull and stimulating the cochlea of the inner ear.

Central auditory processing disorder (CAPD): Difficulty in discriminating speech, often in the presence of background noise, and frequently in the absence of the loss of hearing sensitivity.

Cochlea: A structure in the inner ear that converts the mechanical energy received from the middle ear into an electrochemical code for transmission to the brain.

Conductive hearing loss: A loss of hearing sensitivity caused by damage to the outer and/or middle ear.

Hearing level (HL): The reference that uses normal hearing in the scale of decibels.

Immittance: Measurement of the impedance of the tympanic membrane or admittance of sound to the middle ear.

Mastoid process: The bony protrusion behind the pinna.

Minimal auditory deprivation syndrome (MADS): Difficulty in processing speech because of a central auditory disorder thought to be caused by very mild hearing loss.

Mixed hearing loss: A combination of conductive and sensorineural hearing loss in the same ear.

Myringotomy: Incision into the tympanic membrane with insertion of a small ventilating tube.

Otitis media: Infection of the middle ear.

Otoacoustic emission (OAE): Either spontaneous or evoked sounds emanating from the inner ear.

Otosclerosis: A hearing loss caused by bony fixation of the stapes in the oval window.

Phonetically balanced (PB) word lists: Lists of 50 words that are supposed to contain all the phonetic elements of English speech. These lists are used for testing word recognition.

Sensation level (SL): The number of decibels above the auditory threshold of an individual.

Sensorineural hearing loss: Hearing loss caused by damage to the inner ear and/or auditory nerve.

Speech-recognition threshold (SRT): The lowest intensity at which speech can barely be heard.

Spondee: A two-syllable word pronounced with equal emphasis on both syllables. Used in testing the SRT.

Threshold of audibility: The lowest intensity at which a signal can barely be heard.

Tinnitus: Ringing, roaring, or other sounds heard in the absence of an external sound.

Tympanometry: A pressure/compliance function that reveals the status of the middle ear.

Vestibular mechanism: That part of the inner ear responsible for reporting balance and equilibrium to the brain.

Word-recognition score (WRS): The score, in percent, that reveals the ability to discriminate among the sounds of speech.

7

Audiologic Rehabilitation

John A. Nelson

LEARNING OBJECTIVES

1 To understand the basic components and benefits of personal amplification systems including hearing aids and cochlear implants.

2 To understand what makes some listening environments more difficult than others and how assistive listening devices might assist listening in these situations.

3 To understand the basic audiologic habilitation services for children who have hearing loss.

4 To understand how to empower adults who have hearing losses through audiologic rehabilitation.

CD-ROM

INTRODUCTION

Many different professionals assist individuals who have hearing losses. For example, audiologists fit hearing aids and teach patients how to use the devices. They also provide information about effective communication strategies. Speech-language pathologists teach individuals with hearing impairments how to listen for important speech sounds, how to make their language more informative and complex, and how to produce intelligible speech. Educators of children who are deaf adapt traditional teaching techniques for children with hearing impairments. Psychologists and social workers assist in dealing with the psychological effects of hearing impairment. School administrators can advocate services for children. In many instances, the services are provided by a team of professionals.

The services that these professionals deliver are usually divided into two categories: **audiologic habilitation** and **audiologic rehabilitation.** Audiologic habilitation services are provided to children who are learning to listen and to use speech and language skills for the first time. Audiologic rehabilitation services are provided to adults who need to modify their communication style due to their acquired hearing impairments. Professionals and lay persons often use the term "rehabilitation" to refer to both audiologic habilitation and rehabilitation services.

The first step in audiologic rehabilitation is to increase the individual's ability to hear sounds, usually using amplification. The extent of necessary services following amplification varies from individual to individual. Although follow-up services are beneficial, they are not always provided, an unfortunate occurrence. I first discuss the amplification options that assist individuals in hearing. Following this, I introduce you to the services that are helpful in increasing the quality of life for individuals with hearing impairment.

PERSONAL HEARING DEVICES

As noted in Chapter 2, hearing is a critical part of communication. We rely on hearing for such things as safety, communication, and pleasure. Thus, inventors and researchers have been trying for centuries to help people to hear better. The devices that were developed initially were of limited benefit. The discovery of electricity was an important milestone for the development of hearing aids because it led to the invention of the electrical amplifier.

Nonelectrical Hearing Devices

There are many things that can be done to increase the intensity of sound to make people hear better. For example, you can cup your hand next to your ear. The hand helps to direct sound into the outer ear, leading to a perception of an increase in loudness. This technique provides only a small increase in audibility. Horns and tubes provided an additional increase in audibility. Acoustic horns were used to direct sound from a large area into a small area. The effectiveness of the acoustic horn to direct sound is dependent on its size and shape. These physical properties can be altered to increase the energy applied to the smaller area, the outer ear. Unfortunately, it was awkward to speak into an acoustic horn placed at someone's ear. To rectify this problem, tubes were often used to direct sound from one location to the next. An acoustic horn was attached to a tube, which was then directed to the ear. With this instrument, speakers did not have to talk directly into the listener's ear.

For cosmetic reasons, these devices took many forms. The acoustic horn and tube device, often called the ear trumpet, was often decorated with paintings or jewels. Sometimes the device was hidden in another object. The listening stick was a walking cane that was hollowed out to provide a tube for directing sound. The listening chair had hollowed tubes in the arms and back to direct sound to the listener's ear. Although modern hearing aids use electrical circuits, the physical properties of horns and tubes are still incorporated into their design.

Hearing Aids

With the discovery of electricity, amplification systems have changed dramatically. The original electrical devices were quite large and required a direct line to a power source, for example, an electrical outlet. Thus, these devices were not very portable. Increased developments in technology have provided miniaturization of the electrical circuits as well as their power requirements. During the past few decades, amplification systems have changed tremendously. These devices are now referred to as hearing aids. Every hearing aid requires four basic components: a microphone, an amplifier, a receiver, and a battery (see Figure 7–1).

A microphone converts acoustic signals into electric signals. The changes in the electrical voltage are the same as the changes in the pressure of the acoustic signal. The electrical signals are passed to the amplifier, which increases the amplitude of the electrical signal. The hearing aid does not amplify all frequencies by the same amount. The amount of amplification provided is dependent on the type and extent of the individual's hearing loss.

The amplified electrical signal is then sent to a receiver, which is the third required component of a hearing aid. The receiver converts the amplified electrical signal back into an acoustic signal. The acoustic signal is now more intense than the original acoustic input to the microphone. The receiver can be thought of as a little loudspeaker like the one on your stereo.

These three components require energy. They are powered by a battery, which is the fourth required component of a hearing aid. Currently there are five sizes of hearing aid batteries. Only one battery size will work for a given hearing aid. Each battery has a positive side and a negative side and thus must be inserted in the correct direction for the device to operate.

There are many controls on a hearing aid. The simplest control is the on-off switch. This might be accomplished by flipping a switch, by rotating the volume control wheel, or by opening the battery door. Another user control is the volume control wheel. This allows the hearing aid user to change the

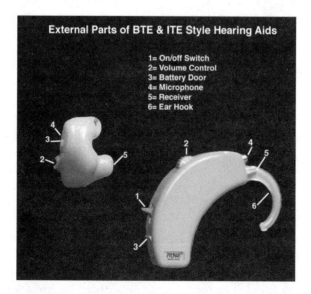

Figure 7–1. External parts of the behind-the-ear (BTE) and in-the-ear (ITE) style hearing aids. (Photograph courtesy of Phonak Hearing Systems and Starkey Laboratories)

intensity of the signal that reaches the ear. Some modern hearing aids do not have a volume control wheel. Instead, there are advanced signal-processing systems within the hearing aid that control the volume automatically.

Another common option on hearing aids is a **telecoil switch** (usually referred to as a t-switch for short). Telephones emit electromagnetic energy that fluctuates in the same pattern as the acoustic signal you hear. When the user flips the t-switch into the telecoil position, the hearing aid microphone is turned off, and the telecoil inside the hearing aid picks up the electromagnetic energy. The telecoil converts this energy to an electrical signal that is delivered to the amplifier.

There are a couple of major advantages to using the telecoil mode. First, it reduces feedback when using the telephone. Feedback is the whistling sound produced from a hearing aid when an object such as a hand or telephone handset is put next to it. By turning the hearing aid microphone off, the hearing aid will not emit feedback. Second, because the microphone is turned off in the telecoil mode, the acoustic signal in the room will not be amplified. Imagine talking on the telephone in a noisy restaurant and being able to "turn off" the noise in the room. The t-switch makes telephone conversations easier.

Hearing aids are available in many different styles. The body type hearing aid was the first mass-produced portable device and, as its name suggests, it is worn on the body. The device consists of a small metal box that contains the microphone, amplifier, battery, and user controls. Attached to the body aid is an electrical cord that extends to the ear and attaches to a button receiver that actually looks like a thick button. The button receiver is attached to an **earmold,** which directs sound into the outer ear.

The earmold is either vinyl or acrylic material that is custom-fit to fill a part of the outer ear. It has a bore or hole to direct sound from the button receiver down the ear canal toward the tympanic membrane.

The original body-worn device was necessary to house the large electronics and battery (see Figure 7–2). With the miniaturization of electronic circuits and batteries, the housing requirements were also reduced. Therefore, body hearing aids are no longer commonly used. The main disadvantage of the body hearing aid involves the microphone. Because the microphone is worn on the chest, body hearing aid users "hear" from their chests instead of their ears. This also makes the microphone susceptible to unwanted noise when clothing rubs against it. One advantage of the device is that it allows for large controls. This is beneficial for individuals with limited dexterity, such as those who are elderly.

The behind-the-ear (BTE) hearing aid is the next smaller hearing aid and, as the name suggests, is worn behind the ear or, more specifically, behind the pinna (see Figure 7–3). The behind-the-ear (BTE) microphone is in the top of the device and is aimed toward the front of the user where the top of the pinna attaches to the head. The device houses the microphone, amplifier, receiver, and battery in one case. The amplified acoustic energy exits the

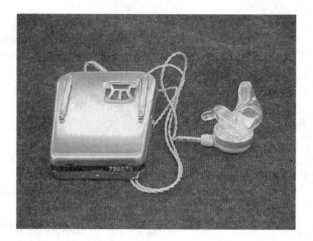

Figure 7-2. A body-worn hearing aid. (Photograph courtesy of Beltone)

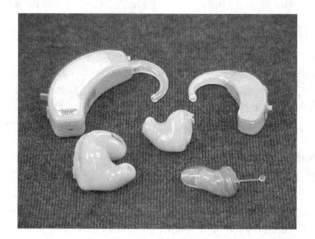

Figure 7-3. Comparison of the ear-level hearing aid styles: behind-the-ear (BTE, large and small), in-the-ear (ITE), in-the-canal (ITC), and completely-in-the-canal (CIC). (Photograph courtesy of Starkey Laboratories, Phonak Hearing Systems, and Rexton, Inc.)

hearing aid at the top and is directed into an earhook. The earhook is a curved, hard plastic tube that directs sound out of the BTE to a flexible tube that is inserted into the earmold. The earhook also helps to hold the BTE hearing aid on the head. The BTE hearing aid is relatively large compared to the other styles, allowing for more circuitry and signal-processing options.

Although some of the BTE hearing aid is often hidden behind the ear, many people feel it is not cosmetically acceptable.

One variation of the BTE hearing aid is the eyeglass device. At one time individuals who needed glasses and hearing aids but wanted to wear only one prosthetic device found the eyeglass hearing aid to be an acceptable option. The bows of the glasses, the side pieces, were hollowed out and hearing aid components were inserted. The portion of the bow that reached behind the ear was the most common place, as this area could easily be enlarged to encase the hearing aid components. Tubing from the glasses' bow was directed to an earmold. As you might imagine, the device required a rather large pair of glasses. Although an admirable idea, the device caused many problems for the people who were responsible for fitting both hearing aids and glasses. People fitting hearing aids usually did not know much about adjusting glasses and people fitting glasses usually did not know much about adjusting hearing aids. Further, if one aspect of the device needed repair, the benefits of both prosthetic devices were unavailable until the complete system was fixed. Today, these devices are rarely seen. Fortunately, with smaller glasses and hearing aids, both devices can be comfortably worn together.

The next smaller hearing aid is the in-the-ear (ITE) hearing aid (see Figure 7–3). All of the components are placed in a plastic shell that is usually custom fit for the hearing aid user. The in-the-ear (ITE) hearing aid fills up the concha as well as part of the ear canal. The microphone, battery door, and volume control are located on the faceplate of the hearing aid. The receiver is located in the canal portion of the hearing aid and delivers the amplified sound into the remaining canal. With this device, the hearing aid microphone is located closer to the area on the head where sound normally arrives. Also, the hearing aid is now contained in one single unit because the earmold and the hearing aid are both part of one device.

The in-the-canal (ITC) hearing aid is even smaller than the ITE and completely fills the outer part of the ear canal (see Figure 7–3). This hearing aid is custom fit for an individual user. Currently, there are some options that are unavailable with ITC (in-the-canal) hearing aids. For example, the telecoil discussed previously will not fit within this device. Also, as hearing aids become smaller, batteries that fit in the hearing aid also need to be smaller. Less energy can be stored by smaller batteries and thus, the battery life is decreased. For those who are concerned about cosmetic issues, the ITC is less noticeable than the ITE hearing aid.

A recent advancement in hearing aids is the completely-in-the-canal (CIC) hearing aid (see Figure 7–3). All of the components of this device fit deep in the ear canal. Like the other types of hearing aids, the CIC (completely-in-the-canal) hearing aid must be custom fit for the individual user. The hearing aid is removed by pulling on a piece of plastic that is similar to a piece of fishing wire. Due to this deep fit, a volume control wheel is not an option. As you might expect, the device is difficult to see when in place, making it desirable by those who are the most concerned about the cosmetics of wearing a hearing aid. The obstacles to fitting this device are twofold. First, the individual must have an average to large ear canal to accommodate the device. Second, as with all hearing aids as they become smaller, the amplification that can be provided is limited. CIC hearing aids are only appropriate for individuals with mild and moderate degrees of hearing losses.

The bone-conduction hearing aid is a special device used for individuals with substantial conductive losses who have difficulty obtaining benefit from amplification that provides a more intense acoustic signal. For example, bone-conduction hearing aids might be a good choice for individuals who do not have an ear canal or those who have constant drainage in the ear canal due to infection. A bone-conduction hearing aid stimulates the cochlea by setting the bones of the skull into motion. The bone-conduction hearing aid consists of a microphone, amplifier, battery, and a bone oscillator. The bone oscillator replaces the air-conduction receiver and is usually placed behind the pinna on the mastoid process. The device is not commonly used today. Because of the introduction of antibiotics, permanent conductive hearing loss is far less common. Plus, other types of hearing aids provide better high-frequency amplification and are smaller and more comfortable to wear.

 CD-ROM

Hearing Aids

CD-ROM segment Ch.07.01 allows you to look at every angle of BTE, ITE, ITC, and CIC hearing aids. After opening the file, click on one style of hearing aid to activate the movie. Then, click and drag the mouse (hold the mouse button down while you are moving it) to rotate the hearing aid to different viewing angles—all 360°! In that segment, the hearing aids are not at the relative scale. To see a size comparison of the ear-level hearing aids, open segment Ch.07.02. Segment Ch.07.03 is an example of a body-worn hearing aid, with an appropriate earmold. The major parts of a hearing aid are labeled for a BTE and an ITE hearing aid in segments Ch.07.04 and Ch.07.05, respectively. The segment Ch.07.06 shows a variety of earmold styles and colors. (Hearing aids courtesy of Starkey Laboratories and Phonak Hearing Systems)

Hearing Aid Fitting

The first step in fitting a hearing aid is to obtain an ear impression from the individual. The process consists of placing soft plastic material into the ear following the insertion of a cotton or foam block into the ear canal so the material does not come in contact with the tympanic membrane. After a few minutes, the material hardens and is removed. If the individual is going to use a body or BTE style hearing aid, the ear impression is sent to a laboratory to make an earmold. If the individual is going to use an ITE, ITC, or CIC style hearing aid, the ear impression is sent to the hearing aid manufacturer to make the custom-fit case that holds the hearing aid components.

 CD-ROM

Taking an Ear Impression

You can watch an abbreviated video of an audiologist taking an ear impression in CD-ROM segment Ch.07.07. As discussed within the text, an ear impression is required to obtain a custom-fit hearing aid earmold. There are a number of steps in taking this impression. These steps follow the video in segment Ch.07.07. This video clip has no audio.

1. An otoscopic examination is required to understand the shape of the external ear, to inspect the external ear for abnormalities, and to look for foreign bodies that might cause difficulties during the impression.

2. An "oto-block" or foam block is placed in the ear canal to ensure the impression material does not flow down the ear canal to the tympanic membrane. A lighted probe is used to insert the oto-block.

3. The material is mixed thoroughly. The impression material used for this video was premeasured for accurate proportions. The mixing must be done quickly, as the material begins to harden during the mixing stage. The mixed impression material is placed in a syringe.

4. The syringe is used to direct the impression material into the external ear. The technique takes practice to ensure a smooth ear impression.

5. After waiting a few minutes for the material to solidify, the ear impression is gently removed from the ear canal.

6. An otoscopic examination is preformed after taking an ear impression to ensure no material was left in the ear canal and that no injury occurred.

There are two main goals in fitting an amplification system. The first goal is to provide audibility for sounds that cannot be heard due to the hearing loss. This is accomplished by the amplifier and is measured in acoustic **gain.** Gain is calculated by subtracting the intensity of sound entering the microphone of the hearing aid from the intensity of sound exiting the earmold. The unit used for measuring hearing aid gain is the decibel (measured by sound pressure level [SPL]). Thus, if the input intensity is 65 dB SPL and the output intensity is 85 dB SPL, the gain is 20 dB.

Fitting hearing aids is not like fitting glasses, where the goal is to achieve 20/20 vision. The audiologist is not trying to achieve hearing thresholds with normal limits. Research has shown that providing gain values that are equal to the hearing loss are often unacceptable to the listener. Therefore, instead of providing enough gain for the individual to hear at 0 dB HL, most audiologists try to achieve gain values that are between one-third and two-thirds of the hearing loss. The gain at each frequency depends on the shape of the hearing loss. A plot of the gain across frequencies is called the frequency response of the hearing aid.

The second goal in fitting a hearing aid is to ensure that the **output** of the device does not reach intensities that cause discomfort or further damage. High-intensity sounds can cause damage to the ear and, thus, hearing aids should not amplify sounds to this level. Additionally, amplified sound can be perceived as too loud, and the hearing aid user will not be pleased with the performance of the hearing aid. It is important to verify that the maximum output of the hearing aid, independent of the input signal, never reaches a level of discomfort. Thresholds of discomfort can be measured with an audiometer and applied to the fitting of the hearing aid. This is commonly done by producing an intense input signal, like speaking loudly into the hearing aid microphone. An annoying loud sound, like shaking a ring of keys by the hearing aid, might also be used. This activity provides the hearing aid user an opportunity to comment on the loudness and annoyance of intense inputs. Because intense sounds can cause damage to the auditory system without being uncomfortable, it is also important to measure the output of the hearing aid in the individual's ear.

The physical measurements of gain and output of a hearing aid can be accomplished in two ways. One way is to obtain behavioral thresholds with and without the hearing aid. The gain, referred to as **functional gain,** is calculated as the difference between the aided and unaided thresholds. A disadvantage to this technique is that it involves a very time-consuming process. Fortunately, real-ear probe-microphone measurements are now available in the audiology clinic.

The alternative to functional gain measures is to obtain real-ear probe-microphone measurements. These measurements allow audiologists to determine the intensity of sound in the ear canal. A small flexible tube is place in the ear canal with the end near the tympanic membrane. The other end of the tube is connected to a small microphone. The **real-ear gain** is the difference between the intensity at the tympanic membrane with and without the hearing aid. This whole procedure takes only a few minutes and yields very useful data.

Hearing aid research laboratories around the world are continually investigating new signal processing techniques. Hopefully, these techniques will increase the quality of life for individuals with hearing aids. One common goal is to increase the ability of the patient to understand speech in the presence of background noise. Although these systems have had some success, the most desirable way is to decrease the level of background noise before it enters the microphone. This is usually accomplished with **assistive listening devices (ALDs),** which are discussed later in this chapter.

Hearing Aid Maintenance

Hearing aids need to be checked daily. First, it is critical that the hearing aid battery has sufficient voltage to power the hearing aid. This can be ascertained with a battery tester. The outer part of the hearing aid should be cleaned of debris, including removal of **cerumen** (ear wax) from the hearing aid receiver. Any part of the hearing aid that has electronic controls cannot be washed with water. Only the earmold of a body or BTE hearing aid can be cleaned with water after it is removed from the hearing aid. If a hearing aid does not amplify with a charged battery, sounds distorted, has intermittent sound, does not make sounds audible, or is uncomfortably loud, the device should be taken to an audiologist to have it checked. The audiologist has the tools necessary to fix many problems, but there are times when the hearing aid must be returned to the factory for repair.

Tactile Aids

Tactile aids are used by individuals who cannot benefit from traditional amplification. These devices contain a microphone that picks up the acoustic signal. The signal is amplified and turned into a vibration that is delivered to the skin. The vibrotactile stimulation is often delivered to the individual's chest, back, or arm. As you might suspect, the sensitivity of the skin to tactile vibrations is not as precise as the sensitivity of the ear to acoustic vibrations. Therefore, one important disadvantage of this device is the limited frequency resolution that can be provided to the listener. In the normal auditory system, very small changes in frequency can be perceived across a large frequency range. The tactile aid is usually limited to coding 10 different frequency bands or ranges. This means less than 10 different "pitches" can be perceived and used for coding speech. Most individuals have experienced difficulty understanding speech with a tactile aid unless it is supplemented with visual and contextual cues.

Cochlear Implants

For individuals with severe-to-profound sensorineural hearing losses, traditional hearing aid amplification provides limited or no benefit. As discussed in Chapter 5, the ear converts an acoustic pressure wave to a mechanical force at the tympanic membrane. This mechanical force is then delivered to the oval window and results in vibration of the basilar membrane. The basilar membrane movement causes electrical activity that can generate action potentials on the auditory nerve. Direct electrical stimulation of the auditory nerve generates action potentials that are perceived by the brain as auditory stimuli. Many individuals with severe-to-profound sensorineural hearing losses have damage within the cochlea. Their hearing mechanisms do not generate action potentials except in response to intense stimuli. If the auditory nerve could be stimulated directly, bypassing the damaged cochlea, individuals with sensorineural hearing losses could hear from direct electrical stimulation to the auditory nerve.

In 1972, after decades of research and product development, the first human received a **cochlear implant** (see Figures 7–4 and 7–5). At first, cochlear implants were only available to adults with profound acquired hearing loss. After many years of clinical investigation, the devices are now available for infants, children, and adults. It is important for readers to know that cochlear implants are not appropriate for every child with a severe hearing impairment. There are guidelines imposed by the Food and Drug Administration regarding candidacy for implants (see Table 7–1).

The implant consists of a microphone (part of a BTE hearing aid case), a signal processor, a transmitter, a receiver, and an electrode array. The acoustic signal is picked up by the microphone and delivered to the signal processor. The electronics of the cochlear implant limit the frequency resolution that can be delivered to the cochlea. Currently, the maximum number of frequency bands that can be provided with the cochlear implant is 22 compared to a normal auditory system that can detect over 10,000 different frequencies.

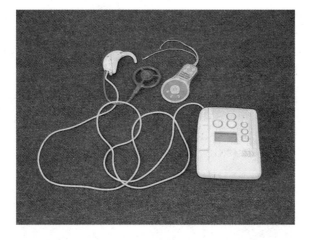

Figure 7–4. A body-worn speech processor and internal components of a cochlear implant. (Photograph courtesy of Cochlear Corporation)

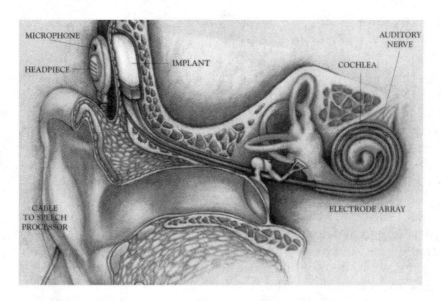

Figure 7–5. A diagram of where the cochlear implant is located in the cochlea. (From *Cochlear Implants for Infants and Children*, by J. G. Clar, R. S. C. Cowan, and R. C. Dowell, 1997, p. 510. San Diego: Singular Publishing Group.)

Table 7–1. Guidelines for Candidacy To Obtain a Cochlear Implant

Children

Bilateral profound sensorineural hearing loss
Limited or no useful benefit from hearing aids
No medical contraindications
High motivation and realistic expectations from both child and caregivers
Educational placement that emphasizes auditory skill development
At least 18 months of age

Adults

Bilateral profound sensorineural hearing loss or bilateral severe-to-profound sensorineural hearing loss if acquired after the acquisition of language
Limited or no useful benefit from hearing aids
No medical contraindications
At least 17 years of age

The signal processor analyzes the input signal and determines how to stimulate the cochlea.

Information about the input signal is coded and is then delivered to the external transmitting device that is worn behind the ear. The transmitting device stays in place by a magnetic force between it and the receiving device that was surgically placed under the skin. The signal is transmitted to the receiver through the skin by means of a radio frequency. The internal receiver delivers the electrical signal to an electrode array within the scala tympani of the cochlea. The electrode array sends electrical current through different regions of the cochlea. This causes the generation of action potentials on the auditory nerve that are perceived by the brain as sounds.

As mentioned earlier, the Food and Drug Administration has specific guidelines for determining candidacy for cochlear implants. These guidelines continue to change with advancements in research and technology. Some of the guidelines include an absence of medical contraindications, bilateral profound hearing loss (or a severe-to-profound loss for adults who lost their hearing after language acquisition), little to no benefit from traditional amplification, a desire to communicate in an auditory mode, high motivation, and realistic expectations. Infants must be approximately 18 months old before they can become candidates for surgery.

There are many reasons why an individual might not want to obtain a cochlear implant. Not wanting to undergo the surgery is a major reason, especially for parents of very young infants. Also, an individual who is deaf might not feel that hearing is critically important to their quality of life. Many deaf individuals live happy, fulfilled lives without hearing. Professionals should respect these personal beliefs, and the rehabilitation team should assist the individual and family members in deciding whether a cochlear implant is an appropriate option.

Most individuals who receive cochlear implants demonstrate a significant increase in their speech perception ability. With the more recent devices, it is common for these individuals to understand speech even without visual cues such as on the telephone. Individuals with cochlear implants often report that nonspeech stimuli, such as music, are also pleasurable. Rehabilitation is nec-

 CD-ROM

Cochlear Implants

The pictures in this section show two example of a cochlear implant. The original speech processor was a body worn unit as shown in CD-ROM segment Ch.07.08. In 1998, the first ear-level speech processor was introduced and is shown in segment Ch.07.09. The device that is implanted in the cochlea is shown with a quarter in segment Ch.07.10. This particular device has an electrode array that is placed in the cochlea and a second electrode that is placed outside of the cochlea. Finally, the placement of the ear-level speech processor and external transmitter is shown in segment Ch.07.11. (Device courtesy of Cochlear Corporation)

essary for the patient to understand how to hear with the cochlear implant signal. Many hours of intensive therapy are usually necessary to develop speech and language skills, especially for individuals who have not heard before. Even with intensive therapy, not all individuals with cochlear implants develop intelligible speech.

DIFFICULT LISTENING ENVIRONMENTS

The main goal of hearing aids is to increase the audibility of the speech signal. Many individuals have difficulty hearing and understanding speech in situations that involve a lot of background noise and reverberation. Reverberations are the sound reflections from hard surfaces. A room such as a bathroom, with tile walls and a tile floor, has considerable reverberation. A living room with carpeting, drapes, and soft furniture has much less reverberation. Reflections of sound overlap and interfere with the original acoustic signal and make it difficult to understand speech. These characteristics of a room are measured as **reverberation time,** which is determined by calculating the amount of time it takes for an intense sound to decrease by 60 dB after it is turned off. Most classrooms typically have reverberation times between 0.4 and 1.2 seconds (Crandell & Smaldino, 1995). Children with hearing loss should be placed in classrooms that have reverberation times no greater than 0.4 seconds (Crandell & Smaldino, 1995). Thus, many classrooms need to be acoustically modified to reduce reverberation.

Listening environments can also be described by the **signal-to-noise ratio (SNR).** The SNR is the signal intensity minus the noise intensity. Positive SNRs indicate that the signal is more intense than the noise; negative SNRs indicate that the noise is more intense than the signal. Talking with a friend in your living room would be an example of a positive SNR; talking to a friend with the fire alarm going off would be an example of a negative SNR. The more positive the SNR, the better the listening situation. Typical SNRs for classrooms have been reported in the range of +5 to −7 dB (Crandell & Smaldino, 1995). Children with hearing loss should be placed in classrooms in which the SNR is greater than +15 dB (Crandell & Smaldino, 1995). As is clearly evident, most public school classrooms are inadequate listening settings for instruction, especially for children with hearing impairments.

Another difficulty in listening to speech in large rooms is that as a listener moves away from a speaker, the intensity of the signal decreases. Thus, for someone to be heard across a large room, the intensity of the signal must increase at the source. This signal might be uncomfortably loud or barely audible at different points in the room.

To improve speech discrimination, it would be ideal to reduce the levels of background noise and reverberation. Unfortunately, this is not always possible. For example, in a restaurant it would be difficult to have all the other

customers sit silently. Or in a school gymnasium that is also used as an audi-
torium, carpeting on the floor would not be an option. A way to compensate
for background noise and reverberation is to increase the intensity of the
speaker's voice (for example, the teacher speaks louder). The disadvantage of
this solution is that the teacher experiences more vocal strain and listeners
near the teacher are in positions of greater intensities compared to listeners
who are further away.

A better way to increase the signal-to-noise ratio is to use an **assistive
listening device (ALD).** These devices pick up the sound at the source and
transmit it directly to the listener without sending intense sound waves
through the air. Frequency Modulated (FM) systems constitute one example
of an ALD that are often used in school settings (see Figure 7–6). Teachers
wear a microphone that is attached to an FM transmitter. The transmitter
acts as a miniature radio station. It broadcasts the FM signal to an FM receiver
(just like an FM radio) that is worn by a student. The receiver converts the FM
signal back into an acoustic signal with the help of devices such as headsets
or personal hearing aids. Wherever the student is in the classroom, he or she
can listen to sounds that come directly from the microphone worn on the
teacher's chest, and the signal intensity and SNR are both increased.

Other ALDs (assistive listening devices) use different technology to deliver
the signal across distances. For example, the signal might be transmitted by
infrared signals or light frequencies that cannot be seen by the human eye.
The benefit of such systems is that the signal cannot travel beyond a room,

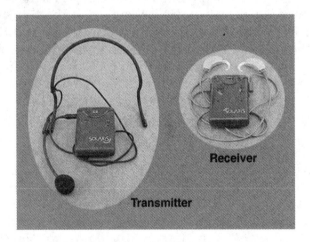

Figure 7–6. An example of an FM system. In
this situation, the transmitting unit is connected to
a head-worn boom microphone and the receiving
device is connected to BTE-microphones that direct sound to an earmold. (Photograph courtesy of
Phonic Ear)

CD-ROM

Personal FM System

A picture of a personal FM system is shown in CD-ROM segment Ch.07.12. The transmitter is connected to a head-worn boom microphone; the receiver is connected to BTE microphones that direct the sound into an earmold. The four video clips demonstrate the advantages of listening with a FM system. Segments Ch.07.13 and Ch.07.14 describe the listening environment. The audio was recorded from the back of the classroom using ear simulators. You will notice that the signal is more intense and clear with the FM system (segment Ch.07.13) than without the FM system (segment Ch.07.14). The second pair of movies, segments Ch.07.15 and Ch.07.16, demonstrate not only the decrease in intensity, but also when the students are making a variety of distracting noises. It is important to note that I was speaking at a normal conversational level. If I were to increase my voice for the size of the room, I could experience vocal fatigue and possibly vocal abuse. (Personal FM device courtesy of Phonak Hearing Systems)

thereby denying the signals to unintended listeners. As you know, FM broadcasts can travel through walls just like the FM radio signals. Therefore, if the message to be transmitted is confidential, the use of an infra-red signal would be a logical choice compared to an FM system.

Another way to transmit signals is by electromagnetic fields. Recall that electromagnetic fields can be generated by telephone handsets and that a hearing aid in the telecoil mode can pick up these signals. Electromagnetic fields can also be produced by running electricity through a special cable. The cable is placed around the section of room where the electromagnetic field is necessary. This is referred to as "looping" a room. The talker speaks into the microphone of the ALD, the signal is delivered through the "loop," and an electromagnetic field is generated. Hearing aid users can set their hearing aids to the telecoil position to pick up the speaker's voice.

These examples of ALDs require that the individual with a hearing loss have a receiving device or a hearing aid to pick up the signal. There are some systems that support multiple users. For example, various individuals using FM receivers can tune to the same transmission frequency, or they can all use hearing aids in the telecoil position. Some of these systems can be adapted to benefit every individual in a room. In group amplification systems, the speaker wears a microphone and the signal is transmitted, amplified, and delivered to loudspeakers placed around the room. You might be familiar with these as public address (PA) systems. These systems are beneficial in places like classrooms so that the teacher is heard above the noises of the room, the SNR is improved, and the teacher's voice is more intense and thus has increased audibility. Teachers like this experience because they have less vocal strain.

ALERTING DEVICES

Alerting devices help individuals hear important sounds such as fire alarms, a baby's cry, the telephone, or an alarm clock. Alerting devices have the ability to increase the intensity of the signal. Sometimes, they alter the frequency range of the signal so that it is in the audible range of the listener, for example, a low-frequency telephone ringer for an individual with a high-frequency hearing loss. Another way to alert someone who has difficulty hearing would be to use flashing lights or vibrotactile stimulation. In this case, an alarm clock might be hooked up to cause lights to flash or the bed to shake. In some instances, dogs are trained to inform the individual of a sound. These wonderful, dedicated animals are called "hearing dogs."

CD-ROM

Assistive Listening Device

The CD-ROM segment Ch.07.17 demonstrates a door knocker assistive listening device. The vibrations to the door due to knocking cause a light on the back of the door to flash. To enhance this experience, there is no sound on this video. (Assistive listening device courtesy of Global Assistive Devices)

Audiologic Habilitation

Audiologic habilitation services are provided to individuals who have not yet mastered oral communication. The first step in audiologic habilitation is the diagnosis of a hearing loss. Until recently, it was difficult to identify hearing loss in young children because testing results were based on limited behavioral reactions to sound. Many times the hearing loss was not documented until several years into the child's life. As explained in Chapter 2, normal language development begins at birth, and a number of major milestones are accomplished by the first year of life. Infants with hearing losses might not hear the speech of their caregivers and parents or even their own attempts at babbling. If this is the case, the development of speech and language skills will be delayed. Sometimes these delays are never overcome, and children do not reach their full spoken language potential. Fortunately, auditory brainstem response (ABR) and otoacoustic emission (OAE) testing, as discussed in Chapter 6, have decreased the delay in documenting the hearing sensitivity of infants. In previous decades, successful early identification of hearing loss was measured in years; today it can be measured in days. This allows infants to be fitted with hearing aids as early as 1 month of age.

Part of the success of early identification is due to infant hearing screening programs that are encouraged or mandated in many states. It is estimated that hundreds of thousands of dollars can be saved by early amplification. If a child can hear during the early years of speech and language development, that child might not need as many services to "catch up" later.

Hearing Aids for Children

There are many special considerations when amplifying the hearing of infants. The primary considerations are with the main two goals of amplification: gain and output. When fitting a hearing aid, it is helpful to know the threshold of hearing at each frequency. The hearing threshold for each frequency is then used in calculating the hearing aid gain. Auditory brainstem response (ABR) and otoacoustic emission (OAE) testing provide estimates of hearing thresholds, but these estimates are not always specific in the degree of hearing loss at particular frequencies. Therefore, the hearing aid gain used with an infant may not be adjusted to the ideal setting. The child will need multiple visits to the audiologist for more diagnostic testing to specifically define the hearing loss and to adjust the hearing aid appropriately.

The second goal of fitting hearing aids in children is appropriate output. Since an infant cannot directly convey when a hearing aid is too loud, it is difficult to ensure that the maximum output of the hearing aid will not cause discomfort. One way that the infant might express loudness discomfort with the hearing aid is by crying. However, infants use this expression for many reasons, and it is difficult to determine the meaning of the cry. Therefore, it is important that the caregiver reports the infant's reactions to the hearing aid to the audiologist. Another reason to check the maximum output levels of a hearing aid is to avoid causing additional hearing loss from exposure to intense sounds.

When fitting hearing aids on infants, there are special considerations in addition to gain and output. As infants grow, so do their ear canals, conchae, and pinnae. Thus, the hearing aid will need physical modifications to continue to fit the ear. If an in-the-ear (ITE), in-the-canal (ITC), or completely-in-the-canal (CIC) style hearing aid was used with an infant, the hearing aid would need to be sent back to the manufacturer to be recased for the growing ear. Thus, the infant would be without a hearing aid during those few weeks. With a behind-the-ear (BTE) style hearing aid, a new earmold can be ordered when necessary and replaced in the audiologist's office. Thus, the infant is not without a hearing aid. Further, a new earmold is a less expensive option than recasing a hearing aid. For the first few years of life, a child outgrows an earmold almost every 6 months.

The BTE (behind the ear) style hearing aid allows the most flexibility for necessary changes in gain and output as the hearing loss is documented more precisely. The BTE hearing aid is also the most flexible device to be used with ALDs. The BTE style hearing aid decreases expenses, duration without amplification, and allows the most flexibility in amplification procedures.

The caregivers of children with hearing losses are responsible for ensuring that the child's hearing aids are functioning and worn properly. As infants cannot voice their concerns about the functioning of their hearing aid, the caregiver must check the battery, listen for clarity of the output signal, and clean the hearing aid. It is often a major task just to keep the hearing aid on an infant. Caregivers have come up with many ways to accomplish this. Sometimes a soft rubber ring is attached to the BTE hearing aid and is wrapped around the pinna. Another option is to use toupee tape to adhere the hearing aid to the skin with minimal irritation upon removal. As children grow older, their responsibility for their hearing aid care should increase. During the school-age years, teachers, school nurses, principals, and speech-language pathologists might assist them during the daytime hours. These individuals require training in hearing aid care as well as ALD care and maintenance.

Communication Mode

The communication mode is another choice that must be made for the child with hearing loss. There are three communication modes: oral, manual, and total communication. The decision of communication mode can be difficult to make. Many parents want their children to communicate in a mode they feel proficient using. When hearing parents have children with severe or profound hearing losses, it is difficult for them to change from speaking to signing. It is important to decide on a communication mode early to initiate the learning process. If this mode does not prove successful, caregivers can reevaluate the decision.

An oral-communication mode uses only auditory signals for the transfer of messages. The underlying assumption of oral communication training is that children will communicate in an auditory world and with individuals with normal hearing. To be able to communicate with the most people, children need to be able to hear and speak messages. In oral-communication education settings, children with hearing impairments are taught to rely only on auditory signals. The facial cues and visual speech movements are eliminated from the message during therapy to force the child to listen more carefully. Although this therapy technique is not an accurate representation of communication, it forces children to maximize their residual hearing in order to understand auditory signals. Oral communication becomes more difficult with increased amounts of hearing loss.

A manual-communication mode uses hand shapes and movements to communicate a message. In this mode, no auditory message is communicated. American Sign Language (ASL) is the sign language system most often used in the Deaf culture of the United States. Like any language, ASL has conventions that are accepted and followed by the people who use the language. ASL uses hand shapes and movements as well as movements of the eyes and mouth to communicate the message. ASL is usually used by individuals with profound hearing losses who have joined the Deaf community. Since these individuals do not use hearing for communication, they do not receive audiologic habilitation. The subject of ASL and the Deaf culture is covered in greater detail in Chapter 8.

In a total-communication mode, speech and language are learned using both oral and manual methods. The sentence structure for ASL is not parallel to English and therefore the messages cannot be spoken and signed simultaneously using ASL. Other manual-communication systems have been developed for use with spoken English. For example, 26 hand shapes have been developed that correspond to the letters of the alphabet. This allows for words to be spelled with the hand and is known as finger spelling or the Rochester Method (see Figure 7–7). Other manual systems have hand shapes and movements that represent words and inflectional morphemes, including plural and verb tense inflections found in standard English. An example of this system is Signed Exact English. Cued Speech uses hand shapes that provide information about manner, place, or voice of a sound. Cued Speech has been beneficial in teaching children how to produce their own speech. It helps them to remember how and where the sound is produced. Advocates of total communication realize that the general public does not know the manual communication systems but feel that the supplement is beneficial for teaching and learning the rules of speech and language as well as other educational subjects such as reading, writing, and arithmetic.

Learning To Hear

For most individuals, learning to hear requires minimal effort. Hearing and the knowledge of sounds is something that individuals with normal hearing take for granted. Learning to hear with an impaired auditory system is a complicated process. Three levels of auditory processing must be obtained before auditory comprehension.

The first level is **detection.** This level is fairly simple to understand. If a sound is not heard, it cannot be processed by the auditory system. Thus, the first step in audiologic habilitation is to document the softest sound that is audible with and without amplification.

The second level of auditory processing is **discrimination,** which is the ability to determine if two or more sounds are the same or different. This level of auditory processing can often be learned. It is important to realize that the impaired auditory system might not be able to code some sounds. Two sounds

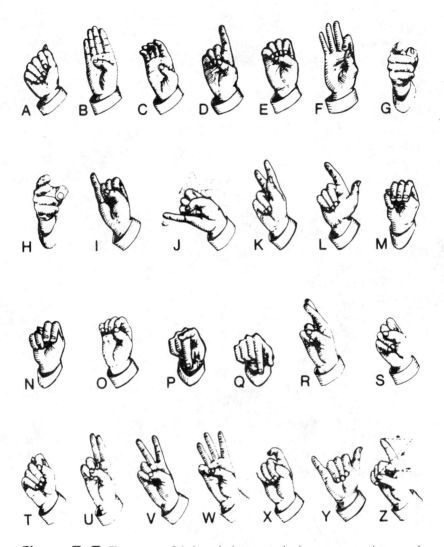

Figure 7–7. There are 26 hand shapes, which correspond to each letter in the English alphabet. (From *Audiologists' Desk Reference, Volume II: Audiologic Management, Rehabilitation, and Terminology,* by H. G. Mueller, III, and J. W. Hall, III, 1998, p. 557. San Diego: Singular Publishing Group.)

that are inadequately coded might sound the same. Children who cannot discriminate between two important sounds cannot advance to higher levels of auditory processing. When this is the case, the use of nonauditory cues, such as visual cues, becomes critical.

If children can detect a sound and discriminate it from other sounds, they can begin to identify the sound. **Identification,** the third level of auditory processing, occurs after the child has learned a symbolic representation for the sound. By representation, we mean categorization within the auditory system. If all four phonemes of the word "cats" have been coded and processed as a meaningful unit, the child can begin to comprehend "cats" as multiple, four-legged animals that purr. This subject is discussed in greater detail in Chapter 16.

It is critical to ensure each level of auditory processing is accomplished before expecting the child to reach higher processing levels successfully. Consider a child who cannot hear the sound /s/. Instead of hearing "cats," the child would hear "cat." This problem with detection would interfere with the child's ability to learn the plural morpheme in English (see Chapter 2 for an explanation of morphemes and inflections). Children might use nonauditory cues in this situation. For example, the placement of the lips might provide a visual cue of an /s/ at the end of a word. Contextual cues also become important for the child. If contextual cues were understood, the phrase "five cats" would allow the child to "fill-in" the undetectable /s/ sound at the cortical level.

Educational Environments

Audiologic habilitation services are provided in various settings. The diagnostic evaluation and hearing aid fitting are usually done in an audiologist's office. Some audiologists operate their own private practice in medical or professional buildings. Other audiologists see clients in hospitals or provide services as part of a team working out of a physician's office. Sometimes, the audiologist might provide these services in a quiet room in a school. In 1975, Public Law 94-142, the Individuals With Disabilities Education Act, was the first of many laws requiring that children be educated in the "least restrictive environment" following amplification. The concept of a least restrictive environment is discussed in more detail in Chapter 18. The educational environment that should be the most beneficial for the child is determined by the caregivers and the habilitation team.

Success of audiologic habilitation is achieved when children have integrated what they have learned into their daily lives. Therefore, although services are usually provided in a classroom setting, these skills must also be reinforced outside the school. Parents, grandparents, siblings, babysitters, and other caregivers need to be included in the process. They need to know how to reinforce effective communication as well as to understand realistic expectations.

AUDIOLOGIC REHABILITATION

Audiologic rehabilitation is provided to individuals who need to modify their communication style due to hearing loss. Hearing loss is often difficult for individuals to accept. To many people, a hearing loss represents getting older. It is often difficult to get adults to undergo a hearing test and to understand the results. Sometimes, a great deal of encouragement is required before an individual will try a hearing aid. Fortunately, many people realize the benefits of audiologic rehabilitation. It is rewarding to be told by a new hearing aid user "I can hear my grandchildren," "I enjoy the symphony again," or even "I had a great conversation with my spouse at dinner last night." These individuals are benefiting from amplification.

Communication Breakdown

The main speech communication loop consists of speakers who produce an acoustic signal and listeners who receive that signal. When an individual has a hearing loss, part or all of the acoustic signal may be inaudible and therefore unavailable for auditory perception. One way to compensate for hearing loss is to have people speak louder. In some situations, speakers might find themselves shouting to be heard. Although the message might be heard, shouting also carries a message, often felt as anger. The message "Good Morning" has a different tone when you are shouting it into someone's face. These communication situations can cause tremendous distress in a relationship.

Imagine a couple who has been married for many years. Over the years either one or both of the individuals have developed hearing losses as a result of the normal aging process. A simple whisper in one's ear of "I love you" might receive a response of "What?" After a few repetitions, with each getting louder, the communication might result in "Never mind" or "You don't have to yell at me!" These situations can cause emotional strain on a relationship. Further strain on the relationship might also occur due to one person not responding because he or she did not hear the other. This can be internalized by the speaker as being ignored or even being unimportant.

The hearing loss might also cause miscommunication. For example, if you did not hear the grocery list correctly, you would not get the items which were requested. These errors might result in feeling the loss of cognitive ability and memory. As this type of hearing loss usually progresses slowly, individuals might not realize that it is hearing loss and not memory loss. If you cannot hear the message, you certainly cannot remember it. Paranoia can also develop from these miscommunications.

When each of a couple's hearing is not similar, other problems can also occur. For example, the person with a greater hearing loss might want the television or radio set at a greater volume. One spouse might consider this volume setting comfortable while the other considers it too loud. Depending on the communication difficulties, adult rehabilitation should include more than fitting amplification. These topics are often addressed within an adult rehabilitation group.

Adult Rehabilitation Groups

Aural rehabilitation groups are designed to empower individuals who have hearing losses. The discussions are tailored for adults with hearing losses and their significant others to learn more about hearing loss. Group sessions usually focus on understanding the hearing mechanism, types of hearing aids, communication strategies, and assistive listening devices. Some of this information will have been presented during the audiological evaluation and the hearing aid fitting, but the group sessions allow for further clarification.

The Hearing Mechanism

Many individuals with hearing losses do not understand how sound travels from the mouth of the speaker to the brain of the listener. Thus, the first topic for an adult rehabilitation group is the nature of the communication channel. The discussion begins with how sound travels through the air and is directed into the hearing system by the outer ear. Then the basic mechanics of the middle and inner ear, including the neural auditory pathways, are presented. When the concept of how sound travels through a normal functioning auditory system is understood, the discussions turn to understanding the impaired auditory system. The different types of hearing losses are discussed and the audiogram is explained. Finally, group members learn to interpret their own audiograms. At this point, individuals should begin to understand why they are having difficulty communicating.

Hearing Aids

Another session of an adult rehabilitation group might focus on how hearing aids work. The components of the hearing aid are reviewed as well as how to care for them. Tips on how to fix a hearing aid problem are also provided. It is important to discuss during these sessions the realistic benefits to expect from amplification. Many individuals have difficulty accepting that hearing aids do not fix the hearing loss. Questions also arise about hearing aid advertisements and modern technology. Advertisements often stir hope of better hearing aids, and this might not always be feasible.

Communication

As amplification is only the first step in rehabilitation, effective communication using hearing aids must be discussed. Most individuals develop poor communication strategies during the years prior to amplification. Often, they do not try to seek clarification of a misunderstood message, as it might be too difficult or perceived as weakness. Assertiveness training is often beneficial.

Assertiveness interactions allow for each individual's needs to be met while respecting the feelings of others.

For example, an individual with a hearing aid might say, "I have difficulty understanding you when I cannot see your face. It would be helpful if you would get my attention before speaking." In this situation, the individual has stated the problem and requested, but not demanded, a solution. It is also important during communication to realize that it is not the sole responsibility of one person to set up ideal listening situations. Both participants need to actively use effective communication strategies. It is not effective when people communicate between different rooms. They need to decide together how they are going to get to the same room. These are a few of many possible improvements in communication styles.

Assistive Listening Devices

As discussed earlier, ALDs can be beneficial for the adult population. Group sessions are good opportunities to demonstrate and practice using such systems. As there are many of these systems available, the hearing aid user is unaware of different possibilities and might become overwhelmed when investigating them without assistance. Adults often find benefit from infrared systems that are used in connection with their televisions. These systems increase the intensity of the television to the listener without needing to turn up the television volume. Individuals also benefit from ALDs that are available at public theatres. The Americans With Disabilities Act (1990) requires public theaters to have ALDs available. The FM system is most commonly used in these settings. Group sessions increase the awareness of these systems and are used to teach participants how to use them.

Empowerment

The adult rehabilitation group is one way to empower individuals with hearing losses. These sessions might be held during one afternoon or occur one evening a week. The Self-Help for Hard-of-Hearing People (SHHH)[1] is a national organization with many local chapters. The organization has regularly scheduled meetings, national conventions, and publishes a magazine (*Hearing Loss: The Journal of Self Help for Hard of Hearing People*). The focus of the group is the empowerment of individuals with hearing losses through educational and support meetings.

Although adult rehabilitation groups are important in the rehabilitation process, the individual might need some extra assistance. For example, indi-

[1]Self-Help for Hard-of-Hearing People (SHHH) can be contacted at 7800 Wisconsin Avenue, Bethesda, MD 20814 or (310) 657-2248.

viduals with severe hearing impairment might require individual sessions to work on monitoring articulation, nasality, or vocal intensity. These individual sessions would also be helpful for adults who have recently obtained a cochlear implant.

SUMMARY

Audiologic habilitation and rehabilitation services are critical to effective communication for individuals with hearing impairments. These services can be divided into two areas: amplification devices and communication strategies. Amplification devices include hearing aids, tactile aids, cochlear implants, and assistive listening devices, which assist individuals to hear the acoustic signal. Communication strategies teach individuals how to decrease the obstacles due to a hearing loss. Although devices and counseling are quite different, both are necessary to empower individuals with hearing impairments. Most importantly, audiologists should make sure that individuals with the hearing impairment and the significant people in their lives play an active role in decision-making processes.

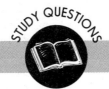

STUDY QUESTIONS

1 List the four major components of a hearing aid. Describe what each component does.

2 What are the major considerations in candidacy for a cochlear implant?

3 In a classroom situation, what degrades the signal and makes it difficult to hear the teacher? How might the listening environment be improved?

4 Discuss the four-stage hierarchy of auditory listening skills. Provide an example of each stage.

5 Discuss the effects of hearing loss on communication with adults. How might an audiologist or speech-language pathologist empower this individual in these situations?

REFERENCES

Americans With Disabilities Act. (1990). (Public Law 101-336) USC Sec. 12101.

Crandell, C. C., & Smaldino, J. J. (1995). Classroom acoustics. In R. J. Roeser & M. P. Downs (Eds.). *Auditory disorders in school children* (3rd ed., pp. 217–234). New York: Thieme.

Education for all Handicapped Children Act of 1975, Public Law 94-142. (1975 November 29). United States Statutes at Large, 89, 773–796.

SUGGESTED READINGS

Ross, M. (Ed.). (1990). *Hearing-impaired children in the mainstream.* Timonium, MD: York Press.

Roeser, R. J., & Downs, M. P. (1995). *Auditory disorders in school children* (3rd ed.). New York: Thieme.

Ross, M. (Ed.). (1992). *FM auditory training systems: Characteristics, selection, & use.* Timonium, MD: York Press.

Sanders, D. A. (1993). *Management of hearing handicap: Infants to elderly* (3rd ed.). Englewood Cliffs, NJ: Prentice-Hall.

Schow, R. L., & Nerbonne, M. A. (1996). *Introduction to audiologic rehabilitation* (3rd ed.). Boston, MA: Allyn & Bacon.

Tye-Murry, N. (1998). *Foundations of aural rehabilitation: Children, adults, and their family members.* San Diego: Singular Publishing Group.

Tyler, R. S. (Ed.) (1993). *Cochlear implants: Audiological foundations.* San Diego: Singular Publishing Group.

Wayner, D. S., & Abrahamson, J. E. (1996). *Learning to hear again: An audiologic rehabilitation curriculum guide.* Austin, TX: Hear Again.

GLOSSARY

Alerting devices: Devices that change auditory alerting signals that are inaudible for individuals with hearing losses into audible acoustic, visual, or vibrotactile stimuli

Assistive listening device (ALD): Devices that transfer an acoustic message over distance so the listener can hear the signal with greater intensity and signal-to-noise ratio.

Audiologic habilitation: Amplification, auditory training, and speech-language services provided to children with a hearing loss.

Audiologic rehabilitation: Amplification and coping strategies.

Cerumen: Earwax.

Cochlear implant: A device that is surgically placed in the cochlea and provides auditory stimulation for individuals with severe-to-profound hearing loss.

Detection: The ability to hear if a sound exists, the first level in auditory processing.

Discrimination: The ability to hear two sounds as different, the second level in auditory processing.

Earmold: Vinyl or acrylic material that is custom-fit to fill part of the outer ear. A hole in the earmold directs sound from the receiver to the ear canal. When fitted properly, the earmold prevents feedback.

Functional gain: The increase in sound intensity provided by a hearing aid (in decibels) calculated by subtracting behavioral thresholds without a hearing aid from behavioral thresholds with a hearing aid.

Gain: The increase in sound intensity provided by an amplification system and measured in decibels.

Identification: The ability to associate a sound with a symbolic representation, the third level in auditory processing.

Output: The intensity of the acoustic signal produced by an amplification system.

Real-ear gain: The increase in sound intensity provided by a hearing aid (in decibels) calculated by subtracting the intensity at the tympanic membrane without the hearing aid from the intensity at the tympanic membrane with the hearing aid, by using a probe microphone.

Reverberation time: The amount of time (in seconds) it takes a signal that was abruptly turned off to decrease in intensity by 60 dB.

Signal-to-noise ratio (SNR): A representation of the signal intensity compared to the background noise intensity calculated by subtracting the intensity of the noise from the intensity of the signal (in decibels).

Telecoil switch (t-switch): An option on a hearing aid to use electromagnetic energy as the input instead of the microphone

8

The Habilitation of Children With Severe-to-Profound Hearing Loss

Mark E. Bernstein

LEARNING OBJECTIVES

1 To understand and describe the possible developmental consequences of prelinguistic severe-to-profound deafness.

2 To differentiate communication development in deaf children who have parents who are deaf from those with parents who have normal hearing.

3 To learn about speech and language development in children with hearing impairments.

4 To learn about the communication options available for children with hearing impairments, including the use of speech, listening, writing, and sign communication.

5 To understand and describe the concept of "bilingual-bicultural" education for children who are deaf.

6 To learn about approaches to assessment and intervention in speech and language for children with hearing impairments.

Sally always sits in the front of her second-grade classroom and watches the teacher intently. Her hearing aids are barely visible beneath her hair, and almost no one in the class pays attention to them. Sally is just one of the kids. When the boy next to her starts a conversation with their neighbor, she turns to him and says, "Shush, it's hard for me to listen!"

David watches his algebra teacher demonstrate how to work an equation on the board. The teacher never utters a word; his hands do the communicating, showing how to move elements of the fractions and group them. David isn't sure about something, so he raises his hand, and in the spatial eloquence of the sign language he learned growing up, asks his question.

Wendy also sits near the front of Ms. Smith's classroom, her gaze following Julie, the Signed English interpreter. Julie converts Ms. Smith's spoken words into manual gestures, so Wendy can listen to Ms. Smith and also "see" her words. Wendy and Julie have become close, because Julie accompanies Wendy throughout the school day.

Ricky stands up in front of the class and takes the microphone proffered by his teacher. He reads his poem to his classmates, and they watch closely and listen carefully through the miniature radio receivers that pick up Ricky's speech. Ricky's speech is somewhat strange sounding, but intelligible. His deaf classmates watch his face, "read" his lips, listen to his voice, and enjoy the poem.

Katie's teacher accompanies her speech with manual signs as she discusses the types of birds found in the nearby park. Katie has a question about blue-jays, so she, too, uses her speech and signs. Her five other classmates are also deaf and use sign and speech simultaneously in the classroom. At play in her neighborhood, Katie mostly talks with her friends; in the school cafeteria she will sign with her classmates. If her friend Jan, who hears normally, comes over, she'll start to talk, too.

INTRODUCTION

The previous examples depict a few children with hearing impairment in our schools. The life experiences of such children vary tremendously, as do their educational experiences. This chapter explores the relationship between serious hearing impairment and a child's development and education and introduces the range of possibilities for educational intervention. As we shall see, despite a long history of striving, educators are still challenged to provide a completely effective education for all children with hearing impairment.

As noted in Chapter 4, there is tremendous variation in type and degree of hearing impairment. Many children with mild to severe hearing impairment benefit greatly from personal amplification systems such as conventional hearing aids. With a modicum of special attention, these children can function socially and educationally, essentially as if they have normal hearing. This is true primarily for children whose hearing impairment was detected early (within the first 2 years or so) or whose hearing loss occurred after the development of speech and language. Such a child might be like Sally, who must sit near the teacher, and must listen very carefully, but who otherwise differs little from her peers with normal hearing.

This chapter focuses on children like David, Wendy, Ricky, and Katie, whose hearing impairment has a much greater impact on their lives and who present the biggest challenge to educators, audiologists, and speech-language pathologists (SLPs). These children have severe-to-profound hearing losses, typically of a sensory or sensorineural nature. This is not to suggest that children with less severe hearing losses require little or no intervention. On the contrary, such children (and their families) may require a fair amount of attention, especially with regard to management of hearing aids, speech training, and the like, in order to ensure optimum growth and development. Most of these children's needs will be met by the procedures discussed in Chapter 7. But severe-to-profound hearing loss typically represents a quantum leap in developmental consequences and professional intervention, and children with such losses are those most typically served in special education programs for the "deaf" or "auditorily impaired." I will refer to such children as "deaf," always bearing in mind, however, that these children represent a variety of hearing levels and communication abilities.

We will take up, in turn, the impact of deafness on a child's development and family; communication choices; and assessment and intervention, including speech, language, and literacy development. The habilitation of most deaf children is by no means a simple matter.

HEARING IMPAIRMENT AND DEVELOPMENT

Communication Development

One can ask people whether they would choose to have been born deaf or blind (not that we have this choice!). Most people would respond that they would rather be born deaf; we find it difficult to imagine life without sight, unable to read, to drive, and so on.

But those familiar with deaf children might disagree sharply, for the primary consequence of **prelinguistic** deafness is that it prevents the normal, spontaneous acquisition of speech and language skills in the early childhood years, the so-called **critical period** for language acquisition. It is not hard to imagine how this might affect a child's growth, development, and socialization.

It is generally accepted that more than 90% of deaf children are born to parents who have normal hearing (the remaining children are born into families in which at least one parent is deaf; these children will be discussed later in this chapter). Prelinguistic deafness is a relatively low incidence condition (various estimates put it at no more than 2 to 3 per thousand children), and newborn hearing screening is far from universal as of this writing. As a result, the assumption is usually made that an infant has normal hearing, and parents do not worry about it until given some reason to do so. This is made easier, of course, by the fact that in most ways, infants who are deaf act no differently from those who have normal hearing. While it is true that there may not be appropriate responses to environmental sounds (or voices), this may not be readily apparent to hearing parents who have no reason to suspect a problem with their child's hearing.

It might not be until the child is 12 to 18 months old that many hearing parents would even suspect a problem, usually because most children with normal hearing begin to use recognizable words at this time, but the child with a significant hearing loss will not. There may in fact be a protracted period of parental suspicion, then perhaps some denial ("He's just a late talker"), then only belatedly a hearing assessment and diagnosis. It is not unusual for a deaf child to be as much as 2 to 3 years of age upon diagnosis.

This, of course, is highly significant, because until that time the deaf child of hearing parents typically has had only minimal (if any) stimulation of the speech and language components of their cognitive system (see Chapter 2). Parents and others in the child's environment may interact with her; they may talk with her. But little or no language-related input actually "gets into" the child's system because the child cannot hear it; in effect, throughout much of the critical period for language and speech acquisition, the system lies essentially dormant. It simply does not receive the "linguistic data" that is required for it to undergo normal development. A child in this situation, if left untreated, may end up with profound delay and deviance in language and speech acquisition to the extent that there is effectively no functional communication method other than idiosyncratic gesture for basic needs, if that.

Socialization

The absence of a common communication medium between child and caregiver potentially has grave consequences in the domain of socialization. Numerous researchers have studied interactions between deaf children and their hearing mothers and have often reported a lack of reciprocity, of joint engagement (McCarthy, 1996). It is obviously difficult to instruct a child in even the simplest things if there is no shared medium of communication. Social and cognitive structuring can suffer, and the imaginary domain can become severely constricted. To complicate matters, parents often carry intense feelings of guilt associated with their deaf child, and have been observed to go through what may be a long emotional roller-coaster ride. It can be said that the child's deafness is in some sense "owned" by the whole family, which can feel quite powerless in connection with this, which in turn creates additional dysfunction of communication and socialization (Schlesinger, 1985). Obviously families differ greatly in their response to their child's deafness, but the "worst-case" scenario is unfortunately not at all rare.

Academic Development

It is obvious that a child with no functioning language system will find it next to impossible to derive any benefit from the school setting. As we will see, in the United States at least, virtually all deaf children receive special services once they are diagnosed, so almost no children arrive at school *totally* unprepared to engage in their education. However, the academic effects of communication deprivation in the early childhood years may be more subtle. Much of what a child brings to the educational process, in terms of his or her general knowledge of the world, is established during the early years, and for most deaf children there will be considerable catching up to do.

INTERVENTION

Establishment of Communication Systems

It should come as no surprise to the reader that the key to intervention with deaf children is to establish, as early as possible, a functional communication system for the child and the parents. We need to find a way to establish *access* for the child's language learning and cognitive systems, a way for the systems to obtain the information they require to function. Ideally, we would like to do this right from the start, but most often this effort can only begin upon diagnosis and a certain level of comfort and adaptation on the part of the parents (see Luterman, 1987). Typically, efforts to intervene communicatively will start considerably later than desirable, thus forcing a "catch-up" environment. We sometimes find it useful to distinguish children's **language-speech age** from their *chronological* ages. The language-speech age can often lag behind the chronological by several years, which underscores the urgency of communication intervention, as the critical period window of opportunity does not extend much beyond middle childhood.

How we help families establish communication, though, is fraught with controversy and has been for as long as there have been efforts to educate deaf children (Moores, 1987). There does not appear to be a single approach that is suitable for all children, and, as we shall see in the next section, the selection of a particular communication method is perhaps the most critical of the decisions facing parents, yet it is also the most difficult.

Components of Communication Systems Used With Deaf Children

Approaches to communication with deaf children can be distinguished by the extent to which the emphasis is placed on **audition** and speech or on the use of **manual systems** for communication. In most cases, there is general agreement that it is highly desirable to attempt to optimize the child's use of **residual hearing.**

Use of Hearing

The primary goal of any communication intervention is to help the child gain access to linguistic (and other) "data," so that the child's own cognitive system can go to work. For a child with a severe-to-profound hearing impairment, the primary obstacle is, of course, the lack of hearing, so at first glance it would seem reasonable to attempt to solve the problem by taking steps to remediate the hearing loss itself.

This is exactly what is done with most children, and it involves the use of modern technologies such as digital and analog hearing aids, wireless FM assistive listening systems, and cochlear implants. These are more fully described in Chapter 7. The idea is simply to make the best use of the child's residual hearing, thus overcoming the access problem. Tremendous strides have been made in the technology of assistive listening devices in recent years, enabling many children (particularly those with considerable residual hearing of high quality) to function quite well relying on their hearing alone.

Oral-Auditory Methods

The use of residual hearing is the cornerstone of the group of communication approaches known collectively as the **oral method.** Within this general group, some advocates emphasize the use of listening skills almost exclusively (hence the term oral-auditory), while others encourage children to follow the speaker's facial and mouth movements as well (now termed **speech-reading,** an update of the older term lipreading). Regardless of their relative emphasis on audition, all oral approaches incorporate intensive speech training and rely exclusively on oral speech for all communication with deaf children.

Oralism, as it is sometimes called, has been deemed a philosophy rather than merely a method of communicating with deaf children (see Mulholland, 1981). The idea is that because this is a world of hearing people, it is critical for deaf children to learn to communicate using the methods used by virtually all others, namely, the spoken language of the culture. Oral advocates do not accept the use of sign language, believing that its use perpetuates a separate subculture of deaf people and inhibits the deaf person's success in the "hearing world." Further, oral proponents believe that the use of sign language in any form will interfere with the child's development of speech and listening skills; because signing is seen as "easier" for the child, the fear is that the child will take the easy road when communicating and not work hard enough at the mastery of speech. The oral approach maintains that although it is quite difficult, most deaf children can develop functional speech and listening skills, if given appropriate support and consistency of teaching. If provided appropriate intervention, it is said, deaf children can "catch up" linguistically, socially, and academically. In this view, there is no *need* for sign language for most deaf children, and the overall goal would be integration into the mainstream "hearing" society, having overcome the barrier posed by the hearing impairment.

This approach to communication with deaf children, understandably quite attractive to many hearing parents, has been in existence for many hundreds of years and has indeed been successful for a number of children (e.g., our young friend Ricky from earlier in the chapter). Clearly, the success of oral methods is directly correlated with, among other things, the amount and quality of residual hearing.

One enhancement to oral methods is the use of Cued Speech (Cornett, 1967). **Cued Speech** uses a system of hand gestures (see CD-ROM segment 8.01) that are displayed near the face. These gestures serve to distinguish (cue) phonemic distinctions that would otherwise be difficult or impossible to perceive by reading a speaker's lip movements (*man* vs. *pan*). Cueing is always used in conjunction with oral speech, and is primarily intended as an adjunct to speechreading, to help children develop a sense for how the speech patterns of the language work. It is not an independent "sign" or "gesture" system that can be used to communicate on its own.

As of this writing, oral methods are in use in numerous day classes in public schools around the United States and in several well-known private schools such as the Central Institute for the Deaf in St. Louis, Missouri, and The Clarke School for the Deaf in Northampton, Massachusetts, among others.

CD-ROM

Cued Speech and Oral Communication Techniques

CD-ROM segment Ch.08.01 is a demonstration of Cued Speech and Oral Communication techniques. Note how the cueing is coordinated with the speech; the user of Cued Speech must be highly aware of the phonemic structure of the words being uttered. Cueing must be performed in accompaniment to speech; it cannot be done in isolation. Cues themselves carry no meaning; what they do is signal (cue) which phoneme is being produced as it is said. A single gesture, however, is used to cue the presence of more than one phoneme. Which one is designated depends on which particular lip configuration the cue is paired with. Would it be possible to use Cued Speech and sign language simultaneously?

Sign Language and Sign Systems

For as long as there have been partisans of oral approaches, there have also been those who have challenged the oral philosophy by advocating the use of manual communication with deaf children (see Moores [1987] for a historical review). These approaches generally fall into two major categories: those that use one or another form of **manual codes** for English, usually performed simultaneously with spoken English, and those advocating the use of **American Sign Language (ASL)** (usually as part of an overall **bilingual-bicultural** philosophy, to be examined shortly).

The basic premise of any of the manually oriented approaches is that the oralists' insistence on the exclusive use of speech is not effective for most deaf children with severe-to-profound hearing losses and is simply inappropriate for most such children. Rather than attempt to communicate with (and educate) deaf children using their "weakest" channels (hearing and speech), the idea would be to use the modes that are (for most deaf children) readily accessible and quite effective, that is, vision and manual gestures.

Total Communication

The first of the two types of approaches using manual gestures is often referred to as **Total Communication** (see Schlesinger 1986), which became fairly widespread in the early 1970s. Proponents of this approach note the relatively poor results of oral methods for most children with severe-to-profound hearing loss (see Moores [1987] for a review); for every success story there are scores of children who do not achieve even basic-level communication skills and end up poorly educated. In this view, oral methods simply do not provide sufficient information, in usable form, for the child's system to flourish.

The basic idea of the most common form of Total Communication is to encourage parents, teachers, and children to use whatever communication method works best. This would include the use of oral modes, American Sign Language (ASL) if appropriate, and most important, the use of manual forms of English. The core idea behind manually coded English is to simultaneously *supplement* the information provided in the auditory-speech channel with a redundantly coded version of the same information in the manual-visual channel. This is accomplished by the use of one or another system of "signed" English (or whatever the language of the culture), in which manual signs are produced for each morpheme of the spoken utterances. The specific signs used in most systems are based to some extent on the sign vocabulary of ASL, although the signs are placed in English word order, as they accompany English. There is some controversy over the "best" method for coding English, and several competing systems have been developed. Some have even argued that a high level of morphological accuracy is not even necessary for the success of these approaches (Maxwell, 1990).

 CD-ROM

Signing Exact English

Signing Exact English (SEE II) is perhaps the most widely-used of the "exact" systems for representing English manually. In SEE II, as in all such techniques, the communicator is required to produce a manual sign for each English morpheme that is spoken, while maintaining normal speech speed and rhythm. Segment Ch.08.02 presents an experienced user of SEE II communicating material that might be found in a high school class of students who are deaf. Notice how there may be numerous gestures accompanying a relatively short English word. Why does this happen? What might be some of the difficulties encountered in trying to use SEE II in some communication situations?

Proponents of Total Communication suggest that parents can fairly quickly learn to pair sign gestures with their speech and can use this as a means for multisensory production-reception of English. The deaf child would be provided with a more adequate input and output because of the multichannel redundancy and thus would have several avenues for stimulation of his or her language and speech learning centers. As in oralism, English would be the language the child is exposed to and developing, which has obvious facilitative value for literacy development. Note that in Total Communication, audition and speech are very much part of the communication mix; the use of sign does not replace oral modes as much as it supplements them in a kind of partnership. It has been estimated that as much as 90% of the severe-to-profoundly deaf children in the United States are educated in Total Communication programs (*American Annals of the Deaf,* 1998). The success of such programs is, as might be expected, difficult to gauge, because there are numerous variables affecting the outcomes of any intervention with deaf children. There seems to be general agreement, however, that for most deaf children the use of sign in some form is more beneficial than the use of oral-only methods.

American Sign Language (ASL) and Bilingual-Bicultural Programs

Since the early 1990s, there has been a growing interest, particularly in residential schools for the deaf, in what is generically known as **bilingual-bicultural** approaches to communication and education of deaf children. These philosophies typically involve either an American Sign Language first, English as a second language (ESL) approach, or a more concurrent bilingualism approach utilizing both ASL and English.

American Sign Language (ASL) is a manual-visual language utilizing gestures created by the hands, face, head, and body to communicate. ASL is a natural language that, in its general form, appears to have evolved from a combination of French Sign Language and an indigenous sign language used by deaf people in the United States at the beginning of the 19th century. One of the first teachers of the deaf in the United States was a deaf man named Laurent Clerc, a French national, who had been brought to Connecticut in 1816 to teach at the newly established school for the deaf in Hartford. Clerc brought with him teaching methods that had been developed at the school for the deaf in Paris, including the French method for using sign language in education of deaf children. American Sign Language seems to have evolved rather quickly through the 19th and 20th centuries and, at this time, bears only a familial resemblance to French Sign Language, including some cognate signs and other features.

The grammar of ASL is quite unlike that of English, making effective use of the three dimensional space in which it is created, particularly in case assignment and complex verb inflection processes (see CD-ROM video sample segment Ch.08.03). It is not possible to sign ASL simultaneously with English speech, because of the vast differences between the grammars (to sign along with your speech you may use ASL *signs* for English lexical items, but not the grammar). ASL has been extensively studied since the early 1960s and has been recognized as a critical component of the culture and community of most deaf people (at least, that vast majority of deaf people who are not primarily oral in communication).

CD-ROM

American Sign Language

CD-ROM segment Ch.08.03 demonstrates the way American Sign Language (ASL) grammar utilizes the three-dimensional space in which the articulators (hands, arms, body, face, head) operate to produce grammatical utterances. The signer locates points in space (called "index points" by sign language linguists) which serve as pronouns. Verbs can be inflected for direction, number, and other features through changes of direction or modification of the hand shapes used to form the sign utterances. In the early stages of sign language linguistics, researchers had a difficult time figuring out what to even look for, because the grammar of ASL is so different from that of English or other languages that have been studied extensively.

Critical to the bilingual-bicultural philosophy is the firm belief that it is important for most deaf children to develop a first language that is best suited to their sensory capabilities (i.e., one that uses the visual-manual modality), coupled with the belief that it is crucial that this signed language be a "natural" sign language (such as ASL) rather than one of the artificial manual coding systems for English used in Total Communication. In addition, proponents of the bilingual-bicultural philosophy explicitly acknowledge the likelihood that the child will eventually become a fully actuated "Deaf" adult, that is, one who is a member of the Deaf community and shares in its language, culture, and mores.[1]

This *cultural* aspect of the bilingual-bicultural educational philosophy revolves around the recognition that there is a distinct community and culture of Deaf people within a larger society in which the vast majority of people have normal speech and hearing skills. Descriptions of this community and its culture have emerged in recent years (see, for example, Lane, Hoffmeister, & Bahan, 1996). Central to Deaf culture and community is the idea that deafness should not be viewed as a "defect" or pathology, but rather, as a *difference* (some have deemed it akin to ethnicity). In this view, to be Deaf is to have a personal identity *as a Deaf person,* not as a person with impaired hearing. It is less a matter of one's actual level of hearing (in audiological terms), than it is the belief system and behaviors one demonstrates. "Being" Deaf includes the use of ASL for most daily communication; extensive social networking with other Deaf individuals; and shared patterns of beliefs,

---

[1] The capitalization of the first letter in "Deaf" is a convention signifying a reference to the cultural identity, in contrast to the more common use of the term "deaf" in reference to serious hearing loss in the audiological sense only.

values, and rules for social interaction. It has been suggested that there is a characteristic "Deaf" world view, which is different from that shared by most people with normal hearing (although it would be prudent to be cautious about the stark "either-or" character of some of the descriptions). Obviously, members of the Deaf community share much in common with those with normal hearing, as well; Deaf people shop in the same stores, work in the same offices and factories, participate in the same recreational activities and sporting events, and so forth. But, in the same sense as do members of other minority groups in our society, many Deaf individuals feel a distinct difference of identity and culture as well, a special kinship that cannot be shared fully by those with normal hearing. One major aim of bilingual-bicultural programming in education of deaf children, then, is to help them to learn about and participate in this special community and culture.

The keystone of any bilingual-bicultural program is the early and consistent use of ASL as a medium of communication with the child (and for all academic instruction, once the child gets to school), keeping it separate from the use of English. Some bilingual-bicultural advocates reject outright the notion that a deaf child should develop oral speech skills, while others build such skill development into the English component of the program. In one influential version of the ESL approach (Johnson, Liddell, & Erting, 1989), there is no attempt to use English "through the air" at all; face-to-face communication takes place only in ASL, and English instruction is provided solely in the form of reading and writing, and only once the child has mastered the "first" language (ASL), say, around the age of 6 or 7 years. Other, more "concurrent" approaches allow for natural code switching, using both ASL and English (in simultaneous manually coded form as well as print). There may be some individuals (teachers, aides, parents) who use ASL with the child, others who use English, or some of the day may be devoted to ASL, while English is used at other times.

Bilingual-bicultural methodology is still so new that there is little evidence bearing on its effectiveness. Unfortunately, many programs have been started but without much attention to efficacy research, so it is difficult to tell what, if any, long-term educational impact this approach may have.

The Future of Communication With Deaf Children

The "methods" issue is vexing; it will not go away. Few would deny that a most appropriate goal for the communication education of deaf children would be the development of what might be termed **multimodalism.** In this view, the objective of intervention efforts would be to help each child to develop, to the extent possible, skills in both oral and sign communication, and full English literacy.

The dilemma is that we have no reliable way to tell which approach is "best" for any particular child. This is further complicated by a kind of path-dependence in the choices. If one chooses a particular mode, one is buying into a package that requires some period of time to develop. This creates some potentially sticky problems. For example, some educators advocate starting all children off using oral methods only, in the hopes that they will respond well and not require the use of manual communication. Recall that strict adherence to the oral philosophy precludes any use of manual modes; this may lead to greater success in educating some deaf children, but what of those for whom it doesn't work well? These children will have lost valuable time during the critical period, and it may not be possible to make up that deficit. On the other hand, the more radical proponents of bilingual-bicultural approaches tend to alienate those—including the vast majority of parents—who do see much value in helping deaf children to integrate into the mainstream of society. The middle ground, that is, the use of Total Communication methods including various forms of signed English, tends not to satisfy partisans of both extremes and may represent some compromises that undercut their effectiveness.

Parents and professionals alike must work their way through these issues individually, often under circumstances that are trying, at best. It is simply not possible to arrive at a conclusion that fits all children, all families, and all circumstances, despite the confident pronouncements of advocates of all stripes. Ultimately, the decision must be made in a collaborative approach involving the parents and professionals who know the child best.

Speech and Language Teaching

Regardless of the particular approach taken to communication with the child, in most cases the mere establishment of a viable communication system upon diagnosis will not be sufficient to allow the child to catch up to his or her hearing peers in the domains of speech and language. Centuries of work with deaf children have yielded a variety of methods for dealing with instruction in these areas.

For both speech and language, intervention approaches may be characterized as primarily "bottom-up" or "top-down." Bottom-up methods are characterized by highly structured developmental[2] sequences of instruction, attempting to break down goals for learning into smaller parts in specific sequences, building toward the eventual mastery of the system. Top-down methods tend to be more holistic in nature, relying on a more "natural" approach, stimulating the child's own developmental system through rich interactive input and exchange, but without the relatively rigid stepwise structure of bottom-up methods.

[2] The term "developmental" is used with caution. It is not always the case that a bottom-up developmental approach follows observable natural developmental patterns.

Speech Development

In the area of speech development, the most widely used approach is the method developed by Ling (1976, 1989), which is essentially bottom-up in nature. Ling outlines a sequence of developmental steps in the acquisition of specific speech skills, working from the bases of vocalization through the production of consonant clusters, in a highly specific developmental hierarchy that uses primarily drill and practice skill development through the use of isolated nonmeaningful syllables (combinations of target sounds with those already acquired). Ling's approach is relatively easy to use and is spelled out clearly in his books. It is not clear, however, that it is any more effective than other methods; research in the area of speech development of deaf children is notoriously difficult to do well, and despite over 25 years of practice, it is unclear whether this approach is significantly more effective than any other.

 CD–ROM

The Ling Method

The most widespread approach to speech development is that developed by Ling (1976, 1989). As CD-ROM segment Ch.08.04 demonstrates, the Ling method focuses on the child's development of individual phonemes in isolated syllables, working toward fluency by extensive practice producing the target in single syllables, repeated syllables, and in syllables alternated with another target. Ling claims that mastery at this, the "phonetic" level, will lead, with relatively little direct instruction, to the use of the speech skill in communicative speech (the "phonological" level).

Alternative approaches to speech development are more top-down in nature, with the goal being to stimulate the child's own speech development system (the lack of hearing does not automatically mean that the child has no intrinsic cognitive system devoted to speech development). It is felt by some that the relative rigidity of bottom-up developmental sequences may work at cross-purposes to the child's own internal system, to the detriment of the child's acquisition of the speech system. One influential example of a top-down approach would be that of Calvert and Silverman (1983), in which the primary method for early speech development work is the provision of a rich interactive communication environment to stimulate the child's own system. Calvert and Silverman also offer a somewhat more bottom-up component in their approach, to be used with children for whom the general stimulation approach does not seem to be as effective as it should be. This "multisensory syllable unit" approach, though, is still grounded in communicative interaction, in that the syllables used for specific intervention and practice are derived directly from words the child is using (or attempting to use).

 CD-ROM

Conversational Interaction

Quite different from the Ling (1976, 1989) approach to speech development is the method proposed by Calvert and Silverman (1983), which suggests that speech development is best achieved through extensive meaningful conversational interaction based on the child's interests, rather than in exercises involving isolated syllables. Note in segment Ch.08.05 how the clinician focuses the communication interaction in such a way as to engage the child's interest and how she makes sure the child is able to receive the input both auditorily and visually. Approaches such as this use a multisensory approach and attempt to ensure that speech development work takes place only in meaningful contexts.

English Language Development

The relatively few deaf children who grow up with deaf parents who use ASL acquire that language naturally and spontaneously, much as any child with normal hearing acquires his or her first language. Most deaf children, however, will need intervention in order to acquire their first language. The history of educating deaf children is replete with a variety of methods for language instruction, also characterized as primarily top-down or bottom-up. There is a cyclical aspect to this, as the history over the past several hundred years reveals a pattern of pendulum swings, from structured, bottom-up methods to more naturalistic, top-down philosophies.

Through much of the 20th century, the predominant orientation for language instruction was highly analytic and bottom-up, as exemplified by the *Fitzgerald Key* (Fitzgerald, 1929), which employs a template, slot-filling approach to the construction of "straight," grammatically correct English sentences in which children select words from different grammatical classes to fill slots in left-right order. To this day, many classrooms in the United States have a "key" (template) prominently displayed, perhaps above the chalkboard. In the 1970s, such analytic approaches were updated by the incorporation of linguistic concepts such as transformational grammar (e.g., Blackwell, Engen, Fischgrund, & Zarcadoolas, 1978).

Such analytic, bottom-up approaches have their limitations, however, in ways similar to those of the overly structured approaches to speech development and have not yielded the successes hoped for. In structured-analytic language methods, much of what might be expected developmentally is inextricably tied to the adequacy of the linguistic models employed and the extent to which their developmental progression matches that of the child's own developing system. Accordingly, top-down models have been developed, in many ways similar to, and linked with, such models in the speech domain. These are devoted to providing a rich interactive communication environment for the child in which his or her natural language development system may be activated and do much of the work on its own. Obviously, for any such effort to succeed, there must be in use a fully effective communication system, whether oral, signed, or in some combination.

Overall, many educators have found it most effective to employ top-down, naturalistic approaches to language development in the early years, especially while the child is in the critical period for language acquisition. The more analytic, bottom-up methods are then employed as a supplement to the naturalistic method (which is continued throughout the child's education) to work on details and to teach aspects of the language that were not spontaneously acquired by the child.

Assessment and Team Approaches to Intervention

This chapter would not be complete without a consideration of assessment of communicative functioning, which is best carried out in a collaborative team approach. As we have seen, the habilitation of a deaf child is a multidimensional problem, and effective assessment and intervention will require the involvement of a number of professionals. It is imperative that there be close cooperation between the audiologist, speech-language pathologist (SLP), teacher, and parents, in addition to such professionals as counselors, occupational and physical therapists, and others as required.

The audiologist will be the individual most responsible for management of the child's use of his or her hearing, from assessment of residual hearing and fitting of hearing aids, to consultation with regular school personnel on optimizing the acoustic environment. The SLP may take primary responsibility for assessment of the child's speech and language development. Depending on the academic setting, the SLP may take the lead role in development activities (often, if the child is in a mainstream setting) or will work closely with the classroom teacher of the deaf in jointly implementing an approach to speech and language development.

It is critical that all involved in assessment and program development for deaf children be familiar with the concepts and issues associated with the development of deaf children (which we have only touched on in this chapter). The use of standard speech and language assessment instruments, for example, must be considered quite carefully, as deaf children's *language* (or *speech) ages* often lag considerably behind their chronological ages, as discussed earlier in this chapter. Some speech assessment instruments are simply unsuitable for children with limited vocabularies and/or relatively unintelligible speech, often found among deaf students. Some of the approaches used in assessment of individuals with different cultural backgrounds have been found useful.

Luetke-Stahlman and Luckner (1991) provide a useful guide to English language assessment of deaf children, focusing on separate analyses for language use (pragmatics), content (semantics), and form (morphology and syntax). Emphasis is placed on the use of language samples, analyzed with reference to developmental taxonomies (as revealed in the research literature) of both hearing and deaf children's language acquisition. Among the standard tests, many have found the various levels of the Grammatical Analysis of Elicited Language (GAEL) (Moog & Geers, 1985) to be valuable. Other approaches to language assessment are presented in Kretschmer and Kretschmer (1988). In the speech domain, we have found it useful to go beyond such commonly used instruments as Ling's (1976) phonetic and phonological analyses of deaf children's speech. We combine standard articulation testing (e.g., Goldman & Fristoe, 1986), phonological process analysis (e.g., Hodson, 1986), and intelligibility (Monsen, 1981) and suprasegmental measures (Subtelny, Orlando, & Whitehead, 1981) with the information provided by Ling's instruments to provide a full picture of the child's emerging speech capabilities.

SUMMARY

We have explored the impact of serious hearing impairment on the early development of deaf children, in particular, insofar as communication development is concerned, and examined the consequences of the lack of hearing for socialization and academic development. Prevention of negative consequences depends in large part on the establishment of an effective communication system as early as possible. We discussed several major approaches to communication with deaf children, including oral and manual methods. Regardless of the communication method chosen, there are issues involved in speech and language development that were discussed in terms of their relation to the child's naturally operating system.

There is no question that great strides have been made in habilitation and education of deaf children over the years, but there is still quite a bit of work to be done. It is incumbent on all communication disorders professionals to work closely with parents in as professional and empathetic a manner as possible in order to help them make the choices that are most appropriate for their individual children.

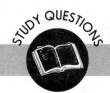

1 What are the primary consequences of prelinguistic deafness if left "untreated"?

2 Explain the ways in which prelinguistic deafness affects the parent-child relationship.

3 What are some of the differences between deaf children who have deaf parents and those with normal-hearing parents? What would be the key educational consequences of these differences?

4 Why do deaf children still require special intervention for speech and language development despite the great advances in hearing aid technology over the past few decades?

5 Compare and contrast the oral and Total Communication approaches to communication development with deaf children. On what factors might one base a decision to follow one path or the other with a particular child?

6 What is the relationship between "bilingual-bicultural" approaches and other communication philosophies used in deaf education?

7 Compare and contrast "top-down" and "bottom-up" approaches to speech and language teaching with deaf students.

8 What are some of the special considerations for assessment of deaf children's speech and language?

REFERENCES

American Annals of the Deaf. (1998). Reference Issue. *143, 2.*

Blackwell, P., Engen, E., Fischgrund, J., & Zarcadoolas, C. (1978). *Sentences and other systems.* Washington, DC: Alexander Graham Bell Association for the Deaf.

Calvert, D., & Silverman, S. R. (1983). *Speech and deafness* (2nd ed.). Washington, DC: Alexander Graham Bell Association for the Deaf.

Cornett, R. O. (1967). Cued speech. *American Annals of the Deaf, 112,* 3–13.

Fitzgerald, E. (1929). *Straight language for the deaf.* Staunton, VA: McClure.

Goldman, R., & Fristoe, M. (1986). *Goldman-Fristoe Test of Articulation.* Circle Pines, MN: American Guidance Service.

Hodson, B. (1986). *Assessment of Phonological Processes-Revised.* Austin: Pro-Ed.

Johnson, R., Liddell, S., & Erting, C. (1989). *Unlocking the curriculum: Principles for achieving access in deaf education* (pp. 89–103). Washington DC: Gallaudet Research Institute Working Paper.

Kretschmer, R., & Kretschmer, L. (Eds.). (1988). Communication Assessment of Hearing-Impaired Children: From conversation to classroom. Monograph Supplement, Volume XXI, *Journal of the Academy of Rehabilitative Audiology.*

Lane, H., Hoffmeister, R., & Bahan, B. (1996). *Journey into the deaf-world.* San Diego: DawnSign Press.

Ling, D. (1976). *Speech and the hearing impaired child.* Washington, DC: Alexander Graham Bell Association for the Deaf.

Ling, D. (1989). *Foundations of spoken language for hearing-impaired children.* Washington, DC: Alexander Graham Bell Association for the Deaf.

Luetke-Stahlman, B., & Luckner, J. (1991). *Effectively educating students with hearing impairments.* New York: Longman.

Luterman, D. (1987). *Deafness in the family.* Boston: College-Hill Press.

Maxwell, M. (1990). Simultaneous communication: The state of the art and proposals for change. *Sign Language Studies, 69,* 333–390.

McCarthy, M. (1996). *Mother-infant communication patterns: Impact of deafness.* Unpublished doctoral dissertation, The University of Texas at Austin.

Monsen, R. (1981). A usable test for the speech intelligibility of deaf talkers. *American Annals of the Deaf, 126*(7), 845–852.

Moog, J., & Geers, A. (1985). *Grammatical analysis of elicited language.* St. Louis: Central Institute for the Deaf.

Moores, D. F. (1987). *Educating the deaf* (3rd ed.). Boston: Houghton Mifflin.

Mulholland, A. (Ed.) (1981). *Oral education today and tomorrow.* Washington, DC: Alexander Graham Bell Association for the Deaf.

Schlesinger, H. (1985). Deafness, mental health, and language. In F. Powell, T. Finitzo-Hieber, S. Friel-Patti, & D. Henderson (Eds.), *Education of the hearing-impaired child.* San Diego: College-Hill Press.

Schlesinger, H. (1986). Total communication in perspective. In D. Luterman (Ed.), *Deafness in perspective.* San Diego: College-Hill Press.

Subtelny, J., Orlando, N., & Whitehead, R. (1981). *Speech and voice characteristics of the deaf.* Washington, DC: Alexander Graham Bell Association for the Deaf.

SUGGESTED READINGS

Lane, H., Hoffmeister, R., & Bahan, B. (1996). *Journey into the deaf-world.* San Diego: DawnSign Press.

Luetke-Stahlman, B., & Luckner, J. (1991). *Effectively educating students with hearing impairments.* New York: Longman.

Moores, D. F. (1987). *Educating the deaf.* Boston: Houghton Mifflin.

Paul, P. V. (1997). *Literacy and deafness: The development of reading, writing, and literate thought.* Boston: Allyn & Bacon.

Ross, M. (Ed.). (1990). *Hearing-impaired children in the mainstream.* Parkton, MD: York Press.

Yoshinaga-Itano, C. (1999). *Language development of deaf and hard of hearing children.* San Diego: Singular Publishing Group.

GLOSSARY

American Sign Language (ASL): A gestural language used by most deaf individuals in North America for everyday communication. It is produced in three-dimensional space by the hands, arms, face, and body, and has a complex grammar quite different from that of English.

Audition: The use of residual hearing as an input mode in communicating with deaf children. *See* Residual hearing.

Bilingual-bicultural: A general term to describe a number of related yet distinct approaches to help deaf children acquire communication facility in both sign language and spoken language, while also helping deaf children discover their cultural identities in both the hearing and deaf communities.

Critical period: That period of a developing child's life, usually the early childhood years, in which the child's neurological and cognitive systems for language and speech learning are both ready and most active. The critical period may be thought of as a window of opportunity for language-speech learning, one, which typically closes due to neurological maturation by early puberty.

Cued Speech: A gestural system, unrelated to sign language, used to signal (cue) distinctions among spoken phonemes by use of particular hand configurations and positions that accompany speech. Cued Speech is often accepted as a gestural supplement to oral communication methods with deaf children.

Language-speech age: For a particular child, the time elapsed (months, years) since the first provision of auditory amplification and speech-language intervention (including signed and/or oral modes). A child of chronological age 3 years and 6 months, who was first diagnosed as hearing impaired and for whom intervention started at age 2 years, may be considered to have a speech-language age of 1 year and 6 months.

Manual codes, manual systems: Systems of manual gestures (often adapted from existing sign languages) that are used simultaneously with speech to present a redundant representation of the spoken signal in another mode. These are typically used in the practice of Total Communication. Manual codes are not sign languages; the codes merely offer a way to make the spoken language more accessible to the deaf "listener" as it is produced, and the grammar is still that of the spoken language. *See* Total Communication.

Multimodalism: The approach to communication that supports the deaf person's development of a variety of speech, sign, and writing methods for communication, depending on the communication demands of the situation, rather than being restricted to one mode only.

Oral method: The approach to communication with deaf individuals that fosters the exclusive use of speech, speechreading, and hearing; sign language is not permitted.

Prelinguistic: Prior to the natural acquisition of spoken language in early childhood and typically taken to mean before approximately 3 years of age. Prelinguistic deafness, therefore, is deafness that occurs earlier than the child's third birthday.

Residual hearing: The hearing ability "left over" despite the hearing impairment. Hearing impairment is rarely total; there is usually some amount of "residual" hearing that might be used by the individual if appropriate amplification is provided. Residual hearing varies greatly in quantity and quality from individual to individual.

Speechreading: Sometimes called "lipreading," speechreading is a method used by people with hearing impairments to "read" the movements of a speaker's face and mouth in order to understand what he or she is saying. Speechreading is an art not easily acquired by all deaf individuals and at best is notoriously unreliable.

Total Communication: A philosophy of communication with deaf children and adults that advocates the use of multimodalism, including speech, sign, writing, and anything else that would facilitate the communication process. In practice, Total Communication typically involves the use of speech accompanied by one of the manual codes for English.

SPEECH AND
SPEECH DISORDERS

9

Speech Science

Thomas P. Marquardt

LEARNING OBJECTIVES

1 To learn the major structures and functions of the central and peripheral nervous systems.

2 To learn the localization of speech and language functions of the cerebrum.

3 To understand the basic processes of respiration, phonation, resonation, and articulation for speech production.

4 To learn the acoustic properties of the speech sounds of English.

5 To learn how speech sounds are categorized based on voicing, place, and manner of production.

INTRODUCTION

Speech production for most individuals requires little effort. We can speak for long periods of time without undue fatigue. The reason is that the physiolog-

Table 9–1. Orientations in Anatomic Descriptions

Superior: toward the top	**Inferior:** toward the bottom
Posterior: toward the front	**Anterior:** toward the back
Medial: toward the middle	**Lateral:** toward the side
Ventral: toward the belly	**Caudal:** toward the back
Superficial: near the surface	**Deep:** away from the surface
Proximal: toward the middle	**Distal:** away from the middle

ical effort for speech production is minimally taxing. Biting to open a difficult candy wrapper or blowing up a balloon may be more physically demanding.

Speaking involves the interaction of respiratory, laryngeal, and articulatory structures, all governed by the nervous system. We will consider each of these components in turn but with the understanding that they do not function independently but rather as a whole during speech production.

Locational terms helpful to understanding the relationship among structures of the body (Table 9–1) need to be reviewed first. These terms provide an orientation of structures of the nervous system as well as respiratory, laryngeal, and articulatory systems. Take a moment to review them before we continue.

Nervous System

The nervous system is composed of a series of complex, densely connected structures that make speech and language possible. The vital building blocks of the systems are neurons supported by an infrastructure of other cells essential to their operation.

 CD-ROM

Overview of CD-ROM Segments for Chapter 9

The CD-ROM segments show several views of the brain including:

Ch.9.01: Cerebral hemispheres and longitudinal fissure.

Ch.9.02: Lobes of the cerebrum.

Ch.9.03: Neuroimages from computerized tomography and magnetic resonance imaging.

The Neuron

The nervous system contains as many as 10 billion neurons and perhaps many more. The neurons differ in size and shape, depending on their location and function. Most often we think of these cells as being microscopic and densely packed. In some cases, however, neurons are very long. If we considered the unusual example of the giraffe, there are neurons that extend from the surface of the brain to the tail end of the spinal cord, a total distance of perhaps 14 feet.

Regardless of the size, shape, or function of neurons, they have common architectural features. If we examine the neuron shown in Figure 9–1, we can identify a cell body, a nucleus and nucleolus, dendrites, and an axon. Neurons may have many dendrites, but only one axon. They also may or may not have **myelin,** a fatty insulator covering the axon that speeds transmission of impulses, and *neurilemma,* a covering of the axon that allows it to regain function after being damaged. Only nerves of the peripheral nervous system have neurilemma, so they are the only neurons that can effectively reestablish function after damage to the axon.

Neurons can be described by their function. A neuron is termed an **efferent** if it conveys impulses from higher to lower structures. In most cases, efferent neurons are *motor* and make up the nerves that carry impulses to muscles and glands from the brain and spinal cord. Neurons that bring information to a higher structure of the nervous system are termed **afferent.** Afferent neurons are *sensory* and bring information, for example, from the

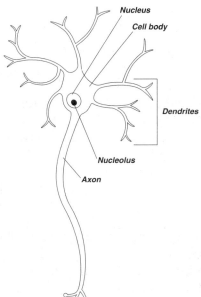

Figure 9–1. The neuron. (From *Speech sciences* [p. 234], by R. Kent, 1997, San Diego: Singular Publishing Group. Copyright 1997 by Singular Publishing Group. Reprinted with permission.)

ear, eye, and nose to the brain. *Interneurons* make up the neural tissue of the brain and spinal cord. They are far more numerous than the sensory and motor neurons combined.

Neurons communicate with one another by means of synapses, functional gaps between the axon of one neuron and the dendrites and cell bodies of surrounding neurons. When excited, a wave of electrical activity (depolarization) sweeps down the axon to end branches where **neurotransmitters** are released to excite or inhibit the response of surrounding neurons. Neurotransmitters are the chemical messengers of the nervous system. There are a large number of different types of neurotransmitters that facilitate or inihibit responses and make a complex functional networking of groups of neurons possible. Networks of neurons work together in a group, but a single neuron may be involved in more than a single network. In fact, neurons may be influenced by hundreds of other neurons due to varied synaptic relationships.

There is also another important group of cells in the nervous system, **glial cells.** Glial cells perform a number of functions: (1) they form the fatty myelin covering of axons that affect the speed of transmission of an impulse down the axon, (2) they serve as a blood-brain barrier for nutrients delivered to neurons, and (3) they remove dead cells from the nervous system.

The brain has characteristic areas of gray and white matter. The gray matter is composed primarily of neuron cell bodies. White matter is given its appearance by the myelin covering on axons that make up the projections or transmission lines between different parts of the brain.

Central Nervous System

The central nervous system includes the cerebrum, brainstem, cerebellum, and spinal cord (Figure 9–2). It is encased within the skull and spinal column, covered by tissue layers **(meninges),** and surrounded by circulating cerebrospinal fluid. The *cerebrum* has two **cerebral hemispheres** that are similar but not identical in appearance. There are differences in the size of the areas of the two hemispheres but the functional importance of the differences is not fully understood.

Cerebrum

Each hemisphere has four lobes: frontal, parietal, temporal, and occipital (Figure 9–3). The lobes of the hemispheres have unique but not exclusive functional roles. The frontal lobe is responsible for motor planning and execution, the temporal lobe is important for auditory processing, the occipital lobe for visual processing, and the parietal lobe for sensory association and spatial processing.

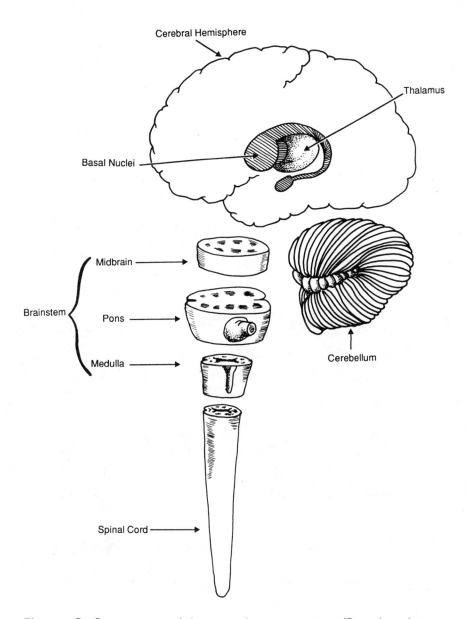

Figure 9-2. Structures of the central nervous system. (From *Introduction to communication sciences and disorders* [p. 318], by F. Minifie [Ed.], 1994, San Diego: Singular Publishing Group. Copyright 1994 by Singular Publishing Group. Reprinted with permission.)

The surface of the cerebrum is folded with prominences **(gyri)** and depressions **(sulci).** The gyri and sulci are idenitified most typically by brain lobe and position. For example, three gyri of the frontal lobe are the superior, middle, and inferior frontal gyri (Figure 9–4).

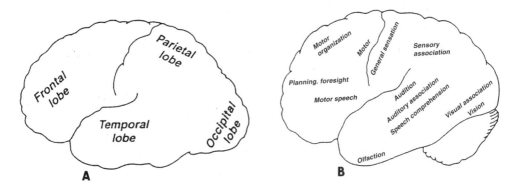

Figure 9–3. Lobes of the cerebrum (A) and selected localization of functions (B). (From *Speech sciences* [pp. 247 and 248], by R. Kent, 1997, San Diego: Singular Publishing Group. Copyright 1997 by Singular Publishing Group. Reprinted with permission.)

 CD-ROM

The Brain

On the CD-ROM, view the pictures of the two cerebral hemispheres and the lobes of the cerebrum:

Ch.9.01: Cerebrum

Ch.9.02: Lobes

The two hemispheres are separated by a deep longitudinal fissure, but are joined by a series of connecting pathways that form the **corpus callosum.** The frontal lobe is demarcated by the lateral **(Sylvian) fissure** and by the central **(Rolandic) fissure.** The Sylvian and Rolandic fissures serve also as landmarks for the anterior border of the parietal lobe and the top of the temporal lobe. The occipital lobes lie at the back of each hemisphere.

The surface of the cerebrum is gray matter, that is, neuron cell bodies. Deep to this mantle of gray matter is white matter given its appearance by the presence of myelin on the neuron axons. Lying within each hemisphere are groups of cell bodies (nuclei) important for sensory and motor processing, the **basal ganglia** and **thalamus.** The basal ganglia are important for the control of movement. Damage to these structures results in involuntary movements like tremors that you might observe in an elderly person with Parkinson's disease or writhing arm movements in a child with cerebral palsy. Sensory information is projected to the cortical surface through the thalamus.

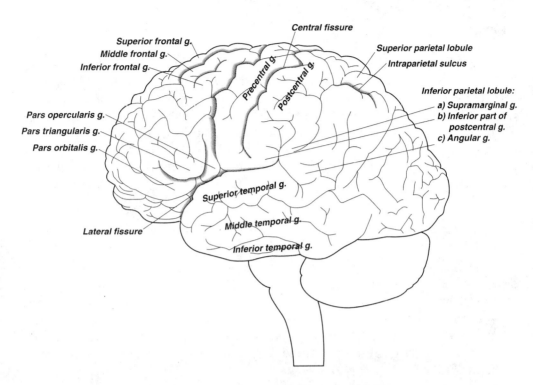

Figure 9–4. Major gyri of the cerebral cortex. (From *Speech sciences* [pp. 246], by R. Kent, 1997, San Diego: Singular Publishing Group. Copyright 1997 by Singular Publishing Group. Reprinted with permission.)

What this means is that all the information from our senses, with the exception of our sense of smell, is routed through the thalamus on its way to the surface of the cerebrum. An example of a nucleus of the thalamus is the medial geniculate, a structure within the auditory pathways described in Chapter 5.

Brainstem

The **brainstem** lies at the base of the brain in front of the cerebellum and includes in descending order the *midbrain, pons,* and *medulla.* The brainstem is a conduit for sensory information coming from the receptors of the body for touch, temperature, pain, and pressure as well as vision, hearing, balance, and movement, and for motor pathways to the muscles of the body. The strategic position of the brainstem is clearly evident in Figure 9–2. Many of the nerves that bring sensory information from the head and neck and that project to the muscles of this region are located in the brainstem, so these structures are important to speech production.

Cerebellum

The *cerebellum* lies in back and on top of the brainstem and includes two hemispheres. The cerebellar cortex is highly convoluted such that its surface area is large. It is connected to the brainstem by three pathways that allow for the (1) input of sensory information from the body, (2) output of signals for motor execution to the body musculature, and (3) input from the cerebrum for control of cerebellar function. The cerebellum is important for balance and for ensuring coordination of various body movements, specifically, the timing, amount, and speed of movement.

Spinal Cord

The *spinal cord* lies within the vertebral column. In contrast to the cerebrum and cerebellum, the outer part of the cord is composed of white matter with a butterfly-shaped area of gray matter in the interior. Areas of the spinal cord are identified by the surrounding vertebrae. There are 7 cervical, 12 thoracic, 5 lumbar, and 5 sacral vertebrae plus a coccyx. The spinal cord has enlargements at the cervical and lumbar levels for sensory and motor innervation of the arms and legs

Peripheral Nervous System

Groups of nerves extending from the central nervous system make up the *peripheral nervous system*. The nerves can be divided into highly specialized cranial nerves that extend from the cerebrum and brainstem, and the spinal nerves that extend from the spinal cord.

There are 12 pairs of *cranial nerves* specialized for sensory, motor, or sensory and motor functions (Table 9–2). The cranial nerves most important for speech production include the trigeminal, facial, glossopharyngeal, vagus, accessory, and hypoglossal that innervate the musculature of the head and neck. It would be helpful at this point to review each of the nerves to learn their names and function.

There are 31 pairs of *spinal nerves* that arise from the spinal cord and innervate sensory and motor functions of the body below the level of the neck. In contrast to the cranial nerves, the spinal nerves are not specialized for sensory or motor functions but innervate specific areas of the body. They carry general sensory information from specific areas of the body, such as the side of the leg or bottom of the arm, and serve as a final common pathway for motor impulses from the central nervous system to the muscles. In general, input from the cervical level is to the hands and arms, from the thoracic level to the trunk of the body, and from the lumbar, sacral, and coccygeal levels to the front and back of the legs and the feet.

Table 9–2. Cranial Nerves

Number	Name	Function
I	Olfactory	Sensory for smell
II	Optic	Sensory for vision
III	Oculomotor	Motor for eye movement
IV	Trochlear	Motor for eye movement
V	Trigeminal	Motor for mastication (chewing) Sensory for face, maxillary teeth, and eyes
VI	Abducents	Motor for eye movements
VII	Facial	Motor for facial movements Sensory for taste for front of tongue
VIII	Vestibulocochlear	Sensory for hearing and balance
IX	Glossopharyngeal	Motor for pharyngeal movements Sensory for taste at back of tongue
X	Vagus	Motor for intrinsic laryngeal and pharyngeal movements Sensory for motor for thoracic and abdominal viscera
XI	Accessory	Motor for shoulder movements
XII	Hypoglossal	Motor for tongue movements

Hemispheric Specialization/Localization of Function

The two cerebral hemispheres are specialized in terms of the types of information they are most adept at processing. The left hemisphere is specialized for sequential functioning; the right hemisphere for wholistic processing. Since speech and language are processed over time, the left hemisphere has a dominant role in this aspect of communicative functioning. The right hemisphere's wholistic processing makes it more adept at face recognition, comprehending and expressing emotion, and music. This functional asymmetry is true, in most cases, whether the person is right or left handed.

Although the two hemispheres are specialized for the types of information they are best able to handle, it is clear they work together during communication. When talking with a friend, for example, you listen not only to what he says, but how he says it, his facial appearance, the intonation of the phrases, and the gestures used. What the friend communicates is more meaningful than simply the words he uses.

Earlier, we mentioned that the lobes of the cerebral hemispheres differ in the types of functional responsibilities they hold. For example, we mentioned that the temporal lobe is responsible for auditory processing and the occipital lobe for visual processing. More specific functional roles can be assigned to cortical areas of the left hemisphere, not like a mosaic, but more like an increased role of one area compared to another in carrying out a particular processing task.

Localization of function for the left hemisphere based on the Brodmann numbering system is shown in Figure 9–5. Obviously, we will not discuss the functional specialization in detail, but rather will focus on sensory and motor behaviors and speech and language representation. Both anatomic and functional descriptions may be employed for this purpose. Anatomically, particular gyri are identified; in functional terms, Brodmann's areas are described. Brodmann's numbers demarcate areas where specific types of processing take place (Figure 9–5). An example may be helpful. The area responsible for programming speech movements is Brodmann's area 44; it also could be described as the posterior part of the third (inferior) frontal gyrus.

The frontal lobe has important representation of motor functions for the opposite side of the body on the precentral gyrus (Brodmann's area 4), which lies just in front of the frontal fissure. More than 50 years ago researchers studied this area while doing brain surgery. They found they could cause movements of various parts of the left side of the body by stimulating this "motor strip" on the right side of the brain. Stimulating the gyrus near the top of the brain caused movements of the lower limb, stimulating the gyrus at a

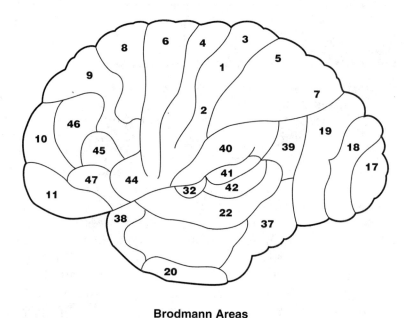

Brodmann Areas

Figure 9–5. Brodmann areas of the cerebral cortex. (From *Speech sciences* [p. 247], by R. Kent, 1997, San Diego: Singular Publishing Group. Copyright 1997 by Singular Publishing Group. Reprinted with permission.)

lower point caused arm and tongue movements They also observed that a larger area could be stimulated to obtain tongue or thumb movements than arm movements. They demonstrated that the representation for body movements is in the form of an inverted and distorted body image, with the feet and legs located on the medial aspect of the hemisphere with the body, neck, and head, and then hand represented laterally. The body scheme is distorted because there are a larger number of neurons that project to areas with highly developed motor skill like the tongue and thumb. This "motor strip" is the primary origin for direct motor pathways to the muscles of the body.

Just in back of the lateral fissure is the postcentral gyrus of the parietal lobe (Brodmann's areas 1, 2, 3). Here is where there is a sensory representation of the body in a form similar to the motor strip. That is, the feet and legs are represented near the top of the gyrus with the trunk, face, and hands along the side. Broad areas of the frontal and parietal lobes, like the other lobes of the brain, contain association cortex. These are areas that do not have highly specialized functioning, but are involved in processing various types of information.

There are several areas of the left side of the brain that are important to speech and language. **Broca's area** (area 44) and surrounding tissue of the posterior part of the inferior frontal gyrus are important for the programming of movements for speech production. Damage in this location causes problems in the planning and carrying out of speech movements

The temporal lobe includes an area critical for understanding auditory information **(Wernicke's area).** This area (Brodmann's area 42) is located on the back part of the first temporal gyrus. It is linked to the supramarginal and angular gyri that are important to language interpretation. Damage to Wernicke's area results in a marked deficit in understanding what is heard. There also are other areas of the temporal lobe that are important for reading.

The cerebrum could not function unless there were pathways that carry information from one place to another within and between the hemispheres of the brain. Particularly important to speech and language is the *arcuate fasciculus* that connects Wernicke's area to Broca's area. Damage to this connecting pathway causes difficulty in repeating what is heard because the information cannot be conveyed efficienctly between Wernicke's and Broca's area. The Broca's area-arcuate fasciculus-Wernicke's area complex is critical to speech and language functioning. Damage to this area produces classifiable types of language disorders in adults, which will be the focus of the chapter on neurogenic language disorders (see Chapter 19).

Motor Pathways

Motor activity is controlled by two major tracts of the nervous system—pyramidal and extrapyramidal. The **pyramidal tract** is a direct pathway from the cortical surface to the peripheral nerves (Figure 9–6). Pyramidal tract

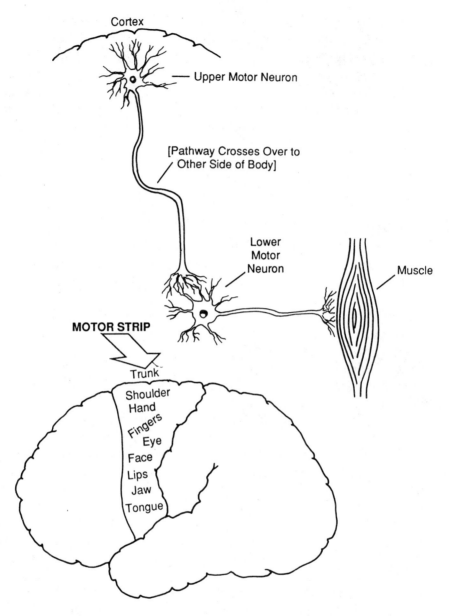

Figure 9–6. Pyramidal motor pathway. (From *Introduction to communication sciences and disorders* [p. 339], by F. Minifie [Ed.], 1994, San Diego: Singular Publishing Group. Copyright 1994 by Singular Publishing Group. Reprinted with permission.)

neurons frequently are referred to as upper motor neurons and peripheral nerve neurons as lower motor neurons. The lower motor neurons that innervate muscles are a final common pathway since all input to the body by necessity must be channeled through these nerves The origin of the pyramidal tract is centered on the motor strip (Brodmann's area 4), approximately the area of the precentral gyrus. Representation of motor function, as we have discussed, is inverted, with the feet and trunk of the body represented on the superior aspects of the frontal lobe, with the face and hand represented on the lateral aspect of the hemisphere. The neurons of the pyramidal tract form pathways that travel through the interior of each hemisphere to either the cranial nerves of the brainstem or to the spinal nerves. Approximately 85% of the fibers traveling to the spinal nerves cross to the opposite side of the body at the medulla. Therefore, the left side of the body receives innervation from the right side of the brain and vice versa.

For the cranial nerves, the innervation is somewhat different. Axons from both the left and right hemispheres innervate the motor cranial nerves with the exception of part of the facial nerve. When an individual has a stroke in the frontal lobe of the left hemisphere, most of the motor functions of the head and neck are spared because innervation from the right side of the brain to these nerves has not been interrupted.

The **extrapyramidal tract** is a complex system important for control of movements. It originates in an area just in front of the motor strip (Brodmann's area 6) but overlaps with the pyramidal tract on the frontal lobes. This tract is indirect to the extent that input is from the cerebral cortex to basal ganglia deep within the cerebrum, with internal loops that project back to the cerebrum and downward to influence lower motor neurons. The extrapyramidal tract's role is to modulate the complex motor activity of the nervous system. Damage to the system results in problems with the level of background electrical activity within muscles and the development of involuntary movements like tremors.

There are a number of modern methods for studying brain anatomy and function including, among others, computerized tomography (CT) and magnetic resonance imaging (MRI). Computerized tomography scans are based on computer processed x-rays; magnetic resonance imaging relies on intense magnetic fields that affect the spin axis of electrons. Other modern techniques such as functional magnetic resonance imaging (fMRI) and positron emission tomography (PET) are important new developments because they allow

 CD-ROM

Neuroimages of the Brain

On CD-ROM segment Ch.9.03, compare the neuroimages from computerized tomography and magnetic resonance imaging in terms of how the brain structures are revealed.

brain activity to be investigated during the performance of speech and language tasks.

The nervous system governs speech production by providing input to the more than 100 pairs of muscles of the respiratory, laryngeal, and articulatory structures with continual on-line sensory monitoring of the process. We will examine each subsystem of speech production and then consider the dynamic process by which these components are used to produce articulate speech.

RESPIRATION

Respiration is the power source for speech production. The primary components of the respiratory system are the lungs, ribcage, and abdomen. The lungs lie within the bony framework of the thorax. They have access to the upper airway by means of the trachea, which is composed of a series of cartilage rings that extend from the larynx to the bronchi of the lungs (Figure 9–7).

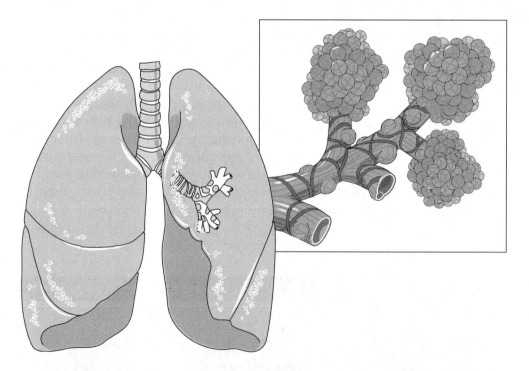

Figure 9–7. The lungs with an enlargement of the alveolar sacs. (From *Speech sciences* [p. 76], by R. Kent, 1997, San Diego: Singular Publishing Group. Copyright 1997 by Singular Publishing Group. Reprinted with permission.)

The lungs are analagous to an inverted tree (Kent, 1997) composed of a trunk (trachea) and a series of branches that end in air-filled sacs *(alveoli)*. The alveoli are the end organs where the exchange of oxygen and carbon dioxide takes place. In their natural state, the lungs are spongy and elastic.

The lungs are surrounded by 12 pairs of ribs that extend from the thoracic vertebrae at the spinal column to the front of the body (Figure 9–8). Seven pairs of ribs attach to the sternum, three additional pairs attach to cartilage at the base of the sternum. Two additional ribs do not attach to the sternum and are termed "floating ribs." Superimposed on the top of the thorax are additional bones, the two scapulas (shoulder blades) and the two clavicles (collar bones) to which muscles attach to effect respiration.

Air pressures and flows result from changes in lung volume. At rest in the body, the lungs are slightly inflated and would collapse if punctured. The thorax, in contrast, is compressed and would expand if unlinked from the lungs. The lungs and thorax are linked by tissues called *pleura* that surround each lung and the interior of the thorax. The pleura of the lungs and thorax are bonded together by negative pressure. At a mechanically neutral point

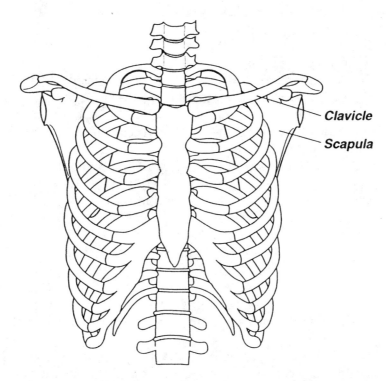

Figure 9–8. The rib cage with clavicle and scapula. (From *Speech sciences* [p. 79], by R. Kent, 1997, San Diego: Singular Publishing Group. Copyright 1997 by Singular Publishing Group. Reprinted with permission.)

(resting expiratory level), the opposing forces of the lungs (collapse) and thorax (expand) are in balance and air pressure in the lungs is equal to the air pressure outside the body (atmospheric pressure). This assumes, of course, that the airway from the lungs is open.

Respiration is the process of moving air in and out of the lungs. We know from elementary laws of physics that for an enclosed gas like air, pressure is inversely related to volume (Boyle's Law) and that air flows from areas of high to areas of low pressure (Law of Gases). An increase in lung volume causes a reduction in the air pressure within the lungs with an inward flow of air (inspiration); a reduction in lung volume causes an increase in air pressure in the lungs and an outward flow of air (expiration).

Changes in lung volume are due to the application of active muscle forces to the respiratory system. Some muscles increase the size of the lungs (expiratory muscles) by pulling them to a larger volume; other muscles decrease the size by compressing the lungs (expiratory muscles). The respiratory system is elastic. When it is moved to a larger or smaller volume by active muscle forces, an oppositional force is stored which, when released, causes the system to return to its rest position (resting expiratory level). This is much like a coiled spring that can be stretched or compressed, but which returns to its original shape when released. Recoil (relaxation) forces of this type in the respiratory system are described as passive.

Primary inspiratory muscles that expand the size of the lungs are the *diaphragm,* a bowl-shaped partition between the lungs and abdominal contents, and the *external intercostals,* a sheet of 11 muscles that lie between the ribs (Figure 9–9). These muscles act to increase the front to back, side to side, and top to bottom volume of the lungs. In effect, they cause an increase in the size of the lungs by pulling them to a larger volume. They are supplemented by other muscles that help to raise the rib cage, sternum, and clavicle during more demanding inspiratory activity, like taking a deep breath.

Expiratory muscles work to reduce the volume of the lungs by pulling down the ribs and by compressing the abdominal contents. You probably have noticed during a demanding singing activity that the muscles of your abdomen were fatigued after a particularly long passage. That is because you were using muscles such as the *rectus abdominis* to push inward on the abdominal contents, which forced the diaphragm upward to reduce lung volume (Figure 9–10). At the same time, the *internal intercostals,* a series of muscles lying between the ribs, pulled down on the ribcage and expiratory muscles of the back pulled down on the back of the ribs to reduce the volume of the lungs.

As you probably have deduced by this point, changes in lung volume are accomplished by application of muscle forces to the respiratory apparatus. With the application of these forces there is a storing up of recoil (relaxation) forces in the lungs, ribcage, and abdomen that have the potential, when released, of increasing or decreasing the pressure within the lungs. When the volume of the lungs is increased from a mechanically neutral point (resting

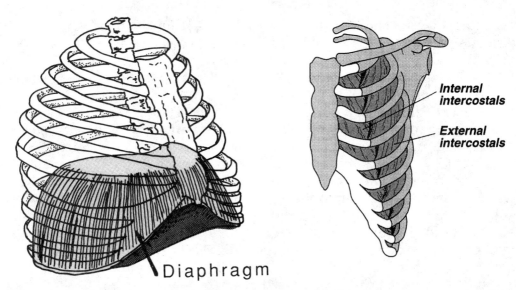

Figure 9–9. The diaphragm and intercostal muscles. (From *Speech sciences* [pp. 76 and 81], by R. Kent, 1997, San Diego: Singular Publishing Group. Copyright 1997 by Singular Publishing Group. Reprinted with permission.)

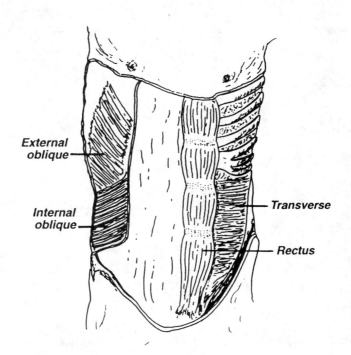

Figure 9–10. The abdominal muscles. (From *Speech sciences* [p. 87], by R. Kent, 1997, San Diego: Singular Publishing Group. Copyright 1997 by Singular Publishing Group. Reprinted with permission.)

expiratory level), relaxation results in a decrease in lung volume, an increase in lung pressure, and an outward flow of air. Compressing the lungs to a smaller volume than at rest stores up recoil (relaxation) forces that will cause the lungs to expand to a larger volume with an inward flow of air when respiratory muscles are relaxed.

The total amount of air in the lungs can be partitioned (Figure 9–11). The air in the lungs after a maximum inspiration is termed the *total lung capacity* and is made up of two components: residual volume and vital capacity. *Residual volume* is the air in the lungs that cannot be expired and is the result of the lungs being slightly inflated within the body. **Vital capacity** is the total amount of controllable air in the lungs. You can get a sense of vital capacity by taking as deep a breath as possible and then forcing all the air out of your lungs. The total volume of air you expired is the vital capacity. **Tidal volume** is the volume of air exchanged during a task. During quiet breathing, it is the air (approximately 500 milliliters) that you inspire and expire, but the amount may increase if you begin a different activity.

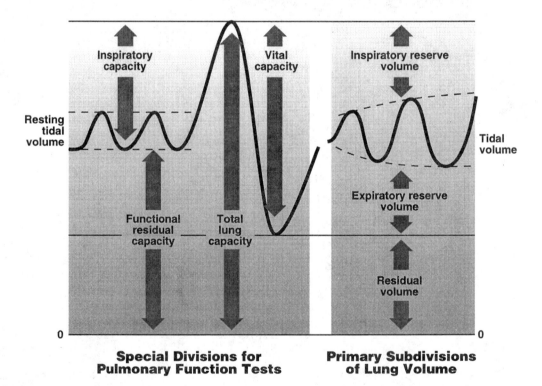

Figure 9–11. Patterns of respiration. (From *Speech sciences* [p. 89], by R. Kent, 1997, San Diego: Singular Publishing Group. Copyright 1997 by Singular Publishing Group. Reprinted with permission.)

During quiet breathing (breathing while sitting quietly), the diaphragm and external intercostals actively increase lung volume to develop an inward flow of air. When the pressure within the lungs is equal to atmospheric pressure, the flow of air stops. The process of inspiration resulted in the storing of recoil forces primarily in the lungs and abdomen. When released, these forces produced a reduction of lung volume and expiration. Note that during this quiet breathing cycle, inspiration was active and expiration was passive. That is, muscles were active in expanding the lungs, but were not active as the lungs collapsed back to their original size because the relaxation forces made the lungs smaller without help from expiratory muscles.

During speech, the respiratory system provides a stable air pressure within the lungs. This activity is accomplished by the balancing of active (muscle) and passive (recoil) forces to maintain a constant pressure while lung volume is decreasing with the loss of air. This maneuver includes the active use of inspiratory and expiratory muscles during the expiratory phase of speech production to act like brakes and accelerators to maintain a constant pressure.

Speech breathing is different in two important respects from quiet breathing—the lungs are increased to a larger volume and the expiratory phase is extended. More air is taken into the lungs while talking. The amount of air inspired is determined by the length and intensity of what the speaker intends to say. Obviously, if you wanted to shout or to read a paragraph aloud without stopping to take a breath, you would take in more air and use a greater portion of the total volume of air in your lungs.

During quiet breathing, inspiration and expiration take about the same amount of time. However, this pattern is altered during speech with an extended expiratory phase in the respiratory cycle. The effect of respiratory activity for speech, then, is to provide an extended stable air pressure to the larynx and upper airway.

PHONATION

The function of the larynx in speech production is to convert respiratory energy into sound energy. The larynx is a structure composed of cartilages, muscles, and membranous and connective tissues located at the top of the trachea. Although vibration of the vocal folds within the larynx is the focus of our discussion, the larynx has other important functions. Perhaps the most critical function it serves is to keep food from entering the lungs. Closure of the folds of the larynx and downward movement of a leaf-like structure called the epiglottis prevents food from entering the trachea and helps to direct it down the esophagus to the stomach. Sometimes, however, food lodges in the larynx, particularly when there is an effort to carry on an enthusiastic conversation while eating. If food enters the trachea, the larynx helps to expel the material by working with the respiratory system. The vocal folds close and are powerfully exploded open to expel the material back to the oral cavity. We also cough to clear our lungs when there is excessive mucous from a respiratory infection. Finally, the vocal folds function to anchor the thorax during heavy lifting. You probably have noticed that when you lift a heavy package, you hold your breath. This maneuver allows the arms to operate against a fixed resistance for load bearing.

The primary cartilages of the larynx are the cricoid, thyroid, and paired arytenoid cartilages (Figure 9–12). There are several other small paired carti-

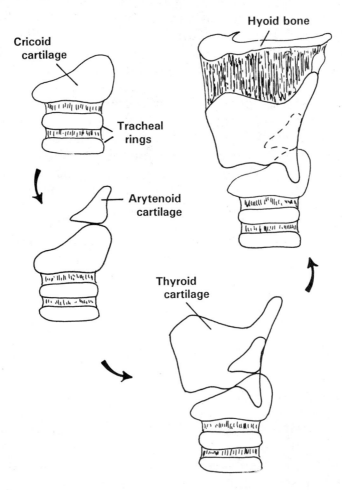

Figure 9–12. Assembly of the major cartilages and bones of the larynx. (From *Speech sciences* [p. 101], by R. Kent, 1997, San Diego: Singular Publishing Group. Copyright 1997 by Singular Publishing Group. Reprinted with permission.)

lages that provide support to the laryngeal structures but that do not contribute significantly to phonation. The *cricoid* is signet ring-shaped and is located at the top of the trachea. It is larger in the back than the front. Superimposed at the top and back of the cricoid are two pyramid-shaped *arytenoid* cartilages that lie in concave indentations of the cricoid and are anchored by ligaments. At the front of the neck is a single butterfly-shaped *thyroid* cartilage that articulates by means of horns (cornu) at the sides of the cricoid and another set of horns that extend upward from the body of the thyroid to approximate a floating bone at the base of the tongue from which the larynx is suspended, the *hyoid bone.* The various cartilages are interconnected and provide scaffolding for the muscles and tissues of the larynx.

There are two pairs of vocal folds. The "false" vocal folds lie above the "true" folds with the two pairs separated by an open space, the laryngeal vestibule (Figure 9–13). The false vocal folds are closed during activities such as heavy lifting. The true folds extend from the arytenoid cartilages in back to a point just below a notch in the thyroid carilage in front. You can locate this front attachment by palpating the neck to find the "Adam's apple" and phonating. The folds are composed of several tissue layers that form a medial *vocal ligament,* but their bulk is formed by the vocalis muscle. The space between the folds is termed the **glottis** and, as we will discuss later in this chapter, is the place of production for one of the consonants of English, the glottal fricative /h/. When brought together **(adduction)** the folds can

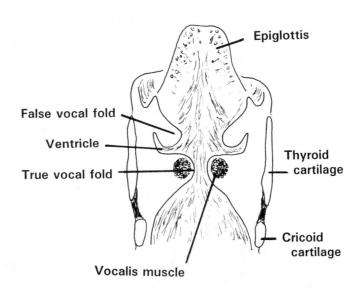

Figure 9–13. Coronal section of the larynx. (From *Speech sciences* [p. 105], by R. Kent, 1997, San Diego: Singular Publishing Group. Copyright 1997 by Singular Publishing Group. Reprinted with permission.)

be vibrated if the pressure below them is large enough to overcome their resistance.

Movements of the vocal folds and positioning of the larynx in the neck are effected by intrinsic and extrinsic laryngeal muscles. Intrinsic muscles (Figure 9–14) have both their origin and insertion within the larynx; extrinsic muscles have only one point of attachment in the larynx. The intrinsic muscles function to close, open, elongate, relax, and tense the vocal folds and are named according to their position and the cartilages to which they attach. The *thyroarytenoid muscles* extend from the arytenoid cartilage to the thyroid and tense the folds. The *posterior cricoarytenoid* opens the folds; the *cricothyroid* elongates and tenses the folds. Other intrinsic muscles, including the *interarytenoids* (not shown in Figure 9–14) and *lateral cricoarytenoids,* function to close and increase the compression of the closed folds.

The extrinsic laryngeal muscles have one attachment at the larynx or hyoid bone and a second to a nearby structure above or below the larynx. Contraction of these muscles of the neck and base of the tongue have the effect of raising or lowering the position of the larynx in the neck to tense or relax the vocal folds. You have probably noticed that the position of the head in an inexperienced singer is raised for high notes and lowered for low notes. This maneuver is carried out to increase or decrease the tension of the folds.

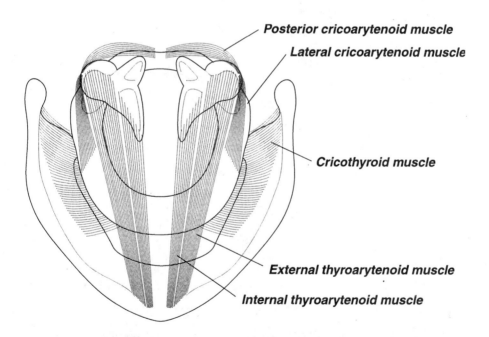

Figure 9–14. Intrinsic muscles of the larynx. (From *Speech sciences* [p. 109], by R. Kent, 1997, San Diego: Singular Publishing Group. Copyright 1997 by Singular Publishing Group. Reprinted with permission.)

When the vocal folds are adducted and air pressure from the lungs (subglottal pressure) is sufficient to overcome their resistance, the vocal folds are set into vibration. The folds vibrate in a relatively complex fashion, opening first at the bottom of the folds with the opening progressing upward to the top. As they are blown apart, they move up and toward the side. The folds then are brought back together again because they are elastic and return to their predeformed state, and because of the **Bernoulli effect.** In essence, the Bernoulli effect is the reduction of air pressure with increases in air flow. As the air rushes through the opening created by the movement of the folds, the air pressure between the folds is reduced and they are sucked back together. The cyclical opening and closing of the folds will continue as long as the subglottal pressure is sufficient to blow them apart. This description is termed the *aerodynamic myoelastic theory of vocal fold vibration,* which suggests that active closing of the vocal folds is not required to accomplish each cycle of vocal fold vibration. Rather, the vocal folds are closed and will continue to vibrate until the subglottal air pressure cannot blow them apart or the vocal folds are opened.

The frequency of vibration is determined by the mass and tension of the vocal folds. Tension is increased by stretching the vocal folds with an increase in distance between the arytenoid and thyroid cartilages with a corresponding reduction in their mass. This is like strumming on a rubber band. As the rubber band is stretched to a longer length and then plucked, the frequency of vibration increases.

Intensity is determined by the force with which air escapes through the glottis and strikes the air mass in the vocal tract above the vocal folds. The force of the air is determined primarily by the amount of subglottal pressure; the greater the pressure, the greater the movement of the vocal folds and the greater the amount of air that escapes through the glottis during each cycle.

The frequency of vibration of the vocal folds is different for men, women and children. Men have vocal folds with greater mass (size) and their vocal folds vibrate, when a large group is considered, at an average frequency of approximately 125 Hz. For women the mean is 225 Hz, and for children it is higher than females. Quite obviously, as children mature the vocal folds become larger and their frequency of vibration decreases.

The opening and closing of the vocal folds produces triangularly shaped airflows that activate the air in the upper airway. The airflow is triangular if viewed over time because the vocal folds are opening and then closing. If the volume of air passing between the vocal folds is measured during the cycle, it increases until the vocal folds are completely open and then decreases until they are fully closed.

The movements of the vocal folds are quasiperiodic and produce a complex waveform with a triangular shape. Recall that complex waveforms were discussed in Chapter 5. Quasiperiodic means that the waveform repeats itself at relatively equal time intervals, but not exactly. The wave shape is important because the triangular waveform has particular properties. It has a

fundamental frequency equal to the frequency of vibration of the vocal folds and a large number of **harmonics;** that is, whole number multiples of the fundamental frequency. The acoustic output of the larynx is one of the sound sources that will be shaped to produce the sounds of the language, a topic we will return to after considering the upper airway.

Articulation

Articulation is the process of forming speech sounds by movement of the articulators (structures used to produce speech sounds). The articulatory system creates sound sources and shapes the resonance of the vocal tract to produce the recognizable speech sounds of the language. This is the primary focus of our discussion.

The *vocal tract* is made up a series of interconnected tubes from the larynx to the opening of the mouth and nose (Figure 9–15). The *oral cavity* extends from the lips to the back of the throat. The *nasal cavity* extends from the

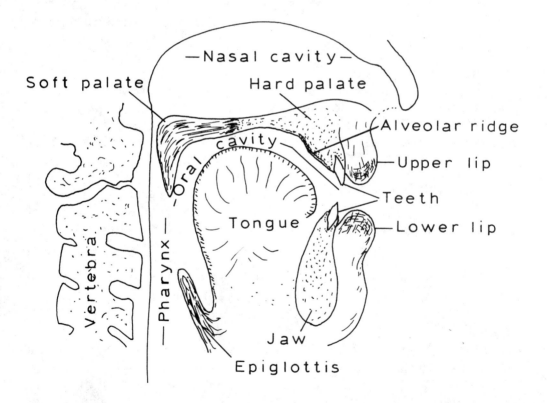

Figure 9–15. Anatomy of the vocal tract. (From *The acoustic analysis of speech* [p. 6], by R. Kent and C. Read, 1992, San Diego: Singular Publishing Group. Copyright 1992 by Singular Publishing Group. Reprinted with permission.)

opening at the nares to the *velopharynx,* the opening between the nose and mouth where the oral and nasal cavities are joined. The shape and size of the oral cavity is highly malleable and constantly changing during the course of speech production due to movements of the tongue, lips, jaw, and velum. The configuration of the nasal cavity, in contrast, is fixed. The *pharynx* is the portion of the vocal tract that extends from the vocal folds to the nasal cavity and is subdivided into the laryngopharynx, oropharynx, and nasopharynx.

Articulation requires the coordinated movement of structures for the production of speech sounds. The articulators can be considered as fixed or mobile. Fixed structures include the teeth, the alveolar ridge, and the hard palate. Mobile articulators are the jaw, tongue, face, and structures of the velopharynx.

The teeth are embedded in the alveolar ridge of the *maxilla* (upper jaw) and *mandible* (lower jaw). The chisel-like incisors are important to the production of sounds in English such as the voiceless and voiced /th/ sounds and sounds produced between the lower lip and upper incisors such as /f/ and /v/ in which contact is made between a mobile structure, like the tongue and lips and the teeth. The alveolar ridge, the bony semicircular shelf of the upper jaw, is important to the production of sounds such as /t/, /d/, /s/, and /z/. Extending from the alveolar ridge is a inverted bowl-shaped hard palate formed by the palatine processes of the maxilla and the horizontal plates of the palatine bones. The hard palate is important as a contact point for multiple sound productions that involve the tongue such as articulatory contacts for the formation of the /sh/ at the midpalate and /k/ at the back of the palate.

The face is important to communication beyond the production of individual speech sounds. Expressions of anger, happiness, surprise, and fear are difficult to envision without the facial posturing that accompanies the emotion. The facial muscles are similar in function to a purse string used to gather the opening for closure. The primary rounding and closing muscle is the *obicularis oris,* a tear-shaped muscle that forms the interior of the upper and lower lip in circular fashion. Other facial muscles work in opposition to the obicularis oris to retract and open the lips. Primary movements of the face during speech production provide a point of closure for the stops /p/ and /b/ as well as the fricatives /f/ and /v/.

A second mobile articulator is the mandible. The mandible has the largest mass of any of the articulators and functions as a platform for the tongue. The mandible lowers or raises the tongue depending on the height of the vowel produced. For example, if you produce the vowels "eee" and "ahh," you will notice that the jaw is raised for the the first vowel and lowered for the second. The jaw also is raised to make it easier for the tongue to make articulatory contacts.

The upward and downward movements of the jaw are different during chewing and speech production. While chewing food, the jaw moves asymmetrically as food is ground between the teeth; during speech production the mandible moves up and down symmetrically.

Mandible movements are accomplished by muscles that extend between the sides of the jaw and the skull and between the mandible and the hyoid bone at the base of the tongue. Some muscles connect to a midline connective tissue structure extending posteriorly from the mandible to form the floor of the mouth. You can identify two muscles responsible for jaw closure quite easily. If you bite down and place your fingers at the angle of the jaw approximately an inch below the outer ear, you can feel the *masseter* muscle flex. Now repeat this action but place your fingers on the lateral aspect of the forehead to palpate a muscle, the *temporalis,* that extends from an attachment on the mandible to insert broadly on the temporal area of the skull.

The tongue is perhaps the most important articulator. It is composed of intrinsic muscles that allow it to change shape. It can be shortened, lengthened, widened, narrowed, flattened, and made thicker. The extrinsic muscles of the tongue anchor it to the hyoid bone, mandible, temporal bone, and pharynx and position the tongue in the mouth. The tongue may be protruded, retracted, raised, or lowered depending on the speech sound being produced. The tongue has several identifiable parts including the root, body, dorsum, blade, and tip (from back to front), which are important in the description of the production of speech sounds. Since many speech sounds are produced by constriction (narrowing) of the vocal tract, the tongue has a strategic role in their formation within the oral cavity.

The speech sounds of English, with several exceptions, are nonnasal, meaning they are produced with the opening between the oral and nasal cavities closed. The opening is closed by raising the velum and inward movement of the sides of the pharynx. Upward and backward movements of the velum are accomplished by the *palatal levator muscle* that inserts into the central sheet of connective tissue of the velum and extends upward and backward to insert on a prominence of the temporal bone. Additional muscle fibers may aid in tensing the velum. During speech production, movements of the velum are actively utilized to open and close the velopharyngeal port for nasal and nonnasal speech sounds.

To this point, the fixed and mobile articulators have been viewed independently and their actions considered in isolation. It is important to remember that respiratory, phonatory, and articulatory movements are overlapping and conjoined in a complex series of actions during the production of speech. We will consider this topic after a discussion of sound sources for speech.

Speech Production

The vocal tract serves as a resonator or filter and as a site for the development of sound sources for speech production. We previously described the complex acoustic waveform created by movements of the vocal folds. Additional noise-like sound sources are created in the vocal tract during speech production.

Acoustic resonance is the response of air within an enclosed space such that some components of the sound are amplified (increased) while others are attenuated (decreased). In other words, there is a redistribution of acoustic energy.

The complex periodic sound produced at the larynx is comprised of a **fundamental frequency** equal to the frequency of vocal fold vibration and **harmonics,** that is, whole numbered multiples of this frequency. If the fundamental frequency is 100 Hz, then energy also is present at 200 Hz, 300 Hz, 400 Hz, and so forth up to 4000 Hz but not at frequencies in between these points. The waveform is filtered by the acoustic resonant characteristics of the vocal tract. We have some experience with this type of filtering. If you watch a trombone player, she moves the slide to make the instrument longer or shorter. With increases in the length of the tube and total volume of the tube, there are reductions in the pitch of the instrument. With a shortening of the tube and reduction of the volume, the pitch is higher. The sound source for the instrument is produced by a "buzzing" of the lips, which activates the enclosed volume of air whose response is determined by the size and shape of the instrument. A longer tube with a larger volume responds best to low frequency; a shorter tube with smaller volume responds best to higher frequency components of the complex waveform created by the lips.

The vocal tract is a more complex resonator than a band instrument. It is open at one end and closed at the other and varies in important respects from the hollow pipe that we may blow across to produce sound. First, the vocal tract is not a hard-walled tube, but rather is lined with muscosal tissue that serves to absorb part of the sound energy and is shaped like a cavity than a tube. Second, the vocal tract can be constricted at more than a single point to form more than a single volume and may be used to create more than a single sound source. Finally, coupling of the nasal cavity with the oral and pharyngeal cavities produces a complex filtering that produces a reduction of energy within some frequency regions.

Consonants are classified uniquely on the basis of three parameters—the place of constriction, the manner of production, and whether or not they are voiced. (See Chapter 4 for a discussion of this classification.) The place of articulation can be described, for example, as bilabial, lingualveolar, lingua-palatal, or some other point of constriction in the vocal tract. The manner of production addresses how the sound is produced, as a stop, nasal, fricative, affricate, and so on. Consonants can be described as voiced, as in the sound /b/, or unvoiced as in /p/. Accordingly, /b/ would be described as a bilabial voiced stop, /s/ as a lingualveolar unvoiced fricative, and /m/ as a bilabial nasal. All vowels, diphthongs, semivowels, and nasals are voiced; fricatives, stops, and affricates may be voiced or unvoiced.

Vowels are produced with vocal fold vibration (voicing) and with a relatively open vocal tract; that is, there are no points where the flow of air is obstructed. The resonances for vowels, termed **formants,** are determined by the place of constriction or narrowing in the oral cavity (front, central, back), by the degree of constriction, and by lip rounding. For front and central vowels, the place and degree of constriction is a good approximation to predicting the formants. The degree of lip rounding primarily affects back vowels in English.

The **source filter theory** of vowel production proposes that sound energy produced by the vocal folds is modified by the filter characteristics of the vocal tract. The vowels of English have different formants, then, because of different filtering characteristics determined by the vocal tract shape. **Diphthongs** are speech sounds produced by movement from one vowel position to a following vowel position while maintaining vocal fold vibration in words such as *buy* and *toy*. They vary based on regional dialects. In some cases, particularly in the southeastern United States, words like *white* and *oil* are produced with long vowels rather than diphthongs.

Semivowels are consonants produced with greater constriction of the vocal tract than for vowels but less than for other consonants. These sounds, /l/, /r/, /j/, and /w/ are characterized by a rapid transition from a vowel position to a following vowel. An example is the cartoon hero Popeye whose motto "I yam what I yam" typifies this rapid transition. *Nasals* such as /m/ and /n/ are produced with an open velopharyx that results in the creation of anitresonances, areas in the acoustic spectrum where there is a marked reduction in intensity of the sound produced in the oral cavity.

Aperiodic sound sources are produced when airflow becomes turbulent at a constriction. There are two types of noise-like sound sources of this type produced in English. If a narrow constriction is created in the airway, the airflow becomes turbulent and a friction noise is created. In English, these sounds, like /s/ and /z/, are termed *fricatives*. A second type of turbulence occurs when the flow of air through the oral cavity is stopped and then suddenly released. A burst of noise is created that characterizes sounds like /p/ and /b/, which are termed *stops*. There also are two sounds in English, termed *affricates,* that are produced as a stop combined with a fricative, the *ch* sound in *church* and the *j* sound in *judge*.

Speech sounds are not produced in isolation; the unit of programming is most likely the syllable. If you produce the word *construe* you will notice that the lips begin to round for the *-ue* before the vowel is produced. This anticipation of upcoming sounds to be produced is a form of **coarticulation,** the overlapping of articulatory movements for the production of sounds. Coarticulation suggests that more than one sound at a time is being programmed for production.

Speech production is accomplished by a series of overlapping articulatory movements that have sufficient specificity to allow individual speech sounds and syllables to be perceived. In this process there is a specification of aero-dynamic and structural targets but the goal of the system is to accomplish auditory goals. These auditory goals can be gained from more than a single underlying vocal tract shape or sequence of shapes. Try this for yourself. Produce the word *Albuquerque* with your teeth clenched on a pencil. You will notice that you can produce the word almost identically with or without your jaw included within the articulatory program because you have an intimate knowledge, gained through years of practice, of what shapes of the vocal tract will give you similar acoustic output. *Motor equivalence* is based on the observation that an auditory goal can be reached with various combinations of articulatory movements that shape the vocal tract.

Suprasegmentals

Suprasegmentals include aspects of speech motor programming that are longer than individual segments and include stress, intonation, and rhythm. Stress that signals a distinction between a verb and a noun (con-TRACT vs. CONtract) is termed lexical stress. Stress marking that denotes important aspects of the meaning of a phrase ("John caught a FISH" vs. "JOHN caught a fish") is called prosodic stress. The intonation of the sentence that is important for signaling a grammatical distinction is called linguistic prosody. For example, we differentiate the declarative compared to the interrogative grammatical form of the phrase "He bought the car" on the basis of the intonational contour of the sentence. Try saying this sentence as a question and as a statement. Notice the difference? Intonation also is important in conveying emotional aspects of the message. Sadness, fear, surprise, sarcasm, happiness, and so forth all are imparted through the intonational contour (emotional prosody) and facial expression of the speaker.

SUMMARY

Speech production is a complex behavior that requires the coordination of respiratory, laryngeal, and articulatory systems. The speech output of this coordinated activity is programmed by the nervous system based on our experience of the relationship between vocal tract shapes and acoustic outcomes. The speech sounds of the language can be described from the vantage point of their manner (how), place of production (where), and voicing (vocal fold vibration), but are programmed in longer units of output including syllables and prosodic elements.

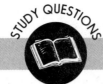

1 Describe three sound sources for speech production.

2 How are consonants different from vowels?

3 What are the parts of the vocal tract?

4 Why does increasing the length of the vocal folds increase their frequency of vibration?

5 What is the difference between static and mobile articulators?

6 What change in respiratory activity would be needed to talk louder?

7 Why is the vocal fold frequency of vibration higher for women than men?

8 What are some functions of the larynx in addition to its role as a sound source for speech?

9 What is a formant?

10 What are the major structures of the central nervous system?

11 Describe the representation of speech and language in the nervous system.

12 How do neurons differ from glial cells?

13 Which cranial nerves are most important to speech production?

14 Compare the functions of the pyramidal and extrapyramidal tracts.

15 Describe three places for consonant production.

REFERENCES

Kent, R. (1997). *The speech sciences.* San Diego: Singular Publishing Group.

Kent, R., & Read, W. (1992). *The acoustic analysis of speech.* San Diego: Singular Publishing Group.

Minifie, F. (Ed.). (1994). *Introduction to communication sciences and disorders.* San Diego: Singular Publishing Group.

SUGGESTED READINGS

Kent, R. (1997). *The speech sciences.* San Diego: Singular Publishing Group.

Minifie, F., Hixon, T., & Williams, F. (Eds.). (1973). *Normal aspects of speech, language and hearing.* Englewood Cliffs, NJ: Prentice-Hall.

Webster, D. B. (1999). *Neuroscience of communication* (2nd ed.). San Diego: Singular Publishing Group.

Zemlin, W. (1968). *Speech and hearing science.* Englewood Cliffs, NJ: Prentice-Hall.

GLOSSARY

Adduction: Movement toward the midline.

Afferent: Axonal fibers that conduct impulses toward the central nervous system.

Basal ganglia: A group of subcortical structures that include the putamen, globus pallidus, and caudate that contribute to control of motor behavior.

Bernoulli effect: As the velocity of airflow increases, pressure decreases with total energy remaining constant.

Broca's area: Brodmann's area 44 located on the third frontal gyrus anterior to the precentral face area.

Cerebral hemispheres: Two major parts of the cerebrum joined by the corpus callosum.

Coarticulation: Overlapping of articulatory and acoustic patterns of speech production due to anticipation or retention of a speech feature.

Corpus callosum: Fiber pathways joining the cerebral hemispheres.

Efferent: Conduction away from a central structure.

Extrapyramidal Tract: Indirect motor pathway made up of networks of neurons.

Formant: A resonance of the vocal tract.

Fundamental frequency: The lowest frequency (first harmonic) of a complex periodic waveform.

Glial cells: Support cells of the nervous system.

Glottis: Opening between the vocal folds.

Gyri: Folds of the cerebral cortex

Harmonic: An integer multiple of the fundamental frequency.

Meninges: Tissue coverings overlying the central nervous system.

Myelin: White fatty covering of an axon.

Neurotransmitters: Chemical messengers of the nervous system

Prosody: The intonation and rhythm of a spoken language.

Pyramidal tract: Major motor pathway from cerebral cortex to brainstem and spinal cord.

Resting expiratory level: Mechanically neutral position of the respiratory system.

Rolandic fissue: Fissure that divides posterior frontal lobe from anterior pareital lobe.

Source-filter theory: An acoustic theory of speech production that states a sound energy source is modified by the filter charactertistics of the vocal tract.

Sulci: Furrows of the cerebral cortex

Sylvian fissure: Horizontal fissure superior to the temporal lobe.

Tidal volume: Quantity of air exchanged during quiet breathing.

Thalamus: Structure located at either side of the third venticle; responsible for sensorimotor integration and sensory projection to the cerebral cortex.

Vital capacity: Controllable air in the lungs; total volume of air that can be expired after a maximum inspiration.

Wernicke's area: Posterior part of first temporal gyrus important for auditory processing and comprehension.

10

Articulatory and Phonological Disorders

Barbara L. Davis and Lisa M. Bedore

LEARNING OBJECTIVES

1 To understand the distinction between an articulation disorder and a phonological disorder.

2 To understand the causes of articulation and phonological disorders in children and adults.

3 To learn what factors are important in describing the severity of articulation and phonological disorders.

4 To understand how articulation and phonological disorders are related to language disorders in children.

5 To differentiate between organic and functional articulation and phonological disorders.

6 To learn how articulation and phonological disorders are identified and treated.

INTRODUCTION

We are all capable of making many different types of sounds by changing the configuration of the articulators (the lips, tongue, teeth, jaw, and velum). When we communicate our ideas about the world around us, we produce specific kinds of sounds, called **phonemes** (e.g., /b/ or /a/), that we sequence together in a variety of ways to form words. Recall from Chapter 2 that **phonology** is the term for the language conventions (or rules) that govern how phonemes are combined to make words. The *ability* to produce sounds in sequence by moving the articulators is referred to as **articulation.** Articulation is somewhat different than other motor activities such as skiing, where Olympic athletes are always better than the rest of us at performance. With respect to speech production, nearly all normal adult speakers of a language are proficient at producing strings of speech sounds that are correct and easily understood by others.

People with articulation and phonological disorders produce words that sound different than the words that are produced by most other speakers of a language. Because language is most often expressed through speech, severe difficulties with articulation can negatively affect the way linguistic knowledge (phonology, morphology, semantics, syntax, and pragmatics) is expressed. As you might expect, this has a negative affect on communication. That is why speech-language pathologists (SLPs) are interested in describing, assessing and treating people with articulation and phonological disorders.

Articulation and phonological disorders are among the most common types of communication disorder treated by speech-language pathologists (SLPs). As a result, articulation and phonology are considered core aspects of the scope of practice of certified speech-language pathologists. Few of these professionals will deliver assessment and intervention services in any work setting without a portion of the caseload being comprised of clients with some component of their communication disorder characterized as articulation or phonological impairment.

Our primary interest in this chapter is children, but we discuss aspects of speech sound production disorders that are equally applicable to children and adults. First, we describe the population of interest. Next, we discuss the tools for describing speech disorders, including a framework for understanding what is normal in speech development. Last, we provide an overview of assessment and treatment procedures for individuals with speech disorders.

CD-ROM

Overview of CD-ROM Segments for Chapter 10

In the CD-ROM segments for this chapter you will view examples of children with articulation and/ or phonological disorders.
Ch.10.01: A child with an expressive language disorder that co-occurs with a speech disorder.
Ch.10.02: A child with a mild speech sound production disorder.
Ch.10.03: A child with a severe speech disorder.
Ch.10.04: Use of gestures by a child with a severe speech disorder.
Ch.10.05: A young child with delayed speech development.

DEFINITION AND INCIDENCE

It is important to distinguish between an articulation disorder and a phonological disorder because this distinction is critical for the way speech production problems are assessed, described, and treated. Children or adults may have difficulty producing the sounds and sound sequences of their language (an **articulation disorder**) or with understanding and implementing the underlying rules for producing sounds and sequences (a **phonological disorder**). An individual with an **articulation disorder** may have difficulty with the movements of the vocal folds, lips, tongue, teeth, and jaw that are necessary for the production of understandable speech. An example of a simple articulation disorder would be the substitution of a /w/ where /r/ is expected (e.g., *wed* for *red*). An example of a more complex articulation disorder would be the person with cerebral palsy who has difficulty coordinating and controlling respiration, phonation, and articulation. This person may know exactly what she wants to say. Nevertheless, she may not have adequate control over the movements of her articulators, causing most sounds to be produced in an unusual manner. She may also have breath support for only one or two words at a time. As a result, listeners may have a difficult time understanding what this individual is saying. These types of disorders are discussed in greater detail in Chapter 14.

A **phonological disorder,** in contrast, is considered to be a deficiency in the abstract system of knowledge that forms the rule system for sounds and sequences needed to convey a message in a given language. That is, a person may not have developed adequate mental representations of the sound system of the language that surrounds him. An example of a simple phonological disorder would be the English-speaking child who thinks that the affricate *ch* (/tʃ/) and the fricative *sh* (/ʃ/) are completely interchangeable. (These sounds are interchangeable in some languages, but not in English.) The child can produce both sounds correctly, but he mistakenly uses one for the other, saying *shair* for *chair* or *choe* for *shoe*. An example of a more complex phonological disorder would be the child who represents the fricative sounds (/ʃ/ (sh), /θ/ (th), /s/, /z/, /f/, and /v/) with the stop /t/, but uses fricatives like /ʃ/ (sh) to represent the affricates /ʤ/ (j) and /ʧ/ (ch). The child might say the word *ship* as *tip,* but he would say the word *chip* as *ship*. We know this is a phonological problem and not necessarily an articulation problem because the child demonstrates the ability to produce fricatives. Yet, he represents fricatives with stops when he produces words.

Some children have difficulty with both articulation and phonology simultaneously. For example, a child with a history of chronic otitis media accompanied by a mild hearing loss may not have been able to hear speech clearly. Such a child may not develop the same mental representation of speech sounds as a child with normal hearing. At the same time, this child will not have been able to monitor her productions and thus may not know if she is producing sounds or sound sequences correctly. Other children with both articulation and phonological disorders are those with severe limitations in the number of sounds they can produce. We have seen 5-year-old children whose inventory of speech sounds include only the nasals /m/ and /n/, the stops /p/, /b/, /t/, and /d/, and a few vowels. As a result of producing so few sounds, these children have developed unusual representations of the phonology of the language.

It can be quite difficult to determine whether a child has difficulty with articulation alone or with both articulation and phonology. However, as we discuss later, many assessment and intervention approaches are specifically designed to evaluate or treat either articulation problems or phonological problems. We use the term *articulation disorder* when we are referring to difficulties producing speech sounds and the term *phonological disorder* when we are referring to difficulties with phonological rules.

A FRAMEWORK FOR UNDERSTANDING ARTICULATION AND PHONOLOGY

Two scientific perspectives have been utilized for understanding individuals who have difficulty with speech production, speech perception, and phonological knowledge. Physiological systems for producing and perceiving speech have been the focus of phonetic science. Speaker knowledge of speech sounds in a language has been studied as an aspect of phonological science. The most salient difference between these perspectives is that phonetic science emphasizes the physical ability to produce speech, and phonological science emphasizes the acquisition of the rules for combining sounds to produce words in a specific language such as English or French. Both perspectives on understanding of speech have been employed by SLPs in assessment and treatment of clients with speech production deficits.

Phonetic Science

The discipline of phonetic science studies the three major subsystems of the body that are involved in producing speech: the respiratory system, the phonatory system, and the articulatory system. Chapter 9 provides an in-depth look at speech production processes. In addition, speech is served by perceptual processes of audition (hearing sounds) and discrimination (sorting sounds into recognizable categories). Perception is crucially important for acquisition of speech production skills as well as for ongoing speaker self-monitoring of the adequacy of speech production. Recall that speech perception was described in Chapters 6 and 7. Individuals with difficulty in the physiological processes involved in producing and perceiving speech are usually termed articulation disordered.

Phonological Science

Speech is a system that is used to relate meaning with sounds. For meaning to be conveyed in a message, the speaker and listener must share a common understanding of how specific sounds and sound sequences are combined to form words. Recall from Chapter 2 that the individual sounds in a language are called **phonemes.** A phoneme is the smallest unit in a language that conveys meaning (i.e., /p/ and /b/ are phonemes used to convey the difference between *pig* and *big*). Two different types of phonemes, consonants and vowels, were discussed in Chapter 2. Recall that consonants are described by where they are produced (place of articulation) and how they are produced (manner of articulation), in addition to whether they are voiced or not (i.e., are the vocal folds vibrating). Vowels (e.g., /a/, /i/, /o/, etc.) are made with a relatively open vocal tract and alternate with consonants to create syllables (see Tables 2–1, 2–2, and 2–3 in Chapter 2).

A variety of systems of analysis have been employed to describe difficulties in using the sounds and sound sequences of language. **Distinctive features** (Chomsky & Halle, 1968) reflect the underlying units of knowledge that are used to construct sounds in words. There are 15 binary ($\pm$) features in Chomsky and Halle's system, and each phoneme has it own "distinctive" set of features. For example, the sound /n/ is termed a nasal sound because air moves through the nose. In distinctive feature terminology, /n/ is +nasal, meaning that it is stored mentally as a +nasal sound. The other features of /n/ include +sonorant (spontaneous voicing is possible), +consonantal (there is obstruction in the oral cavity), +anterior (the obstruction is at the alveolar ridge), +coronal (the front part of the tongue is raised), and +voiced (the vocal folds are vibrating). The phoneme /n/ also has a minus (−) value for mean features. For example, it is −syllabic (it's not a vowel), −strident (the airstream does not produce a high frequency noise), and −lateral (it is not produced by lowering the sides of the tongue). From a distinctive feature perspective, an individual with a phonological disorder or delay may have difficulty retrieving and using the mentally stored units that specify sounds. In addition, the individual may not have figured out one or more of the important features of the language he speaks.

Another system for describing mental representations of sound is called **phonological processes.** Phonological processes are variations in the way phonemes are combined. For example, when two sounds are produced in rapid sequence, they become more like each other. This is the process of assimilation. For example, vowels that are followed by nasals tend to become nasalized. This happens because the velum lowers for the nasal consonant while the vowel is still being produced. Say the words *fan* and *fad*. Can you hear how the vowel in *fan* is more nasalized? Another common phonological process is called deletion. In English, the last phoneme in a consonant cluster like /st/ is deleted when the cluster appears at the end of a word that is followed immediately by a word that begins with a voiceless consonant. For example, the final /t/ in the word *most* and the initial /t/ in the word *teams* are rarely produced separately in the phrase *most teams*. Unlike distinctive features that describe differences between the individual phonemes in a language, phonological processes are ways to describe phonological rules that operate above the level of the individual phoneme.

ARTICULATION AND PHONOLOGICAL DISORDERS

There are a number of important factors to consider in understanding and treating articulation and phonological disorders. In this section, we consider the concepts of disorder versus delay, the severity of disorders and delays, issues related to dialects, the etiology of articulation and phonological disorders, and the co-occurrence of articulation and phonological disorders with other types of communication disorders.

Delay Versus Disorder

Description of articulation and phonological development as disordered or delayed is based on comparison of the child's speech to the articulation and phonological patterns of children of a comparable age who are developing normally. Recall the discussion of early, middle, and late developing sounds in Chapter 2. Children who are considered to have delayed articulation development have speech production patterns that typically occur in children who are younger. For example, a 5-year-old child may produce all the sounds of English but may have difficulty using them at the ends of words, resulting in a pattern where *top, cat,* and *kiss* are produced as "to_," "ca_," and "ki_." Normally developing children between the ages of 24 and 36 months often leave off the ends of words. An older child who presents this pattern would be considered to have an articulation delay because she is producing speech like a child who is chronologically 24–36 months old. A 38-month-old child who produces only one-syllable words beginning with "b" and "d" (i.e., "ba" for *ball* and "da" for *doll*) and no consonants at the end would also be considered to be speech delayed. She would be described as speaking like a child 12–15 months old who normally might use few different consonants and produce mainly one-syllable words.

 CD-ROM

Brian

In CD-ROM segement Ch.10.05, Brian, age 5, demonstrates delayed speech production abilities for his age. In talking with his clinician about the "good guy and the bad guy cars," he is difficult to understand. His most obvious error is the use of a "t" sound where he should use a "k" sound. View segment Ch.10.05 again and see if you can understand Brian now that you know which sound is substituted. His delay is considered moderate because he is talking in long sentences and is somewhat difficult for an unfamiliar listener to understand.

In contrast to children with a **speech delay,** children with a **speech disorder** do not produce speech that is like children who are developing normally. A 10-year-old child who produces speech that is whispered and contains mostly vowels with only a few consonants shows skills that are not like a normally developing child of any age. She would be described as disordered. Adults who lose speech or phonological abilities after having intact skills are always designated as disordered because their speech production skills are not like the skills seen in other adults.

Severity of Involvement

The severity of a speech delay or disorder is related to several important aspects of speech production:

1. the number of sounds produced correctly (e.g., If the child is saying the word *watermelons,* how many of the sounds does she say correctly?),

2. the accuracy of production (e.g., saying "*dall*" for "*ball*"),

3. the ability to produce sounds in different word positions (saying "l" in both *like* and in ki*ll*),

4. the ability to produce sound sequences (saying *blu* instead of the simpler *bu*), and

5. the ability to produce various types of words (saying *top* as well as *marginal*).

Each of these factors is related to speech intelligibility. **Intelligibility** is the understandability of spontaneous speech, and it is a crucial factor for determining the need for and the effectiveness of therapy (Bernthal & Bankson, 1998).

Three adjectives are often used indicate the degree of impairment: *mild, moderate,* and *severe.* Table 10–1 provides examples of how hypothetical children with mild, moderate, and severe speech impairments would produce a list of words of varying complexity. Mildly involved children have problems producing only a few sounds. They are able to produce most of the sounds of their language and can use these sounds in sequences both within words and in varied types of words. Children whose only speech errors are the substitution of /θ/ for /s/ ("thee" for *see*) or the substitution of /w/ for /r/ ("wabbit" for *rabbit*) are considered to be mildly speech delayed. Individuals with mild delays are generally intelligible to most listeners, but their speech errors call attention to the way they speak. Frequently, the sounds that are produced incorrectly by these individuals are those identified in Chapter 2 as in the "late 8" group. Individuals with mild delays or disorders usually have excellent treatment outcomes.

The child with *moderate* impairment has more difficulty producing speech sounds correctly than the mildly involved child. A 4-year-old child with a moderate speech disorder may have difficulty producing all velar sounds where the back of the tongue approximates the top of the mouth (i.e., /k/, /g/, and /ŋ/ as in *k*ite, *g*o and ki*ng*). Moderately involved children may use sounds incorrectly in different word positions such as /d/ in place of /t/ at the ends of

Table 10–1. Examples of How Hypothetical 4-Year-Old Children With Mild, Moderate, or Severe Speech Disorders Might Produce Selected Words

Target Word	Mild	Moderate	Severe
Soup	/sup/	/tup/	/tu/
Rabbit	/wæbɪt/	/wæbɪ/	/æʔɪ/
Yellow	/jɛwo/	/wɛwo/	/ɛo/
Crayon	/kweɪən/	/keɪən/	/eɪə/
Butterfly	/bʌdəfwaɪ/	/bʌfaɪ/	/ʌaɪ/
Refrigerator	/wifwɪdəweɪdə/	/fɪdəweɪə/	/wɪ/

CD-ROM

Alex

In CD-ROM segment Ch.10.02, Alex, age 3, exhibits a mild speech delay for his chronological age. His speech is intelligible, but calls attention to the way he speaks because some of the sounds are missing or incorrect. Here he is looking at a book with the clinician and he says, "A dwaf, a pinwin, teddy beo" to describe a giraffe, a penguin, and a teddy bear. How would you describe his errors?

words (i.e., "po*d*" for "po*t*"). These children often have difficulty producing all the syllables in multisyllabic words (i.e., [pamus] for *hippopotamus*), leave sounds off the ends of words (i.e., "do" instead of *dog*), and simplify some **consonant clusters** (two consonants "clustered" together without an intervening vowel) as in "bu" for *blue*. Children with moderate speech disorders are mostly intelligible to familiar listeners such as parents or family members, but they may not be understood by unfamiliar listeners, especially when the listener is not sure what the individual is talking about. Moderately involved clients have a good prognosis for improvement, although the course of therapy may be longer than for children with mild difficulties.

 CD-ROM

Andrew

In CD-ROM segment Ch.10.03, Andrew, age 7, is talking to the clinician about his dog. He notes that he has a new dog, and his big dog knows how to swim. He is very difficult to understand in this segment. These types of errors in a child age 7 connote a severe speech impairment. What types of errors do you hear?

Severe speech or phonological involvement is found in individuals who are unintelligible to most listeners or who may not be able to use speech consistently to communicate. These individuals usually produce more than six sounds in error. They do not sequence sounds consistently to produce intelligible words. As a consequence, their ability to use sounds to communicate effectively is limited. Children with severe speech disorders may resort to using gestures to get their message across. For example, a 6-year-old child who only produces four different consonants, uses vowels inconsistently, and primarily gestures for communication would be considered to have a severe speech disorder. A 12-year-old child with cerebral palsy who does not have adequate control over breathing to support speech production would also have a severe disorder.

In very severe cases, a speech-language pathologist may decide to use augmentative communication systems (i.e., systems in which the client pushes a button or points to a picture) as an alternative method for communication. Unfortunately, children with severe speech or phonological disorders often have a less positive long-term prognosis than mildly or moderately involved children.

 CD-ROM

Andrew 2

In CD-ROM segment Ch.10.04, Andrew is using gestures to supplement his comments about where he is going. The use of gesture is typical for Andrew and for individuals with severe problems with intelligibility, because it helps to convey the message to the listener. In this instance, Andrew's gestures are not sufficient to help Jena understand exactly what he is trying to say.

Language and Dialect

There are an increasing number of speakers of languages whose rules for producing the sounds and sequences of sounds do not match English. The result is widely differing types of pronunciation found among nonnative speakers of English. Recall from Chapter 3 that speakers who have some competence in English, but who have a different primary language, are termed **bilinguals.** These speakers have the same ability to produce speech sounds and sequences; they simply have different rules for how to produce them based on the requirements of their primary language. If you have tried to learn a second or third language, you might have noticed you do not produce words, phrases, and sentences in the same manner as native speakers of the language you are learning. One reason is that you are not proficient at producing the specific sound types and sequences of sounds of the new language. For example, there are no "b," "d," or "g" sounds at the ends of German words. English speakers learning German may use these sounds at the ends of German words since they are present in English (e.g., *mob*). When speaking English, you will not spend time thinking about how to produce sounds or how to order them when you ask your roommate "Where are your car keys?" In contrast, you may labor consciously in German to produce sounds correctly and to put them in order in ways that are different from your English pronunciation patterns.

It is important to discern dialectal differences from speech disorders. If a child's speech errors are related to learning a second language (i.e., the Latino child who says "shiken" for *chicken* because the "sh" is an allophone of the "ch" sound in Spanish), the patterns are considered to be sound differences rather than delay or disorder. Children whose phonological production patterns are different because they are applying the phonological patterns of their first language to their second or third language are not usually placed in speech therapy. Children who have adequate speech production abilities and good language-learning capabilities often develop production patterns that are consistent with the phonological rules of the second language they are learning.

Adults who learn a new language late in life and who need to master the phonology of the language quickly may seek the assistance of SLPs in order to improve their intelligibility. For example, a Japanese businessman who needs to be more intelligible to accomplish his business goals in the United States may seek the assistance of an SLP. Persons like this are frequently served by SLPs in private practice settings. It is important to remember that dialectal differences are not delays or disorders. However, adults who are trying to master the phonological system of a new language in a short period of time may enroll in speech therapy.

Etiology

Finding a cause for an articulation or phonological disorder in children is often quite difficult. Many children with articulation or phonological impairment are termed as having **functional speech impairment.** A functional impairment indicates that the cause of differences in speech development from normally developing children simply cannot be determined. With these individuals, the SLP describes articulation and phonological skills carefully and works to change deviant articulatory patterns to speech patterns that are appropriate for the child's chronological age. Behavioral description takes precedence over a search for etiological cause. The clinician does not utilize information about possible causes to plan therapy or to predict the child's prognosis for improvement.

Most phonological disorders and delays are considered to be "functional." We do not know why a child has difficulty representing the phonology of the language that surrounds him. Phonological knowledge is based on descriptions of abstract mental representations of language that have no literal reality in brain structures. No information is available to pinpoint possible etiologies for differences in the ways in which children learn the phonology of their language. Phonological perspectives provide rich descriptions of a child's pattern of differences from normal development; they do not provide explanations of *why* these children are different in their development.

Articulation disorders or delays are more likely to have a known etiology or to be associated with a risk factor for developmental delay. In general, the term *articulation disorder* or *delay* is used when the peripheral organs of speech are involved (i.e., the input system of perceptual organs that receive sensation and discriminate sounds and/or the output system of jaw, tongue, lips, etc. that produce sounds and sequences). Etiologies for articulation delay or disorder fall into three major categories: perceptual or input related etiology, structural etiology, and motor or output-related etiology. Table 10–2 lists examples from each of these major etiological categories for articulation delay or disorder.

Co-Occurrence With Other Types of Disorder

Articulation or phonological disorders can co-occur with other types of speech and language problems. For example, children with expressive or receptive language problems and voice and fluency disorders often have articulation or phonological impairment as well. For example, a second grader may have a problem producing speech sounds at the ends of words. This same child would probably omit many grammatical morphemes in English that happen to occur at the end of words, which would affect his ability to express his ideas in complete sentences (an expressive language disorder).

 CD-ROM

Andrew 3

In CD-ROM segment Ch.10.01, notice that Andrew, age 7, is speaking in incomplete sentences. Instead of including all the sentence elements when he expresses himself, his sentences include only the main words. Andrew is telling his therapist about his dog who swims in the river. What sounds are missing?

Another example of co-occurring speech and language disorders is a 32-month-old child who may be using just four or five words to communicate, all of which contain only a consonant and a vowel put together (e.g., "da" for *doll*). This child may also have difficulty with understanding directions from her mother at home (language comprehension), with grammatical morphemes (plural -s, past tense -ed), and with combining words to form sentences. In these cases, the speech-language pathologist must decide whether to work on both deficits at once or whether to work on each deficit separately. With some careful planning, it is usually possible to work on all of a child's problems at once.

Table 10-2. Examples of Common Etiologies That Are Representative of Major Classes of Organic Etiologies

Disorder Type	Definition	Speech Characteristics
Perceptual Etiology		
Prebycusis	Decline in hearing acuity in adults due to effects of aging.	Distortion of high-frequency speech sounds such as /s/ that are outside of the range of the individual's hearing. Generally these difficulties are classified as *mild*.
Otitis media	Middle ear fluid secondary to ear infection. Hearing loss is mild to moderate and duration of loss is variable.	Fluctuating losses as are observed in children with otitis media are thought to put children at risk for delays in speech development. There is not a distinctive pattern of errors that is associated with this risk factor.
Sensorineural loss	Genetic or postnatal disease processes that result in moderate or severe hearing loss	Children with moderate to severe hearing loss do not hear speech sounds adequately. Thus, it is difficult to impossible for children to learn to produce them without prolonged remediation. These children typically demonstrate *severe* difficulties. You can learn more about the impact of sensorineural hearing loss on speech and language in Chapter 7.
Structural Etiology		
Cleft lip and palate	Oral-facial malformations resulting from interruption of development during the prenatal period.	Children's speech may be very nasal even after closure of the palate. Children may have difficulty producing speech sounds that require high pressure such as /s/ or "ch." You can learn more about cleft lip and palate in Chapter 12.
Motor Etiology		
Dysarthria	Neuromuscular impairment resulting in speech disorder.	Speakers with dysarthria have difficulties with respiration, phonation, articulation, resonance, and prosody. Speech involvement is usually *moderate to severe*. You can learn more about dysarthria in Chapter 14 in the section on cerebral palsy.
Apraxia	Neurological damage resulting in inconsistent speech production abilities.	The difficulties observed in the speaker with apraxia are due to the inability to plan or program speech. Apraxia affects speech intelligibility and prosody. Errors are typically inconsistent and more likely to occur as length increases.

ASSESSMENT AND TREATMENT

Infants, children, and adults form a dramatically diverse population of individuals who need assessment and remediation for articulation and phonological delays and disorders. The goal of assessment is to determine the specific nature and severity of the disorder or delay. Specific assessment procedures and materials will be needed relative to the suspected etiology and the chronological and developmental age and the primary language spoken. Using the information gathered, specific analysis procedures are employed to understand the patterns of difference between the individual's productions and the relevant comparison population. Decisions about treatment will be based on results of the assessment and analysis.

Collecting Information

Speech Samples

Suspected articulation or phonological impairment requires analysis of a **spontaneous speech and language sample** to evaluate the use and integrity of speech production skills in communication. Clinicians collect a speech sample by simply talking and playing with the child. The spontaneous sample is analyzed to determine the child's ability to produce consonants, vowels, and sequences characteristic of the primary language community. Children with very severe impairment may not use vocalization consistently to communicate. In these cases, the use of gestures or other ways the person has to communicate and the intentionality of vocalizations needs to be evaluated.

Articulation Tests

If the child is capable of naming pictures or objects, a **single word articulation test** may be administered to assess the ability to produce consonants in varied word positions. The *Goldman-Fristoe Test of Articulation* (Goldman & Fristoe, 1969, 1986), for example, samples the consonants of English in all word positions. Vowels in English are not consistently tested by single word tests however. Very young, very old, and/or very impaired individuals may not be able to participate in a structured single word test of articulation. In addition, individuals who are bilingual may not be tested validly on tests developed for English speakers. In these cases the spontaneous sample is the only source of information for analyzing oral communication skills. Regardless of whether we obtain samples of single word production from an articulation test or from spontaneous speech, we would be interested in several measures of phonological development. We would evaluate the number of speech sounds that are correctly produced or determine if children could use complex phonological structures such as consonant clusters (e.g., str-) or multisyllabic words (e.g., *refrigerator*). We will discuss the ways of analyzing phonological behaviors in more detail in the next section. In Table 10–3, we present a brief case summary. This child's speech was assessed using the *Goldman-Fristoe Test of Articulation* as well as a spontaneous speech and language sample.

Analyzing Speech

In severely impaired individuals, regardless of age or etiology, the range of behaviors used for intentional communication is described (e.g., gestures, sign language, use of vision in gaze, or overall body orientation). In addition, types of behaviors (such as vowel vocalizations or ability to use fingers to point) that are not intentionally used for communication must be described. The presence of these behaviors is important for planning where to start a treatment program designed to move toward intentional communication in these severely involved clients.

In individuals who use vocalization for communication, either phonetic or phonological analysis may be employed, depending on the nature of the child's disorder or delay. The clinician is seeking to (1) describe typical patterns of speech production skills and (2) compare those skills to an appropriate group of speakers to plan treatment. The clinician may also employ information about etiology (if it is known) to understand the nature of the client's production deficits. For example, a child with a high-frequency hearing loss may have difficulty with producing sounds such as "s," which are high in the acoustic frequency spectrum. A child with a cleft palate may have trouble with sounds that require a build up of oral pressure due to impaired ability to close the opening between the nose and mouth during speech production.

As has been noted, articulation and phonological skills consist of sounds and sequences of sounds used to communicate. Speech analysis consists of describing consonant and vowel sounds the client can produce and how they are used in sequences (i.e., "b," "a," and "t" can be combined to produce *bat*). In every case, the client's skills are compared to those of his peer group (i.e., 5-year-olds are compared to other 5-year-olds, adult speakers to other adults) to determine if the patterns are different enough from the comparison group to warrant treatment.

An analysis of articulation skills focuses on how the three major peripheral body subsystems (articulatory, phonatory, and respiratory) work together to produce speech. Articulation skills (articulatory), vocal fold coordination with articulators (phonatory), and breath support (respiratory) for speech are described. Specific to articulation, the way(s) in which the tongue, jaw, lips, and palate work together to produce speech sounds and sequences are recorded in detail, and patterns of differences from the comparison group are described. A clinician may note that all sounds made with the tongue tip are deleted and substituted by sounds made with the lips (e.g., "d," "s," and "r" are produced as "b," "m," and "w"). Traditional methods of describing articulation skills include the descriptors of *substitution, omission,* and *distortion.* **Substitutions** are when one sound is produced or substituted for another sound (i.e., the child says "bog" for *dog*). **Omissions** occur when a sound is left out of a word (i.e., the client says "to_" for *top*). **Distortions** are sounds produced in a recognizable but inaccurate manner (i.e., a "slushy" sounding "s" sound). Regarding phonation, use of the vocal folds to produce sound is described. The client may use voiced sounds (where the vocal folds are vibrating while the client moves the articulators) for all voiceless sounds because she does not have good control in coordinating phonation and articulation. Since the vocal folds are always vibrating, the client produces all voiced sounds. Respiratory or breath support for speech production is also an aspect of analysis. Most clients who have difficulty producing adequate breath support for speaking are more severely involved (e.g., clients with cerebral palsy who have poor general muscle control). In general, an analysis of articulation skills focuses on patterns of difference in the ways the client uses her body to produce sounds and sequences. You can see an example of the results of the analysis of articulation skills in Table 10–3.

Phonological analysis focuses on description of how the client's speaking reflects underlying mental representations and or rules for producing speech. Emphasis is placed on the client's *knowledge* of the speech sound system rather than any deficit in *behavior* implied by articulation analysis. Many systems of phonological analysis are employed currently. Two of the most prevalent analysis systems make use of distinctive features and phonological processes.

In distinctive feature analysis, the clinician describes features (understood to be mental representations of aspects of the sounds) that are in error. An example of feature analysis would be "+nasal" becomes "−nasal" when a client uses oral sounds "b," "d," and "g" instead of nasal sounds "m," "n," and "ng." In nonlinear phonological analysis (e.g., Goldsmith, 1990), features are described for both consonants and vowels as well as for stress differences within a word (i.e., *hot* dog vs. hot *dog*).

Another method of phonological analysis is called phonological process analysis (Stampe, 1972). Recall that phonological processes are phonological rules for the way sounds are combined into words. One example of a phonological process is "final consonant deletion" in which *ball* becomes "ba" because the child is not yet proficient at putting final sounds on words. "Reduplication" is a phonological process in which the child says the same syllable twice in order to produce a word with more than one syllable (e.g., *bottle* becomes "baba"). Phonological process analysis was used with the child in Table 10–3 as a supplement to analysis of his articulation skills.

Table 10-3. Steps Involved in the Evaluation of a Child With an Articulation Disorder

Davey was referred for speech and language evaluation when he was 3 years and 10 months old. His mother's concern was that his speech was difficult to understand. His siblings understood his speech as did his mother. However, his father did not understand his speech nor did his teachers and peers at school. He was becoming frustrated when others did not understand him. A parental interview revealed nothing remarkable in Davey's developmental history except frequent sore throats and ear infections.

Davey's speech evaluation consisted of several parts. The clinician administered the *Goldman-Fristoe Test of Articulation*, obtained a speech and language sample in the context of play with age-appropriate toys, conducted a hearing screening, and an oral mechanism exam. The evaluation confirmed that Davey's speech was unintelligible approximately 70% of the time to the unfamiliar listener. In addition to phonological errors, the clinician observed that Davey's speech was hyponasal. We will discuss the results of the speech evaluation in more detail below.

Davey passed his hearing screening, but in the oral peripheral examination the clinician observed that Davey's tonsils were extremely inflamed and referred the mother to her pediatrician for follow-up.

The clinician analyzed Davey's speech sample in several ways. Davey obtained a score in the 9th percentile for his age on the *Goldman-Fristoe Test of Articulation*. This indicated that his articulation skills were less well developed than other children his age. Some examples of Davey's productions on the Goldman-Fristoe included:

Telephone	/tɛɪwəpod/
Gun	/dʌd/
Cup	/tʌp/
Chicken	/tɪtə/
Zipper	/dɪpə/
Lamp	/wæp/
Plane	/pweɪd/
Drum	/dʌp/

The clinician followed up with analyses of Davey's phonetic inventory and substitution and omission patterns. She found that he did not yet use many sounds that were expected for his age. For example, he did not yet use velar sounds, suggesting that he had difficulty producing sounds that required him to raise the back of his tongue. She also found that he systematically simplified words using several phonological processes including fronting (the substitution of front sounds for back sounds) and consonant cluster reduction (omission of one or more elements from consonant clusters). Most of Davey's errors appeared to be developmental in nature, but some of his substitution patterns could be attributed to hyponasality (e.g., the substitution of /b/ for /m/ and /d/ for /n/).

The focus of intervention with Davey was on the development of velar sounds /k/ and /g/. Follow-up with Davey's pediatrician led to a referral to the ear, nose, and throat specialist. Soon after intervention began, Davey had his tonsils and adenoids removed. After he recovered from his surgery, his speech was no longer hyponasal and the substitution errors that could be attributed to hyponasality were no longer observed in his speech. At age 4 years and 6 months, Davey was dismissed from intervention. His speech was intelligible at least 90% of the time. He did not yet produce sounds such as /r/, /th/, or /th/. However, because these are later occurring sounds, they were not of concern. Follow-up evaluations at 6 months and 1 year later revealed that he continued to develop speech normally and was acquiring the remaining sounds and clusters as would be expected.

Other Testing

In addition to assessment of speech production skills, an **oral-peripheral examination** may be completed to evaluate the structure and function of peripheral articulators (i.e., tongue, lips, and palate), if the client is capable of complying with the tasks. Again, very young, elderly, or severely impaired clients may not be able to comply with the tasks required in the oral peripheral examination. A *hearing test* is essential to rule out sensory deficit as the cause of the speech disorder or delay. A variety of tests and observations of other aspects of language skills may also be administered, depending on the speech-language pathologist's assessment of the client's communication abilities (see the section on co-occurring disorders). In the case study presented in Table 10–3, you can see how the results of the oral peripheral examination and the hearing screening were used in conjunction with the results of the speech assessment.

Treatment

Treatment for articulation and phonological disorders centers on teaching the client to use sounds and sound sequences of his language like that expected for peers in the community. The overall goal of treatment is age-appropriate intelligibility that meets community standards. Assessment data are employed by the clinician to plan specific goals and treatment techniques for remediation. The clinician will employ either articulation or phonologically oriented treatment approaches based on understanding of the nature of the client's disorder determined during assessment and analysis.

Generally, articulation-based approaches focus more on repetitive motor practice with feedback and attention to how the body is used to produce sounds. For example, a child might be provided with cues to help him or her identify the correct place or manner of articulation. Some examples of cues include touching the alveolar ridge with a tongue blade to help children feel where their tongue needs to go in order to produce alveolar sounds such as a "t" or "d." To indicate the length of a sound such as an "s" the clinician may run her finger up the child's arm. Practice of the speech sounds is usually conducted in short words in activities that provide the child multiple opportunities to produce the target sound at the beginning, middle, and end of words. Then, clinicians work with children on saying the target sound correctly in phrases and sentences. This will help the children incorporate their new articulatory pattern into connected speech.

Phonological approaches emphasize the use of speech sounds to communicate ideas. Many phonological approaches de-emphasize repetition and feedback on motor performance. One such approach, the metaphon approach, relies on building children's metaphonological awareness of speech sounds. This is a way of increasing the child's knowledge of the phonological system. For example, if the child had difficulty with sounds such as "s" and "sh" the clinician might use the analogy that these are hissing sounds to help the child focus on the high-frequency, fricative aspect of these sounds. Children would do intervention activities in which they had to identify the target in the context of games with everyday sounds before turning their attention to speech. In another phonological approach, called contrast therapy, children are shown pairs of pictures that differ from each other by one sound. The pictures are usually selected to demonstrate a distinctive feature or a phonological process that has been determined to be deficient or absent in the child's phonology. For example, children who do not have the feature ± voicing might work on producing pairs of words that differ only on the voicing feature such as *pin – bin, pit – bit, fan – van,* and *sip – zip.* Children who present unusual final consonant deletion processes might work on producing pairs that include words with and without final consonants such as *no – nose, see – seed, tea – team,* and *me – meet.* The key to the contrast approach is to select multiple contrastive pairs that demonstrate the distinctive feature or the phonological process that is problematic for the child.

The area of articulation and phonological disorders is one of the oldest within the scope of practice of the speech-language pathologist. The examples here are intended to provide you with a glimpse of the many well-developed intervention approaches available to the clinician. See Bernthal and Bankson (1998) for a review of techniques and approaches.

Service Delivery

In general, service delivery for articulation and phonological disorders differs dramtically depending on the setting and the age and severity of the client. Infants who do not develop consistent use of vocalization abilities for communication are often served in *early intervention* programs for birth to 3-year-old infants. These infants must be helped to begin using their voice to communicate ideas before they can begin to work on specific sounds and to learn how to use these sounds in words. In *public school educational settings* (clients ranging in age from 3–17), a considerable percentage of the caseload may consist of children who have difficulty with articulation or phonological skills. These children need remediation to help build their ability to produce all the sounds of their language. They also need to learn how to combine the sounds they can produce correctly into words. Children served in public school settings may have mild, moderate, or severe disorders, and they may have a wide variety of etiological factors. Children and adult clients of all ages may be served in *medical settings* such as hospital rehabilitation centers. Clients in these settings tend to have more severe disorders and sometimes require a major commitment to intervention services in order to improve their speech intelligibility.

SUMMARY

Articulation and phonological disorders are a core aspect of the speech-language pathologist's caseload regardless of work setting. From infants who do not begin to talk as expected to the 70-year-old who has a "stroke" and is difficult to understand, clients of all ages and severity levels have problems with intelligibility of oral communication. The clinician may be able to link the client's disorder to a specific etiology, or the client may be considered "functionally" disordered if a cause is not apparent. Assessment procedures must be tuned to the age or developmental stage of each client. However, for all clients, it is crucial to assess speech intelligibility in spontaneous communication if at all possible. For every client, it is important for the clinician to describe how the individual produces consonants, vowels, and sequences of sounds in various words. There are different types of treatment approaches for articulation disorders and phonological disorders. In all cases of articulation and phonological disorder, the goal of treatment is for the client to produce speech that is intelligible to everyone in his or her daily environment.

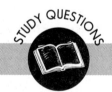

STUDY QUESTIONS

1 What is the difference between articulation disorder and phonological disorder?

2 How do mild, moderate, and severe articulation/phonological disorders differ from each other?

3 What is the difference between articulation or phonological delays and disorders?

4 What are the three possible etiology categories for articulation disorders? Give one example of each.

5 How might articulatory or phonological disorders be related to language disorders?

6 What assessment methods are routinely used during the evaluation of articulatory and phonological disorders?

---

7 Describe an approach to speech analysis that would be appropriate for an articulatory disorder. What analysis approach might be used if the clinician suspects that the child has a phonological disorder?

---

8 Describe one therapy approach for articulation disorders and one approach for phonological disorders.

REFERENCES

Bernthal, J. E., & Bankson, N. W. (1998). *Articulation and phonological disorders.* Boston: Allyn and Bacon.

Chomsky, N., & Halle, M. (1968). *The sound pattern of English.* New York: Harper and Row.

Goldman, R., & Fristoe, M. (1969, 1986). *Goldman-Fristoe Test of Articulation.*

Circle Pines, MN: American Guidance Service.

Goldsmith, J. A. (1990). *Autosegmental and metrical phonology.* Oxford: Basil Blackwell.

Stampe, D. (1972). *A dissertation of natural phonology.* Chicago: University of Chicago.

SUGGESTED READINGS

Ball, M., & Kent, R. (1997). *The new phonologies: Developments in clinical linguistics.* San Diego: Singular Publishing Group.

Bernthal, J. E., & Bankson, N.W. (1998). *Articulation and phonological disorders.* Boston: Allyn and Bacon.

Darley, F. A., Aronson, A., & Brown, J. (1969). Differential diagnostic patterns of dysarthria. *Journal of Speech and Hearing Research, 12,* 246–269.

Vihman, M. M. (1996). *Phonological development: The origins of language in the child.* Oxford, England: Basil Blackwell.

GLOSSARY

Articulation: The physical ability to produce speech sounds. A speaker needs to be able to manipulate the articulators including the tongue, lips, and velum to produce all of the required place and manner distinctions.

Articulation disorder: Difficulty producing speech sounds and speech sound sequences.

Bilingual: Speakers with some competence speaking one or more secondary languages, but a different primary language.

Consonant cluster: Two or more consonants spoken together without an intervening vowel (e.g., *sp*oon, *tr*ee, *bl*ue, *str*ing).

Distinctive features: A system of the component features of sounds (e.g., ± continuant, ± voicing, ± anterior, etc.) that is used for describing the differences between phonemes in a language.

Distortion: A sound is termed "distorted" when the speaker does not achieve the intended articulatory target and the resulting production is not a recognizable phoneme in the child's native language.

Functional speech impairment: The cause of difficulties with speech development cannot be determined precisely.

Intelligibility: The ability to produce speech that someone else understands.

Omission: An articulation error in which a child leaves out a speech sound ("tip" is produced as "ti").

Oral peripheral evaluation: The clinician examines the structures used to produce speech sounds and assesses adequacy of movement of those structures for speech production.

Phoneme: A speech sound that can change meaning (e.g., *p*an – *f*an).

Phonology: Language rules that govern how sounds are combined to create words.

Phonological disorder: Difficulty understanding and implementing the language conventions for producing speech sounds and speech sound sequences.

Phonological processes: Descriptions of variations in the way sounds are produced when they co-occur with other sounds. For example, vowels become more nasal when they are followed by a nasal consonant in words.

Single word articulation test: A test consists of pictures of words. The pictured words usually sample all of the consonants at the initial, medial, and final positions of words. Children are asked to say the name of the object when they see it.

Speech delay: Articulation errors or phonological processes that are often seen in younger, normally developing children.

Speech disorder: Articulation errors or phonological processes rarely seen in normally developing children.

Spontaneous speech and language sample: The clinician gathers a sample of the individual's speech and language in a communication situation that is considered to be the normal way in which the individual communicates using voice, gestures, and nonvocal communication.

Substitution: A speech error in which the child substitutes one sound (usually a sound that is developmentally earlier than the target) for the target sound. Common substitutions are /t/ for /s/ and /w/ for /r/.

11

Cleft Lip and Palate

Rodger M. Dalston

LEARNING OBJECTIVES

1 To understand the embryologic basis of cleft lip and palate.

2 To know the speech consequences of a person's inability to close the velopharyngeal port.

3 To understand the role of the speech/language pathologist (SLP) on a team dedicated to the care of patients with oral-facial clefts.

4 To learn about nasometry and endoscopy and their use in the evaluation of patients seen by speech-language pathologists.

INTRODUCTION

In Chapter 9, you learned about the basic structure and function of the vocal mechanism. That is, you learned how we create an energy source for speech (respiration), change that source from a steady flow to a pulsatile flow

255

(phonation), couple the oral and nasal cavities to ensure appropriate resonance during speech (velopharyngeal activity), and modify the shape of the oral cavity to produce the speech sounds of our language (articulation).

The primary purpose of this chapter is to describe the development and speech consequences of a condition, known as cleft lip and palate, that affects a person's ability to use velopharyngeal movements to control oral-nasal resonance during speech. In Chapter 12, the aim will be to develop an understanding of a variety of disturbances that adversely affect phonation. The latter disturbances are known as voice disorders.

ORAL-FACIAL CLEFTS: AN OVERVIEW

Clefts of the lip with or without associated clefting of the roof of the mouth (palate) are the fourth most frequent birth defect. This condition, which frequently is written "CL ± CP" (Cleft Lip and/or Cleft Palate) occurs in approximately 1 out of every 750 live births among European Americans. For reasons that are not fully understood, CL ± CP occurs about half as often among African Americans and almost twice as often among Asian Americans.

On average, approximately 25% of affected individuals have clefts involving either one or both sides of the lip. If the lip cleft extends all the way up to the base of the nose, there may also be a notch in the alveolar ridge. Even though the alveolar ridge is part of the palate, a child with a cleft of the lip and alveolar ridge is often still described as having a "cleft lip." Other clinicians may describe the same child as having a cleft of the "primary palate." On the surface, that nomenclature seems just as confusing, although there is a reasonable justification for using the latter term. Nevertheless, we will stick with the terms *cleft lip* and *cleft palate* in this chapter.

Approximately 25% of affected individuals have clefts of the palate only. Some palatal clefts are so minimal that special equipment is needed to detect them, whereas others may be extremely wide defects that involve almost the entire roof of the mouth. The remaining 50% of affected children have clefts of both the lip and palate.

Approximately 6 weeks after conception, the structures that will form the roof of the mouth and the face have grown close together and, unless disturbed, will begin the process of uniting with one another to form the palate and lip. The entire process will be completed by the ninth week.

A relatively early disruption of this normally occurring process will result in a complete cleft of the palate that may extend through the lip on one side **(unilateral)** or both sides **(bilateral).** A study model of the palatal vault of a patient with a bilateral complete cleft of the lip and palate is found in Figure 11–1A, and a full-face view of the same (untreated) patient, at a later age, is shown in Figure 11–1B.

Since union of the lip occurs after palate formation begins, it is possible for a child to be born with an intact palate but a cleft of the lip, as noted

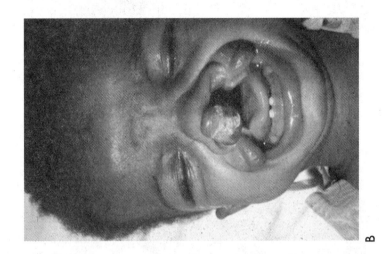

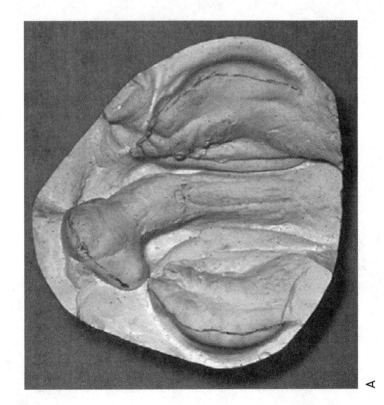

Figure 11–1. Bilateral complete cleft of the lip and palate. **A:** study model of the patient; **B:** full face view of the same patient, at a later age.

previously. Moreover, the extent of lip involvement may be nothing more than a notch in the red part of the lip (vermilion) or it can involve the entire lip, up through the base of the nose and back into the alveolar ridge on one or both sides (Figure 11–2A, B, and C).

Clefts involving only the lip may affect facial appearance and, hence, may have consequences for social interaction. However, they do not adversely affect speech unless the alveolar ridge is involved. On the other hand, unoperated clefts of the palate make it impossible to impound air for the production of pressure consonants. In addition, vowels are compromised by the introduction of unwanted resonances in the nasal cavity. We will return to these issues later in the chapter.

 CD-ROM

An Overview of the CD-ROM Segments for Chapter 11

To enhance your understanding of the structure and function of the velopharyngeal complex and larynx, Volume 1 of the CD-ROM that accompanies this book includes short video segments and some labeled still photographs that enable you to examine these structures using an instrument known as an endoscope. The purpose of this supplemental information is to help you develop a more complete understanding of endoscopy, the nasal cavity, the velopharyngeal area, and the larynx. The video segments associated with the current chapter provide the following information. At appropriate points in the text of this chapter, you will find a suggestion regarding which videos to view.

Segments

Ch.11.01. An ENT (Ear, Nose, and Throat physician) presents information regarding insertion of the flexible nasopharyngoscope.

Ch.11.02. A view of the nasal cavity obtained as the scope is passed through the nose back to the velopharyngeal area.

Ch.11.03. A speech-language pathologist explains normal velopharyngeal closure to the parent of a child with a repaired cleft of the soft palate.

Ch.11.04. The subject demonstrates velopharyngeal movements during normal and simulated hypernasal speech.

Ch.11.05. An image from video segment Ch.11.04 is presented with labels indicating the location of the velum (soft palate), lateral pharyngeal walls, and posterior pharyngeal wall.

Ch.11.06. Laryngoscopic video of velopharyngeal movements during repeated productions of "papa," showing the delineation of hard and soft palate.

Ch.11.07. Velopharyngeal movements during productions of /a/, /i/, /m/, and /p/.

Ch. 11.08. A morphing sequence depicting embryologic development of the human face.

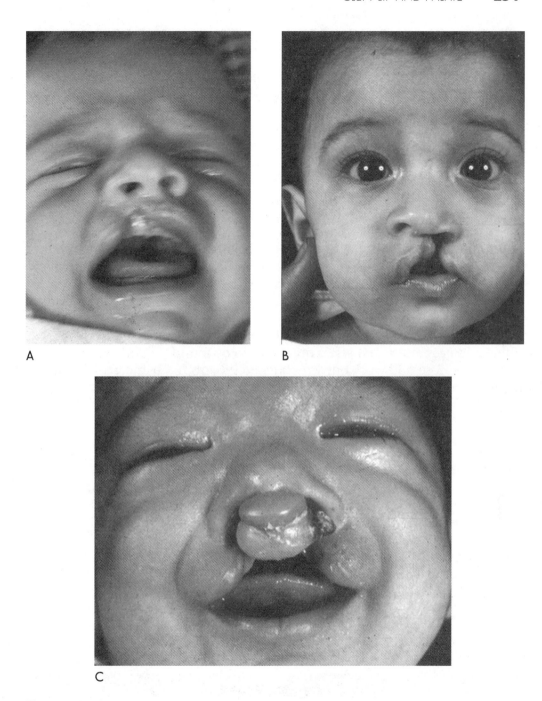

A

B

C

Figure 11–2. Various degrees of lip clefting. **A:** vermilion notch. **B:** Unilateral complete cleft of the lip (through the base of the nose and back into the alveolar ridge area). **C:** bilateral complete cleft of the lip.

THE VELOPHARYNGEAL COMPLEX AND THE LARYNX

Chapter 9 presented a logical sequence regarding the anatomic and physiologic basis of speech production. That presentation began with the creation of an energy source (respiration) followed sequentially by information regarding how the column of air emanating from the lungs during exhalation is modified into a series of air pulses resulting in a spectrum of harmonically related tones (phonation). You learned that this spectrum is modulated to create the vowels and voiced consonants of our language (articulation). In the case of voiceless consonants, the flow of exhaled air is restricted or stopped at specific points of articulation to create the voiceless fricatives and stops. In the case of /tʃ/ (ch) and its voiced cognate /dʒ/ (j), the oral articulation consists of a rapid sequential production of a plosive and a fricative. For the production of the three nasal consonants in the English language, the oral cavity is obstructed at the lips (/m/), alveolar ridge (/n/), or velum (/ŋ/ "ng") and the oral and nasal cavities are coupled to allow for the creation of resonances within the nasal cavity.

The following discussion essentially reverses the sequence just described. That is, in keeping with a series of movies to be found on your CD-ROM, we start at the nose and work our way back to the larynx, using an instrument known as an endoscope. On our journey, clinically relevant information is presented.

Endoscopy

Endoscopy is a general term referring to the use of any instrument to examine a space within the body. The term is frequently modified to provide more specific information about how the scope is used. For example, a scope used to study the nose and velopharyngeal area is typically called a "nasendoscope," while the same instrument is called a "laryngoscope" when used to study the larynx. Speech-language pathologists (SLPs) who work in a medical setting and are called upon to evaluate a patient's speech mechanism may use an endoscope to study the nose, velopharyngeal area, and larynx. In that case, the cryptic term "scope" is frequently the label of choice. Flexible scopes

 CD-ROM

The Nasopharyngoscope

In CD-ROM segment Ch.11.01, an ENT (Ear, Nose, and Throat physician) explains how the flexible nasopharyngoscope is used.

such as the one demonstrated in CD-ROM segment Ch.11.01 consist of two bundles of fiberoptic fibers. One bundle transmits light from a cold light source to the space being examined, while the other bundle provides a visual image of that space to the examiner.

Before discussing the structures visualized using a scope, and the disturbances to function that may affect those structures, clarification of the SLPs role in endoscopy is warranted. First of all, endoscopy typically is preceded by the application of a topical anesthetic. Because of the rare possibility of an exaggerated reaction (anaphylaxis) to the anesthetic, endoscopy that is preceded by application of a topical anesthetic should only be undertaken in a medical setting where a "crash cart" and appropriately trained medical personnel are available. In addition, conducting an endoscopic examination in a medical setting introduces the highly desirable possibility of having a physician present. Such interdisciplinary interaction enhances the evaluation process.

Nasal Cavity

 CD-ROM

The Nasal Cavity

CD-ROM segment Ch.11.02 presents a view of the nasal cavity as the flexible nasopharyngoscope is passed through the nose back to the velopharyngeal area.

The principal biologic function of the nasal cavity is to cleanse, warm, and humidify the air passing through it during inspiration. There is a collection of hairs (cilia) at the entrance of each nostril that serves to capture foreign particles in the air. Once beyond those cilia, air passes between the nasal septum (on the right side of the screen in CD-ROM segment Ch.11.02) and structures that protrude off the side wall of each nasal cavity (on the left side of the screen). These protrusions are called **nasal turbinates** or **nasal conchae** because of their shell-like shape. Their purpose is to increase the amount of warm, moist mucous membrane exposed to the inhaled air. There are three turbinates in each nostril. They are known as the superior, middle, and inferior turbinates or conchae. Only the inferior and middle turbinates are visible in CD-ROM segment Ch.11.02.

Before leaving the nose, we need to discuss how it contributes to the sound of a person's speech. Because everyone has experienced a cold at one time or another, it should not be difficult for you to appreciate that blockages in the nose will make it difficult to produce the nasal consonants of English (/m/, /n/, and /ŋ/ "ng"). That is, the speech will be devoid of the nasal resonances that normally characterize these sounds and the vowels immediately adjacent to them. As a consequence, affected individuals will sound hyponasal (denasal).

One way of simulating a cold would be for you to produce a sentence loaded with nasal consonants but produce all the nasals as "homorganic stops." That is, produce a stop consonant articulated at the same place as the nasal consonant (/b/ for /m/, /d/ for /n/, and /g/ for /ŋ/ "ng"). For example, if you said "Mother knows many songs" in the manner just described, it would come out something like "Buther dowes bedy sogs."

While nasal passage obstructions resulting from a cold are temporary, some individuals have constantly present blockages due to such structural differences as a deviated septum or hypertrophied (enlarged) turbinates. Such disturbances are frequently observed in children born with clefts of the lip and palate.

As we will see presently, children born with clefts of the lip and palate also may have difficulty closing off the nose from the mouth during speech. As a consequence, resonances are produced in the nose during vowel productions when they shouldn't be. That is, affected individuals will sound hypernasal.

Now stop for a moment and reflect on what you just read. Children born with cleft lip and palate may be denasal as the result of nasal structure distortions and may also be hypernasal as the result of inadequate velopharyngeal closure. That is, an affected individual may not be able to produce rich nasal resonances during nasal consonants but also may be unable to keep from producing some nasal resonance during vowels, which should be produced wholly within the oral cavity. That is why some individuals with cleft lip and palate can be both hypernasal (on vowels) and hyponasal (on nasal consonants).

Clinicians in the past were taught that **hypernasality** and **hyponasality** represented polar opposites of a single parameter. As such, a speaker might be either hyper- or hyponasal, but not both. You now know this is wrong. A person who happens to have a compromised nasal cavity and impaired velopharyngeal closure will sound *both* hypernasal and hyponasal.

Velopharyngeal Complex

The floor of the nasal cavity through which the scope initially passes is formed by a bony shelf covered with mucous membrane. This floor is known as the hard palate (see Figure 11–3A and B). As is obvious in Figure 11–3, the

CD-ROM

Velopharyngeal Closure

The reader is encouraged to watch five CD-ROM segments that are related to velopharyngeal closure.

Ch.11.03: A speech-language pathologist explains normal velopharyngeal closure to a parent. The speech-language pathologist actually makes an error in his explanation in Ch.11.03. He says that all sound normally goes out the mouth when counting from 1 to 6. However, the word "one" has a nasal in it, so the velopharyngeal port is opened during production of that particular sound. All other information in that segment is accurate.

Ch.11.04: The pharyngoscopy subject demonstrates velopharyngeal movements during normal and simulated hypernasal speech.

Ch.11.05: An image from video segment 11.04 is presented with labels indicating the location of the velum (soft palate), lateral pharyngeal walls, and posterior pharyngeal wall.

Ch.11.06: Laryngoscopic video of velopharyngeal movements during repeated productions of "papa," showing the delineation of hard and soft palate

Ch.11.07: Velopharyngeal movements during productions of /a/, /i/, /m/, and /p/.

---

hard palate forms the roof of the mouth, or palatal vault, as well as the floor of the nasal cavity. Disturbances to the embryologic development of the hard palate and soft palate, mentioned below, result in the condition known as cleft palate.

Further back in the nasal cavity, the turbinates and septum disappear from view. At that point, the scope is in an area known as the **nasopharynx** (see Figures 11–3 and 11–4). The floor of the cavity in this region is devoid of bone and is, therefore, known as the soft palate. It is also called the velum (Latin, veil) because it serves as a veil to cover the entrance from the mouth into the nose. That is, the upward and backward movement of the velum is of primary importance in closing the velopharyngeal port during production of all English phonemes (speech sounds) except the three nasal consonants ("m, n, ng").

In Chapter 9, you learned that the primary muscle of velar elevation is the levator palatini muscle. Contraction of this muscle causes the velum to move up and back against the **posterior pharyngeal wall (PPW)** (back of the throat). Since the velum is not wide enough to close off the nose from the mouth completely, it is also necessary for tissue on the side of the velopharyngeal opening to move toward midline during velopharyngeal closure.

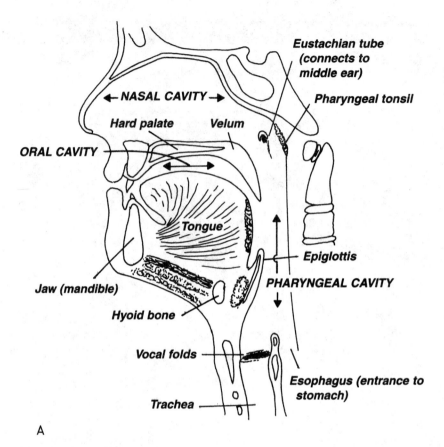

Figure 11–3A and B. Midsagittal views of the vocal tract. (From *Speech sciences* [pp. 142 and 167], by R. Kent, 1997, San Diego: Singular Publishing Group. Copyright 1997 by Singular Publishing Group. Reprinted with permission.)

CLEFT LIP AND CLEFT PALATE

How Clefts of the Lip and Palate Develop

To understand the genesis of cleft lip and cleft palate (Table 11–1), we need to understand what happens during embryologic development of the outer face and palatal vault area. As shown in CD-ROM segment Ch.11.08, tissue in the area that will eventually give rise to the midportion of the upper lip grows downward and laterally to meet tissue growing in from the side. These tissues eventually touch one another and join to form the intact upper lip. If they do not, the result is a cleft on one or both sides of the lip.

The sequential development of the palatal vault begins earlier (week 6) and ends later (week 9) than development of the lip. It begins when a small

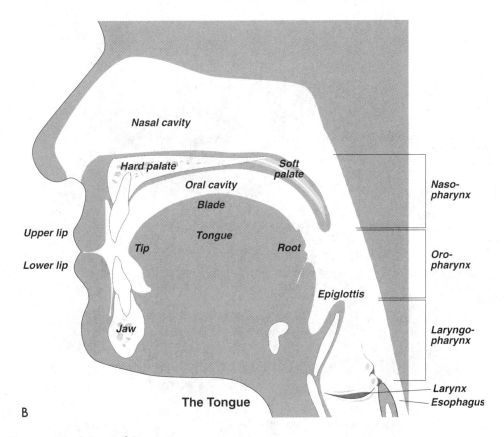

B

Figure 11–3A and B. *(continued)*.

 CD-ROM

Embryologic Development

CD-ROM segment Ch.11.08 will greatly facilitate your understanding of lip formation during embryologic development. This morphing sequence shows the events in formation of the human face that occur between 4 and 8 weeks gestation (during weeks 4 through 8, following conception). The last image in the sequence is of a 1-year-old child. Once the movie has played, you are encouraged to grab the scroll bar tracker with your mouse and move it slowly back toward the left. When you do this, you will be better able to appreciate the fact that some children with disturbed facial development present with widely spaced eyes (hypertelorism) and/or low-set ears. You also can tell that clefts of the upper lip appear to the left and/or right of midline, unlike the naturally occurring cleft in the lip of a rabbit. That is why it is both socially inappropriate and anatomically incorrect to use the term "harelip" to describe a cleft lip.

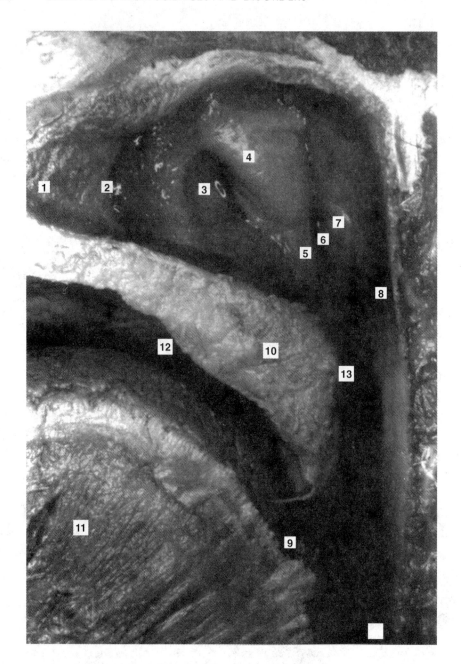

Figure 11–4. Photograph of nasopharynx with muscosal surface intact.
1 = nasal septum, **2** = posterior choana, **3** = eustachian tube, **4** = torus
ubarius (cartilage of the eustachian tube), **5** = salpingopharyngeal fold,
6 = pharyngeal recess, **7** = posteriorlateral pharyngeal wall, **8** =
posterior pharyngeal wall, **9** = posterior faucail pillar, **10** = soft palate,
11 = tongue, **12** = oral cavity, **13** = nasopharyngeal portal, and **14** =
oropharynx. (Courtesy of Joel C. Kahane) (From *Speech sciences* [p. 192],
by R. Kent, 1997, San Diego: Singular Publishing Group. Copyright 1997
by Singular Publishing Group. Reprinted with permission.)

Table 11–1. Malformations Adversely Affecting Velopharyngeal Closure

Cleft Lip
partial
complete
no alveolar ridge involvement
alveolar ridge involved

Cleft Palate
occult submucous
submucous
incomplete
complete

Cleft Lip and Palate
unilateral
  right
  left
bilateral

Congenital Velopharyngeal Inadequacy
congenitally short soft palate without clefting
megapharynx (box-like nasopharynx)
posterior faucial pillar webbing

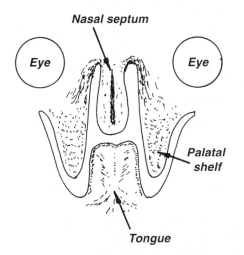

Figure 11–5. Schematic view of the nasal septum, palatal shelves, and tongue in a fetus approximately 6 weeks after conception. (From *Speech sciences* [p. 472], by R. Kent, 1997, San Diego: Singular Publishing Group. Copyright 1997 by Singular Publishing Group. Reprinted with permission.)

triangular wedge of tissue (premaxilla), that will eventually become the area housing the upper four front teeth, fuses with horizontally oriented shelves of tissue known as the palatine processes of the maxilla (Figure 11–5). Behind the premaxilla, these palatine processes fuse with one another in a front-to-back sequence. If this process is disturbed at any time, a cleft of the palate will result. If these processes never begin to fuse, the result will be a complete cleft of the palate. Otherwise, the cleft will be incomplete. If the palatal cleft co-occurs with a cleft of the lip, the lip involvement may either be on one side or the other (a right or left unilateral cleft of the lip and palate) or it may involve both sides of the lip (a bilateral cleft of the lip and palate).[1]

Figure 11–6 shows two subjects who differ in the extent of palatal clefting. Because palatal union proceeds from front to back, the patient shown in the second picture (Figure 11–6B) experienced a disturbance later in development than the patient in the first picture (Figure 11–6A). In fact, almost all of the hard palate and almost all of the soft palate's mucosal covering formed normally in the second patient. This patient has what is known as a submucous cleft, so-called because two of the three signs characterizing this condition are covered by an intact mucous membrane:

1. notch in the hard palate. Not visible to the eye but can be palpated (felt) with a gloved finger.

2. abnormal orientation of the soft palate musculature, causing the middle of the velum to be quite thin and bluish in color. Because that area is rather translucent, it is frequently referred to as a "zona pellucida" (shining zone).

3. **bifid** (split) **uvula** that is the characteristic usually the most apparent to the casual observer.

In rare cases, all the hard palate and the entire mucous membrane have formed completely, leaving only the palatal musculature malformed. This form of cleft is well hidden and, as such, is known as an *occult cleft*. Although the condition is difficult to see, it can result in the same type of speech problems that accompany more involved palatal clefts. That is because the muscular malformation makes it difficult or impossible for the patient to elevate the velum up and back against the posterior pharyngeal wall (PPW).

Palatopharyngeal Inadequacy

Another physical condition that adversely affects speech, but does not involve any of the signs mentioned previously, is congenital palatopharyngeal inadequacy. This problem may be due to a congenitally short soft palate or an enlarged pharynx. It may also be due to foreshortening of the posterior pillars of Fauces (see Figure 11–7), which may tether the velum and keep it from elevating to the PPW (posterior pharyngeal wall). In any of these three situa-

---

[1] The preferred terms used to describe clefts involving the lip and/or palatal vault are clefts of the primary and/or secondary palate, respectively. However, justification for this alternative nomenclature is beyond the scope of this text.

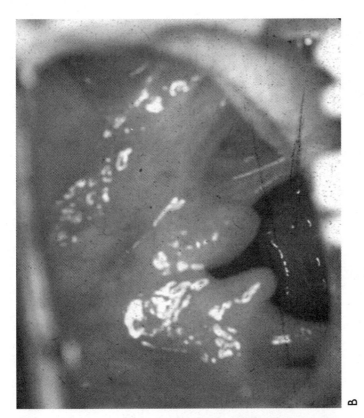

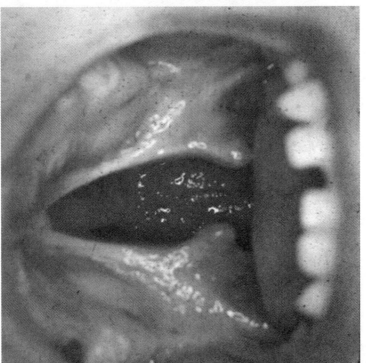

Figure 11–6. Varying degrees of palatal clefting. **A:** Complete cleft of the (secondary) palate. **B:** Submucous cleft.

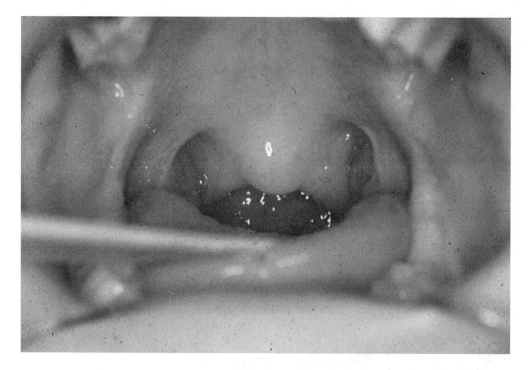

Figure 11–7. Intra-oral view depicting posterior faucial pillars webbing.

tions, the effect upon velopharyngeal closure may be masked early in life by the presence of the adenoid pad (or pharyngeal tonsil; see Figure 11–3) against which the soft palate is able to make contact during the production of nonnasal phonemes. When the adenoid pad disappears naturally, or if it is surgically removed because of recurrent ear infections, the velum may be unable to reach the PPW, thereby making velopharyngeal closure difficult or impossible.

THE SPEECH OF CHILDREN WITH CLEFT LIP AND PALATE

If a child is unable to close off the nose from the mouth during the production of nonnasal speech sounds, two problems will arise. First, the production of the vowels will be accompanied by inappropriate resonances in the nose. That is, vowels will be *hypernasal*. In addition, attempts at producing pressure consonants will result in the audible escape of air through the nose **(nasal emission)**. Take a moment and try to say the word *puppy* while lowering your soft palate. If you are successful, you will hear frictional noise emanating from your nose (nasal emission) during the production of each /p/.

For a reason we still do not fully understand, children with palatal clefts whose primary palatal surgery is not successful typically do not produce /p/ and other pressure consonants in the manner just described. Instead, they tend to occlude the airway behind the velopharyngeal port, producing a plosive release of the air at that point. Thus, these children tend to substitute **glottal stops** or **pharyngeal stops** for all stop (plosive) consonants. Glottal stops are like little coughs produced at the larynx, whereas pharyngeal stops are produced by making and then releasing a contact between the base of the tongue and the back of the throat. Table 11–2 lists a number of speech errors typically seen in the speech of children with cleft lips and palates.

Individuals with velopharyngeal impairment also typically omit fricative sounds (e.g., /s/, /z/, and /ʃ/ "sh") or produce them by retracting the base of the tongue near the back of the throat to create a constriction through which the air is forced, thereby creating fricative noise. To understand the production of this sound, it may help you to know that this sound is part of the phonemic structure of languages such as German and Yiddish. For example, the ("ch") in "ach du lieber" is a **pharyngeal fricative.**

When children develop the above-mentioned consonantal errors, which are examples of **compensatory articulations,** they become the purview of the SLP. However, it is unreasonable to expect a child to develop oral pressure consonants if the velopharyngeal mechanism remains inadequate. By the same token, a child may not even be attempting to close the velopharyngeal port if all pressure consonants are glottals or pharyngeals.

In some cases, a clinician may opt to see a child for therapy in an attempt to establish oral consonants. If oral consonant articulations emerge but are accompanied by nasal emission, secondary physical management would

Table 11–2. Types of **Compensatory Articulations** Frequently Seen in the Speech of Patients With Velopharyngeal Impairment. (Unlike glottal stops, **pharyngeal stops** and **pharyngeal fricatives** may either be voiced or voiceless. Therefore, we use two symbols to denote these phonemes. In the table below, the first symbol in each case indicates the voiced cognate.)

Misarticulation	Phonetic Symbol	Description
Glottal Stop	ʔ	Plosive release of air pressure built up below the **glottis** (similar to a light cough)
Pharyngeal Stop	ʛ	Plosive release of air pressure built up below contact between the base of the tongue and the posterior pharyngeal wall
Pharyngeal fricative	ʕ	Frication caused by forcing air through a constriction between the base of the tongue and the posterior pharyngeal wall

appear to be indicated. If they emerge as acceptable oral productions, then the child has been spared additional surgery or prosthetic management.

MANAGEMENT OF PATIENTS WITH ORAL-FACIAL CLEFTS

The Cleft Palate Team

Children born with cleft lip, cleft palate, or both should be evaluated and treated by a team of specialists with particular expertise in this clinical area. The ideal team is transdisciplinary in nature. That is, the team members work cooperatively and efficiently with one another because each fully understands the treatment priorities of the others. This approach is not an abstract ideal. There are a number of teams in the United States that do, indeed, function in this way. Unfortunately, it is also true that most teams do not.

To be listed as a "cleft palate team" in the directory of the American Cleft Palate-Craniofacial Association (1-800-24-CLEFT), a team need only have an SLP, a surgeon, and a dentist as active members. However, more comprehensive teams include some or all of the specialties included in Table 11–3.

Table 11–3. Clinical Specialties Represented on a Well-Functioning Cleft Palate Team

Audiology
ENT (Ear, Nose, and Throat; Otorhinolaryngology)
Genetic Counseling
Orthodontics
Oral and Maxillofacial Surgery
Ophthalmologist*
Neurologist*
Patient Care Coordinator
Pediatrics/General Medicine
Pedodontics/General Dentistry
Plastic Surgery
Psychology
Prosthodontics
Social Work
Speech-Language Pathology

*Typically, ophthalmologists and neurologists on well-functioning cleft palate teams serve on a consultative basis. That is, they do not see all team patients but are called in on an "as-needed" basis.

Surgical Care and the Role of the Speech-Language Pathologist

Clefts of the lip are usually repaired surgically within the first 3 months of life. The lip surgery **(cheiloplasty)** procedure chosen depends upon the nature of the cleft and the individual preference of the surgeon. There is no single "correct" procedure. Figure 11–8 depicts preoperative and postoperative pictures of a child with a unilateral complete cleft of the lip and palate who underwent a popular lip repair procedure known as the Millard Rotation Advancement. The name indicates the surgeon who originally designed the operation, Ralph Millard, and also describes the basic nature of the procedure in which a portion of the middle of the lip is rotated downward to create a space into which a portion of the side of the lip is rotated.

Clefts of the palate are typically repaired at around 12 months of age. As with surgical closure of the lip, there is no single "correct" procedure. However, most surgeons favor either the Von Langenbeck or the Wardhill-Kilner procedure for unilateral complete clefts. There are theoretical advantages to each, and most surgeons are adamantly in favor of one or the other. Nevertheless, repeated outcome studies by SLPs have failed to uncover any statistically significant difference in the speech outcome of patients who undergo one or the other of these procedures.

In the hands of a competent surgeon, approximately 80–90% of patients who undergo primary repair of the palate (primary **palatoplasty**) will have

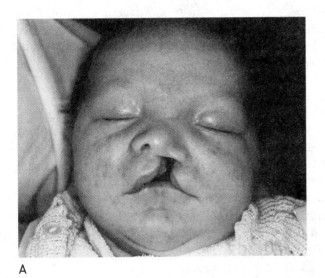
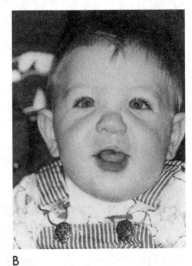

A   B

Figure 11–8. A: Preoperative and **B** postoperative views of a patient who underwent Millard Rotation Advancement repair of a unilateral cleft lip. (From *Diagnosis in speech-language pathology* [p. 340], by J. G. Tomblin, H. Morris, & D. C. Spriestersbach [Eds.], 1994, San Diego: Singular Publishing Group. Copyright 1994 by Singular Publishing Group. Reprinted by permission.)

adequate velopharyngeal closure. The other 10–20% may need to undergo secondary physical management.

Speech Assessment

It is the responsibility of the SLP on a cleft palate team to decide whether a patient with less than optimal speech would benefit most from intensive speech therapy or secondary physical management. Therefore, it is incumbent upon us to make valid and reliable assessments of the speech of children with oral-facial clefts. The three critical elements in cleft palate assessment are articulation testing, examination of the speech production mechanism, and estimates of nasality.

Articulation Testing

As noted in Chapter 10, speech assessments are usually conducted by administering single-word articulation tests and by collecting speech samples during conversations with children. In children with a history of cleft palate, particular attention is paid to the production of speech sounds that require the development of intraoral pressure such as stops, fricatives, and affricates because compensatory articulations like glottal stops and pharyngeal fricatives are expected if there is inadequate velopharyngeal closure. It is important to note, however, that the child may have a phonological delay in addition to difficulty producing speech sounds due to inadequate velopharyngeal closure. The two types of seech sound disorders are not mutually exclusive, and the SLP needs to make a judgment about why and in what ways speech sound development is delayed or deviant.

Examination of the Speech Production Mechanism

Examining the speech structures and their functioning during nonspeech and speech tasks are part of the assessment of all children and adults with articulation disorders. The examination is undertaken to determine the anatomic and functional integrity of the speech production system. The face, teeth, hard palate, tongue, and velopharynx are viewed using a penlight, and judgments are made about individual structures and the relationship between structures at rest and during nonspeech and speech activities to answer the questions "Do the structures appear normal?" and "What is the potential effect of any structural and/or functional deficits on speech production?"

Listener Judgments of Nasality

Most SLPs make perceptual judgments about the acceptability of children's nasal resonance as they listen to their conversational speech. The universal use of listener judgments in clinical settings is due to the fact that these assessments have face validity. That is, they appear intuitively to be a true indicator of the communicative significance of impaired velopharyngeal function. Nevertheless, the recurrent criticism leveled against perceptual evaluations of velopharyngeal function is that they tend to be somewhat unreliable, and the degree of reliability seems to vary depending upon the parameter being assessed. Moreover, listener judgment variability seems to be a particularly troublesome problem in clinical settings, where treatment decisions typically are made. There are a number of reasons why listener judgments may be in error:

- The relationship between perceived degree of hypernasal resonance and the area of velopharyngeal (v-p) port deficit is not linear.

- A speaker's articulation skills may increase a listener's rating of hypernasality.

- A listener's personal biases may contaminate his or her judgments. For example, surgeons who assess the speech effects of their own surgery run an appreciable risk of overestimating their successes or perhaps even underestimating them in an attempt to remain impartial.

- Past experiences can dramatically affect a listener's perceptions. SLPs cannot escape the fact that personal impressions are based in part upon the speech behaviors of patients seen in the past. The clinician who moves from one professional setting to another is perhaps in the best position to appreciate the insidious nature of this phenomenon.

Considering the significant potential for error discussed previously, it is reassuring to note that the reliability of subjective judgments apparently can be improved dramatically by training and by pooling judgments from multiple listeners. Indeed, the intrajudge and interjudge reliability measures reported in clinical research studies typically are quite respectable. However, most clinical assessments are made by a single judge or a relatively small set of clinicians functioning as judges, with varying degrees of vested interest in the outcome of the analysis process. In addition, whatever training clinicians receive typically is of the "on-the-job" type that may not be comparable to the formal training that has been shown to improve listener reliability.

Compensatory articulations usually are easy to discern, although they may be difficult to eliminate. On the other hand, hypernasality can vary over a wide range, and mild degrees of it may be difficult to identify and quantify. Therefore, most clinicians augment their perceptual assessments of speech with information from instruments that are designed to measure nasality.

Instrumental Assessment of Nasality

Considerable research has been conducted in recent years in an attempt to develop valid and reliable instrumental measures of velopharyngeal inadequacy that would overcome the problems mentioned previously. Information obtained from these measures presumably is intended to supplement, rather than supplant, impressions obtained by trained SLPs during the diagnostic process.

One such instrument in wide use today is the Nasometer. This is a computer-based system manufactured by Kay Elemetrics. With this device, oral and nasal components of a person's speech are sensed by microphones on either side of a sound separator that rests on the patient's upper lip. When using the Nasometer to determine the presence and extent of hypernasality, subjects are asked to produce a series of sentences devoid of nasal consonants while wearing the Nasometer headgear. In the absence of nasal consonants, one would expect little acoustic energy to be picked up by the nasal microphone.

Signals from the nasal and the oral microphones are filtered and digitized by custom electronic modules. These data are then processed by the computer and accompanying software. The resultant signal is a ratio of nasal to nasal-plus-oral acoustic energy. This ratio is multiplied by 100 and expressed as a percent, known as a nasalance score. Although nasalance scores vary as a function of English dialect, the score for individuals with normal velopharyngeal function typically falls below 20. Patients with mild hypernasality usually score in the high 20s or low 30s, while those with more significant degrees of hypernasality may receive scores in the 40s or 50s.

Secondary Surgical Management

If, after careful consideration of the perceptual and instrumental data, it is determined that a patient is a candidate for additional surgery, the next step is to choose the most appropriate operation. Two popular secondary procedures in use today are the **pharyngeal flap** and the **superior sphincter pharyngoplasty.** Although many surgeons will use one or the other of these procedures exclusively, there is at least a theoretical basis for using them differentially, depending upon the patient's velopharyngeal structures and function. If you understand normal velopharyngeal function, it should be fairly easy for you to understand the difference.

You already know that velopharyngeal closure involves upward and backward movement of the velum *and* medial movement of the lateral pharyngeal walls. If a patient has a short soft palate, but good lateral wall movement, then it is reasonable to propose that she or he would benefit from a pharyngeal flap, in which a flap of tissue from the back wall of the throat is raised and inserted into the velum. This provides for a constantly present veil over the velopharyngeal port. When the lateral walls of the velopharynx are relaxed, the patient can breathe through the nose and can also produce nasal consonants. When complete velopharyngeal closure is desired, the well-functioning lateral walls can move in against the sides of the velum and flap.

If a patient has good velar length and movement, but reduced lateral pharyngeal wall activity, a superior sphincter pharyngoplasty would appear to be the method of choice. In this case, the posterior faucial pillars are cut free and swung up into the area of velopharyngeal closure. They are sutured together to form a purse string in that area. Their added bulk is intended to ensure that the reduced lateral wall movement is adequate to effect closure.

Prosthetic Management

Most patients requiring additional physical management after primary palate repair are treated surgically in the manner just described. However, some patients, for one reason or another, may not be good surgical risks. In such cases, they may be treated prosthetically.

Patients who have a short soft palate or a deep nasopharynx may be candidates for what is variously known as a "speech bulb" or a "pharyngeal extension appliance" (Figure 11–9). The anterior portion of such an appliance is similar to an acrylic retainer worn by patients who have undergone orthodontic treatment (i.e., who have "worn braces"). Extending back from that retainer portion is a connecting piece off the end of which is placed a mass of acrylic that is shaped to fill the velopharyngeal space that the patient is unable to eliminate during attempts at velopharyngeal closure. Figure 11–9B is a side (sagittal) x-ray view of a patient wearing a pharyngeal extension appliance. The bulb portion of the appliance is visible as a round mass lying in the velopharyngeal port area.

Patients who have adequate soft palate length but inadequate muscle control to effect velopharyngeal closure may be candidates for what is known as a "palatal lift" appliance (Figure 11–10). The primary difference in this appliance is that a broad, spatula-like shelf of acrylic extends back from the retainer portion of the appliance. This lift portion does exactly what its name implies. It lifts the weak (flaccid) velum and places it in a static position against the posterior pharyngeal wall. Figure 11–10B is a sagittal x-ray view of a patient wearing a palate lift appliance. (Yes, we forgot to ask her to remove her earrings.)

The obvious advantages of the prosthetic appliances just described are that (a) the patient does not have to undergo surgery, (b) the appliances can be adjusted as many times as necessary to provide an optimum speech result,

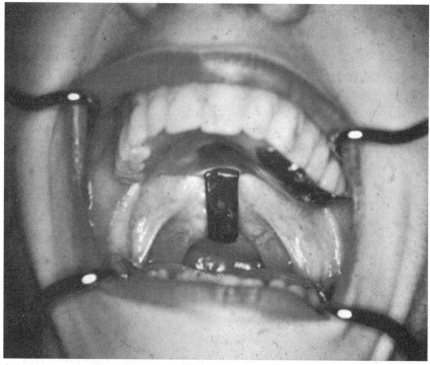

A

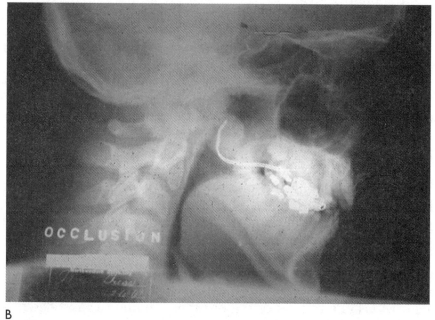

B

Figure 11–9. Intra-oral **(A)** and lateral x-ray **(B)** views of a patient wearing a pharyngeal extension (speech bulb) appliance.

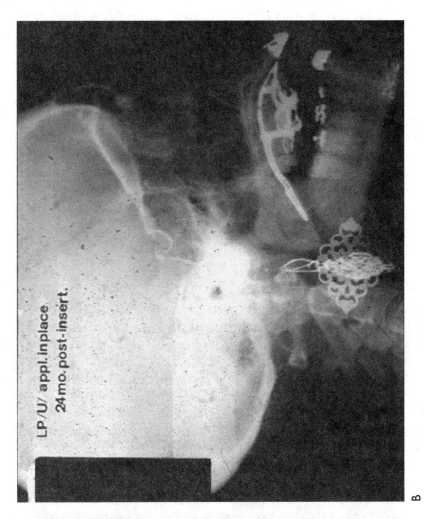

LP/U/ appl. in place
24 mo. post-insert.

B

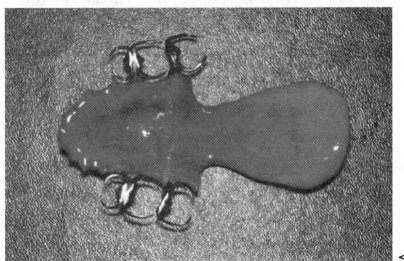

A

Figure 11–10. A palatal lift appliance (**A**) and a lateral x-ray view (**B**) of a patient wearing that appliance.

and (c) the prosthesis can be discarded if the final result is unsatisfactory to the patient. On the other hand, there are a number of disadvantages to prosthetic appliances, including the following: (a) they require daily care for proper oral hygiene, (b) they may be difficult to retain in the mouth if velar movement is extensive, (c) they require periodic follow-up to ensure maintenance of a good fit, (d) they usually cannot be worn while eating, and (e) children frequently take them out and put them in their lunch bag while eating lunch at school and then throw them out with the bag. For these, and other reasons, surgical intervention is usually the preferred method of treatment for patients with velopharyngeal impairment.

SUMMARY

This chapter addressed the evaluation and treatment of disturbances that affect oral-nasal resonance. Extensive information was provided regarding the embryologic basis and speech consequences of a condition known as cleft lip and palate, which occurs in approximately 1 out of every 750 live births. Approximately 25% of these individuals have clefts of the lip only, 25% have clefts of the lip and palate, and 50% have clefts of the lip and palate.

A nasendoscope is often used to examine the nose and the velopharyngeal area, which contain the structures that are involved in clefts of the lip and palate. The principal function of the nasal cavity is to cleanse, warm, and humidify the air. The nose is also needed for nasal resonance for production of the consonants /m/, /n/, and /ŋ/). All the other consonants and vowels should be produced with oral resonance, which is accomplished by actions of the velum and the pharynx. Children with clefts of the palate often have large openings into the nose because of missing palatal bone and/or they may have velopharyngeal insufficiency. These conditions cause varying degrees of hyponasality, hypernasality, and nasal emissions. Children with cleft lip and palate also tend to have difficulties with the production of pressure consonants.

Clefts of the lip and/or palate are repaired through surgical procedures and, in some cases, the insertion of prosthetic devices. Clefts of the lip are usually repaired within the first 3 months after birth. Clefts of the palate are usually repaired around the child's first birthday. Some children require additional surgery to reduce nasality. Two of the most common procedures are the pharyngeal flap and the superior spincter pharyngoplasty. Children who are not good surgical risks can be fitted with pharyngeal extension appliances that fill in the velopharyngeal space.

Speech-language pathologists (SLPs) conduct assessments of children's speech to evaluate the functional outcomes of surgery and to determine whether there is a need for speech therapy. These assessments include articulation testing, behavioral and instrumental examination of the speech production mechanism, and perceptual and instrumental estimates of nasality. When speech therapy is warranted, SLPs typically use a motor-kinesthetic approach to articulation therapy to assist children with the production of pressure consonants.

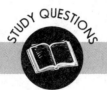

STUDY QUESTIONS

1 What would you expect to hear in someone's speech if the person had extremely large (hypertrophied) nasal turbinates?

2 Which phonemes are easiest to produce for a person with velopharyngeal impairment?

3 What are the three features that characterize a submucous cleft palate? Which is/ are *not* present in occult submucous cleft palate?

4 What are the limitations associated with listener judgments of oral-nasal resonance imbalance?

5 How is a nasalance score obtained?

SUGGESTED READINGS

Shprintzen, R. J., & Bardach, J. (1995). *Cleft palate speech management: A multidisciplinary approach.* St. Louis: Mosby.

Bzoch, K. R. (1997). *Communicative disorders related to cleft lip and palate* (1997). Austin, TX: Pro-Ed.

Moller, K. T., & Starr, C. D. (1993). *Cleft palate: Interdisciplinary issues and treatment.* Austin, TX: Pro-Ed.

Bifid: Divided into two parts.

Bilateral: Pertaining to two sides.

Cheiloplasty: Surgical repair of a lip defect.

Compensatory articulations: Production of a sound utilizing alternative placement of the articulators rather than the usual placement.

Endoscopy: Examination of the interior of a canal or hollow space.

Glottal stops: A plosive sound made by stopping and releasing the breath stream at the level of the glottis; may be a compensatory behavior in the presence of inadequate velopharyngeal closure.

Hypernasality: Excessively undesirable amount of perceived nasal cavity resonance during phonation.

Hyponasality (denasality): Lack of nasal resonance for the three phonemes /m/, /n/, and /ng/ resulting from a partial or complete obstruction in the nasal tract.

Nasal emission: Airflow through the nose, usually measurable or audible and heard most frequently during the production of voiceless plosives and fricatives; usually indicative of an incomplete seal between the nasal and oral cavities.

Nasal turbinates (nasal conchae): Shell-shaped projections of thin facial bone covered by mucous membrane and forming the lateral wall of the nasal cavity.

Nasopharynx: That part of the pharynx above the level of the soft palate and which opens anteriorly into the nasal cavity.

Palatoplasty: Surgical repair of a palatal defect.

Pharyngeal flap surgery: Surgical procedure to aid in achieving velopharyngeal closure; a flap of skin is used to close most of the opening between the velum and the nasopharynx.

Pharyngeal fricatives: Fricative sounds produced by approximating the back of the tongue and the posterior pharyngeal wall and forcing air through the resultant constriction.

Pharyngeal stops: Plosive sounds produced by contacting the back of the tongue to the posterior pharyngeal wall, building up air pressure behind that obstruction and then rapidly releasing it to produce a popping or (ex)plosive sound.

Posterior pharyngeal wall (PPW): Back of the throat.

Superior sphincter pharyngoplasty: Surgical procedure to aid in achieving velopharyngeal closure; the posterior faucial pillars are raised and used to form a bulge that reduces the size of opening between the velum and the nasopharynx.

Unilateral: Pertaining to or restricted to one side of the body.

Uvula: Small cone-shaped process hanging from the lower border of the soft palate at midline.

12

Voice Disorders

Rodger M. Dalston

LEARNING OBJECTIVES

1 To differentiate among disorders that adversely affect phonation.

2 To learn about techniques that may help patients with voice disturbances.

3 To understand the purposes, procedures, and goals of the voice evaluation.

4 To appreciate the problems experienced by persons who undergo surgical removal of the larynx and the ways in which speech-language pathologists (SLPs) can assist in the adjustment process.

INTRODUCTION

You, or someone you know, has probably experienced laryngitis at one time or another. This condition can result from any number of causes, including screaming at a sports event or rock concert. In response to acute traumas of this sort, the vocal folds are swollen (edematous) and red **(erythematous).** Tissue swelling **(edema)** disrupts normal vocal fold vibration, causing a

283

change in voice quality. If severe, the affected individual may experience a total loss of voice **(aphonia).** More often, the voice is hoarse.

Hoarseness is one of a number of judgments people make when assessing the quality of a person's voice. While there is a wide range of vocabulary used to describe voice quality, speech-language pathologists (SLPs) typically use three descriptors: harsh, breathy, and hoarse.

A *harsh* voice is associated with excessive muscle tension. You can simulate this quality by speaking as if you were absolutely furious but wanted to control your temper and not yell. What you would do is press the vocal folds together tightly, releasing them quickly during each vibratory cycle, reduce subglottic pressure so that the abrupt air release did not increase the loudness of your voice, and tighten the walls of the throat (pharynx). Tightening the pharyngeal walls increases their reflectivity and amplifies the high-frequency components of the voice.

A *breathy* voice has been described as a "confidential voice." It is produced with a partial whisper. The vocal folds are brought together so that they vibrate, but a space between the vocal folds remains. Air passing through the space creates a fricative noise that is superimposed on the vocal tone. The larger the space between the folds, the greater the fricative noise and the breathier the phonation. If the space is sufficiently wide, the vocal folds are not drawn into vibration, and the only sound produced is the fricative noise. At that point, the speaker will be whispering, and the term "breathy voice" no longer applies.

A voice that is both harsh and breathy is described as being *hoarse.* It results from irregular vocal fold vibrations, typically due to differential mass and shape of the two folds. Hoarseness can be the sign of a serious laryngeal pathology, or it may simply be due to laryngitis induced by the common cold.

Laryngitis is just one of a host of problems that can adversely affect vocal tone. Some voice disorders result from discrete or diffuse tissue enlargement, while others may be due to a reduction in tissue **(atrophy).** Some are due to increased muscle activity **(hyperfunction),** while others may be due to reduced muscle activity **(hypofunction).** An abnormal degree of muscle activity may be due to brain or peripheral nerve dysfunction (a neurologic problem) or a problem with the muscles **(myopathy),** or it may be due to psychological issues. Each of these categories has a number of conditions associated with it. Moreover, these categories are not mutually exclusive. For example, increased muscle activity may, and frequently does, result in tissue changes. We will return to the topic of voice disorders later in this chapter.

The larynx (pronounced "larinks," not "larniks") is located at the top of the windpipe or trachea and is ideally situated to perform a number of important functions, each of which was discussed in Chapter 9. In the following sections of this chapter, we discuss the evaluation and treatment of difficulties that may arise in the use of the larynx as a sound source. We begin with a discussion of some problems that may be encountered clinically (Table 12–1) and then discuss how such problems are identified and evaluated.

Table 12–1. Various Disorders of Voice

Discrete Tissue Changes
Nodules
Polyps
Papilloma
Cyst
Hematoma
Keratosis
Leukoplakia
Pachydermia laryngis
Cancer
Contact ulcer
Granuloma

Diffuse Tissue Changes
Reinke's edema
Laryngitis
Laryngeal bowing
Sulcus vocalis

Gross Structural Changes
Laryngomalacia
Mechanical, thermal, or chemical trauma
Cricoarytenoid ankylosis
Laryngeal web
Larynx removal (laryngectomy)

Neurogenic Voice Problems
Peripheral paralysis or paresis
Pyramidal disturbances (e.g., stroke, pseudobulbar palsy)
Extrapyramidal disturbances (e.g., parkinsonism, spasmodic dysphonia, essential tremor)

Myopathic Voice Problems
Myasthenia gravis
Myotonic muscular dystrophy

Nonorganic Voice Problems
Stage fright
Muscle tension dysphonia (MTD)
Conversion aphonia/dysphonia
Ventricular phonation
Mutational falsetto (puberphonia)
Paradoxical vocal fold movement (PVFM)[1]

[1]PVFM does not create a voice problem per se. However, patients are often referred to clinicians in our field to extinguish the behavior of partially adducting the vocal folds during inspiration, thereby causing noise (stridor) and impaired respiration during exercise.

CD-ROM

Overview of CD-ROM Segments for Chapter 12

The principal aim of this chapter is to develop an understanding of disturbances that adversely affect phonation. These disturbances are known as voice disorders. To assist in this endeavor, Volume 2 of the CD-ROM that accompanies this book contains the following segments that are intended to help you understand the structure and function of the larynx. The subject used for each of these segments presented with a clinical condition known as gastro-esophageal reflux disease (GERD), a condition that is mentioned later in this chapter. At appropriate points in the text, you will find suggestions regarding which segments to view.

The CD-ROM segments for chapter 12 and all the remaining chapters in the book are located on CD-ROM Volume 2.

Segments

Ch.12.01. An ear, nose, and throat physician (ENT) uses rigid laryngoscopy to view the anatomic structures of the larynx.

Ch.12.02. A frame from the preceding video with various anatomic structures labeled.

Ch.12.03. Flexible laryngscopic view of the subject whispering following by "silent" laughter.

Ch.12.04. Laryngeal activity during whistling (viewed with a flexible scope).

Ch.12.05. Laryngeal compression during simulated weight-lifting maneuvers. These compressions are followed by examples of coughing.

Ch.12.06. Rising pitch (rising glissando) during production of "hey" (viewed with a rigid scope).

Ch.12.07. A frame from the preceding video with various anatomic structures labeled.

Ch.12.08. Rising and falling glissando, including the falsetto register.

Ch.12.09. Breathy phonation observed in real time and using stroboscopy to reveal the presence of a good mucosal wave.

Ch.12.10. Demonstration of one type of artificial larynx.

 CD-ROM

Viewing the Anatomic Structures of the Larynx

CD-ROM segment Ch.12.01. An ENT (Ear, Nose, and Throat physician) uses rigid laryngoscopy to view the anatomic structures of the larynx. As noted previously, the subject presented with GERD. You will see that the posterior portion of each vocal fold is red (erythematous) as a result of irritation by stomach acid.

CD-ROM segment Ch.12.02.	A frame from the preceding video with various anatomic structures labeled.
CD-ROM segment Ch.12.03.	Flexible laryngscopic view of the subject whispering following by "silent" laughter.
CD-ROM segment Ch.12.04.	Laryngeal activity during whistling (viewed with a flexible scope).
CD-ROM segment Ch.12.06.	Rising pitch (rising glissando) during production of "hey" (viewed with a rigid scope).
CD-ROM segment Ch.12.07.	A frame from the preceding video with various anatomic structures labeled.

VOICE ABNORMALITIES UNRELATED TO STRUCTURAL CHANGE

Most phonatory disorders are related to tissue changes in the larynx or abnormal changes in the nervous system. However, there are a number of disturbances that can exist in the absence of underlying pathology. One that you almost assuredly have experienced, perhaps in a public speaking course in high school or college, is the "shaky" voice that accompanies stage fright. It results from a perfectly normal "fight or flight" reaction to danger, whether it is real or imagined. While this condition certainly creates an abnormal voice, it is a transient condition that does not require the services of a speech-language pathologist (SLP).

Conversion Aphonia/Dysphonia

A patient may report a total loss of voice (aphonia) or an extremely abnormal voice **(dysphonia)**, and yet thorough examination by an SLP and an ear, nose, and throat (ENT) physician fails to uncover an organic cause for the problem. The existence of a psychogenic cause for the disorder may be suspected in such cases. This suspicion is particularly warranted if the patient is able to produce normal phonation during such vegetative functions as coughing, gargling, or laughing.

Voice problems of this sort frequently have a sudden onset, and a careful interview of the patient and others in the family often reveals previous occurrences of the problem. In many cases, voice can be restored within an hour or less. However, it is important to note that the underlying cause of the problem is not addressed, and referral to a mental health clinician may be indicated in some, but not necessarily all, cases.

Puberphonia

Puberphonia, also known as mutational falsetto, involves the continued use of a high-pitched voice by a postpubertal male. As with conversion disorders, patients with mutational falsetto typically cough at a pitch level that reflects the more natural vibratory frequency of the vocal folds. The condition may be the result of unresolved psychological issues, or it may be a learned behavior. In either case, the abnormal voice is readily amenable to correction by an SLP. Indeed, puberphonia is one of the most easily corrected psychogenic voice disorders.

Muscle Tension Dysphonia (MTD)

Patients with muscle tension dysphona (MTD) display disordered voices that are due to inordinate tension in the laryngeal muscles. In fact, the condition appears to result from simultaneous contraction of the muscles that draw the folds together **(adductors)** and those that pull the folds apart **(abductors).** Muscles that attach to the larynx and to some other structure **(extrinsic laryngeal muscles)** may also be hypertense and may develop "knots" that can actually benefit from laryngeal massage, much like kneading a muscle during a back rub.

The voice of MTD patients is usually quite hoarse, and patients frequently report fatigue and laryngeal discomfort. The classic description of such patients is hard-driving, upwardly mobile, "Type A" executive types whose hypertensive lifestyles are mirrored in their voices. Of course, many MTD patients do not have such "classic" personality profiles.

Whatever the cause (etiology) of muscle tension dysphonia, voice therapy directed toward facilitating a reduction in muscle tension can have a dramatic effect upon these individuals. However, as with all other voice cases, patients must be motivated to change and be willing to use strategies that they and their therapist have determined work well for them.

VOICE DISORDERS DUE TO NEUROLOGIC IMPAIRMENT

Paralysis

Disturbed function of the cerebral cortex, pyramidal tract, peripheral nerves, neuromuscular junction, or the muscles themselves can cause weakness (paresis) or a total inability to contract one or more muscles (paralysis). Approximately 8–10% of patients seen for voice problems by ear, nose, and throat physicians are found to have a problem of this type. One example of such a disturbance is adductor paralysis resulting from damage to the *recurrent laryngeal nerve* (RLN).

The vagus, or 10th cranial nerve, was discussed in Chapter 9 (Speech Science). The recurrent laryngeal nerve (RLN) of the vagus gets its name from the fact that it runs down past the larynx and then runs back (recurs) to enter the larynx and innervate all the intrinsic laryngeal muscles except the cricothyroid. Because of its location, it is prone to damage during neck and chest surgery. Some diseases also may affect this nerve or its companion, the *superior laryngeal nerve* (SLN). The SLN (superior laryngeal nerve) innervates the cricothyroid muscle and provides sensory innervation to the mucous membranes of the larynx.

Damage to one recurrent laryngeal nerve (RLN) results in one-sided **(unilateral)** paralysis. The affected fold cannot be fully adducted during phonation (see Figure 12–1). Given the three voice descriptors mentioned earlier in the chapter (harsh, breathy, hoarse), which one would predominate in a patient with unilateral RLN paralysis? If you answered breathy, you were right.

Therapy for affected individuals may involve attempts to increase the adductory function of the unaffected fold. Recall that one function of the

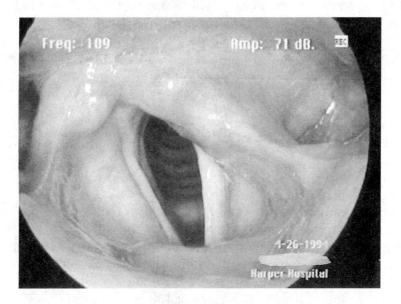

Figure 12–1. Paramedian paralysis of the left vocal fold in a 58-year-old male. Note that the patient's left vocal fold is on your right. (From Dworkin, J. P., & Meleca, R. J., [1996], *Vocal pathologies: Diagnosis, treatment and case studies* [Figure 6-6A, p. 171]. San Diego: Singular Publishing Group. Used with permission.)

larynx is to close off the airway to allow for stabilization of the thorax, and hence the shoulder and upper arm, during attempts to lift a heavy weight. Among patients with a unilateral adductor paralysis, such a maneuver may be of value in stimulating the unaffected fold to "over-adduct" and come into contact or approximation with the paralyzed fold. If this or similar techniques are unsuccessful or inappropriate, patients may be referred for surgical care.

Surgery in the case of unilateral vocal fold paralysis involves physically moving the affected vocal fold closer to midline so that the unaffected fold can contact it during phonation. Such surgery is performed under local anesthesia so that the patient is able to phonate as the fold is moved toward midline (medialized). The surgeon continues to move the fold medially until optimal voice is obtained.

While unilateral vocal fold paralysis is fairly uncommon, it is fortunate that bilateral paralysis is even less frequent. Such a disturbance typically results from central nervous system insult, such as a stroke. If neural input to both recurrent laryngeal nerves is eliminated, both folds assume a static position part-way between fully abducted (open) and full adducted (closed). The folds assume a **paramedian position** in which the space between the two folds **(glottis)** is compromised and may result in difficulty breathing **(dyspnea).** Surgery may be required to create a patent (open) airway adequate for breathing. Patients with bilateral RLN impairment but normal SLN function retain reasonably good voice and vocal range. The paramedian position of the two folds makes it fairly easy for an exhaled airstream to draw the folds into vibration via the Bernoulli effect. In addition, the pitch range tends to remain fairly normal because the SLN innervates the cricothyroid muscle, which is the primary muscle responsible for pitch adjustments.

Spasmodic Dysphonia

Spasmodic dysphonia (SD) is a rare disorder, probably affecting no more than 1 to 2 people per 10,000 in the United States. It was originally thought to be of psychogenic origin because patients with spasmodic dysphonia (SD) often experience an improvement in the voice when the pitch is raised. They also have less difficulty during singing. Moreover, some patients report that the condition arose coincident with an emotional event in their lives.

Nevertheless, SD is accepted as a neurologic problem involving disturbance to a portion of the brain known as the basal ganglia. It is considered to be an example of an organic condition known as **dystonia,** meaning a condition characterized by disordered muscle tonicity.

There are two types of SD. In the more frequent type (adductor spasmodic dysphonia), the patient experiences abrupt, uncontrolled (spasmodic) contractions of the adductor muscles resulting in a "strain-strangle" voice quality.

In contrast, abductor spasmodic dysphonia causes inappropriate contraction of the laryngeal abductor (posterior cricoarytenoid) muscles. Inappropriate abduction of the vocal folds causes the patient's speech to be interrupted by periods of aphonia.

The preferred method of treatment for SD patients is repeated injections of botulinum toxin (BOTOX) into the vocalis (adductor SD) or posticus (abductor SD) muscles. Botulinum toxin (BOTOX) is a neurotoxin that blocks release of acetylcholine at the neuromuscular junction. The treatment reduces contractile activity in the affected muscle but does nothing to address the basal ganglia defect creating the problem. For this reason, once the BOTOX effects disappear, the condition reappears.

Shortly after BOTOX injections for adductor SD, the patient usually presents with a breathy voice quality. Thereafter, the voice normalizes and then eventually reverts to the pretreatment "strain-struggle" quality. The entire cycle from injection to relapse usually occurs over a period of 3 to 6 months, after which another BOTOX injection may be recommended.

The role of SLPs in the care of SD patients frequently involves working with them prior to, and following, medical intervention. The intent of therapy is to help the patient accept the breathiness that occurs following administration of BOTOX and to teach the patient various techniques that may prolong the "normal voice" phase.

VOCAL FOLD ABNORMALITIES THAT AFFECT VOICE

There are a variety of structural changes in the vocal folds that can adversely affect the voice (see Table 12–1). While it is not possible to discuss each of these in detail, we will discuss several that are relatively common and/or have a dramatic effect upon phonation.

Nodules

Nodules are the most common form of vocal fold abnormality seen by ENT physicians and are found in approximately 20% of patients who present with a voice problem. Nodules are frequently called "screamer's nodules" because they are often found in children who scream and mothers who scream at their children. They also are relatively common among coaches and aerobics instructors who do not use any form of amplification. However, it is important to understand that nodules can develop in persons who do not scream but who abuse their vocal folds in other ways (see Figure 12–2). A list of misuses and abuses of the larynx is provided in Table 12–2. Misuses may or may not be traumatic to a particular speaker, whereas abusive vocal behavior almost always is traumatic.

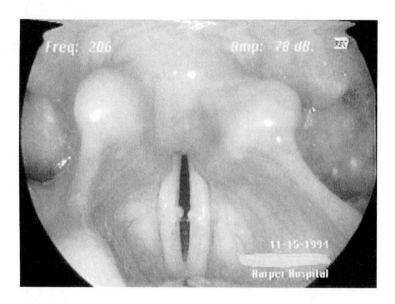

Figure 12-2. Bilateral nodules on the middle one third of both vocal folds in a 52-year-old female. (From Dworkin, J. P., & Meleca, R. J., [1996], *Vocal pathologies: Diagnosis, treatment and case studies* [Figure 3-6, p. 68]. San Diego: Singular Publishing Group. Used with permission.)

It is not unreasonable to think of nodules as calluses that develop on the vocal folds in response to trauma, much as calluses develop on the hands of a day laborer or member of a rowing team. While such growths protect the underlying tissue from further abuse, their presence on the vocal folds adversely affects the voice.

One visually discernible effect of nodules and other solid neoplasms (new growths) on the vocal folds is the tendency for them to dampen a normally occurring mucosal wave. *Mucosal wave* is the name given to the rippling effect that moves across the top surface of a normally compliant vocal fold.

Just as calluses develop in response to tissue trauma, so also do vocal nodules. The point of maximum contact force along the length of the vocal fold is the point of maximum vocal fold movement, which is half-way between the anterior commissure and the anterior end of the vocal process of the arytenoid. It is for this reason that nodules typically develop at this point.

Nodules typically come in pairs. The presumption is that the development of one "callus" will increase trauma to the other vocal fold, thereby precipitating development of a nodule on that fold.

If you think of nodules as a kind of callus, it should be easy to understand that surgical removal is not the preferred treatment of choice. Calluses on the hand, for example, disappear if the abusive behavior is eliminated

Table 12–2. Misuses and Abuses of the Larynx[1]

Misuses (behaviors that may or may not be abusive)

- persistent use of glottal attack
- anterior-posterior (A-P) laryngeal squeezing which is seen as approximation of the epiglottis and the arytenoid cartilages
- puberphonia (maintaining prepubescent voice)
- persistent glottal fry
- speaking with inadequate breath support
- lack of pitch variability
- excessive talking
- ventricular phonation
- aphonia/dysphonia of psychological origin
- loudness variations effected by glottal, rather than respiratory adjustments

Abuses

- excessive, prolonged loudness
- excessive speaking during periods of swelling, inflammation or other tissue changes
- excessive speaking or singing while in a smoke-filled and/or noisy environment
- excessive speaking or singing while using irritants, such as tobacco, alcohol or any number of drugs that affect fluid balance
- prolonged singing without appropriate training;
- excessive coughing and throat clearing (see CD-ROM segment Ch.12.05)
- yelling or screaming
- noise making (e.g., toy or animal sounds grunting (as in exercising and weight lifting) (see CD-ROM segment Ch.12.05)
- grunting (as in exercising and weight lifting) (see CD-ROM segment Ch.12.05)

---

[1]Misuses are vocal behaviors that result in an inefficient use of the laryngeal mechanism. Depending upon a myriad of indeterminate factors, such behaviors may result in laryngeal abuse and consequent structural changes in the larynx. It is unknown why the same behavior or set of behaviors in two apparently similar individuals may result in laryngeal trauma in only one of them.

Source: Adapted from Case, J. L. (1996). *Clinical management of voice disorders.* Austin, TX: Pro-Ed.

and the hand is allowed to heal on its own. One would not consider cutting off the callus of day laborers and then sending them back to the job. Similarly, patients with nodules are almost never considered for surgical intervention. Instead, they are referred to SLPs whose responsibility it is to help the patient alter his or her phonatory behaviors in such a way as to eliminate the vocal abuse. Elimination of the trauma almost always results in the elimination of the "callus."

There are a number of potentially useful techniques that an SLP may employ with a patient with nodules or a variety of other voice problems related to laryngeal hyperfunction. Some of these are listed in Table 12–3.

Seemingly identical patients may respond differentially to one or another of the techniques listed in Table 12–3. It is the responsibility of the SLP and the patient, *working as a team,* to experiment with a variety of these techniques to determine which is most effective. Enlisting the patient as a part of

Table 12–3. Facilitating Techniques That May Be of Value in Extinguishing Inappropriate Laryngeal Behaviors

For All Disorders
Counseling
Ear training
Feedback

For Hypofunction
Altering habitual loudness
Pushing/pulling
Half-swallow, boom
Head positioning

For Hyperfunction
Progressive relaxation
Yawn-sigh
Nasal/glide stimulation
Elimination of hard glottal attack
Chant-talk
Focus:
     Horizontal focus
     Vertical focus
Glottal fry
Massage
Open-mouth approach
Respiration training
Inhalation phonation
Warble
Hierarchy Analysis
Establishing a new pitch

For Psychogenic Problems
Digital manipulation
Masking
Warble

Source: Adapted from Boone, D. R., & McFarlane, S. C. (1994). *The voice and voice therapy.* Englewood Cliffs, NJ: Prentice-Hall.

this exploratory process is empowering for the patient and can be an important part of the therapeutic process. This is just as true for children as it is for adults.

It is not possible to discuss each of the techniques listed in Table 12–3. However, we will describe two in order to give you a sense of how different these techniques can be. First, the *yawn-sigh* technique takes advantage of the fact that the vocal folds are apart (abducted) during a yawn and that they are not fully adducted during a sigh. For an individual who produces inordinate compression of the vocal folds during phonation, a yawn-sigh can be a useful way of enabling the patient to hear, *and feel,* voice produced with little or no untoward tension. Once that is accomplished, the patient works to extend that breathy phonation into a progression of vowels, consonant-vowel (CV) syllables, words, phrases, and sentences. The contrastive use of breathy versus hypertensive voice is frequently useful in enabling the patient to become aware of, and successfully modify, the abusive phonatory pattern.

Vertical focus, by contrast, is an attempt to divert a patient's attention (and hence tension) away from the larynx. One useful approach is to have the patient produce a nasal consonant such as /m/ while lightly touching the sides of their nose with the thumb and index finger. Do it yourself. What did you feel? If you did it correctly, you should have felt the nostrils vibrate in response to the production of a nasal tone. Now remove your fingers and try to perceive that vibration within the nose. Encouraging a patient to do this, using a wide variety of words, phrases, and so on, helps turn their attention away from the larynx, thereby increasing the likelihood that laryngeal muscle tension will diminish. Clinicians often use imagery in eliciting this behavior by asking the patient to "speak into the facial mask."

Polyps

Polyps are another relatively common form of vocal fold abnormality and are found in approximately 10% of patients with a voice problem. If you think of nodules as calluses, then it is reasonable to think of polyps as blisters. As with blisters on the hand, some are "blood blisters" (hemorrhagic polyps) whereas others represent a collection of serous fluid. Unlike typical hand blisters, polyps assume one of two basic shapes (see Figures 12–3 and 12–4). Some are akin to small balloons connected to the vocal fold by a narrow stalk or foot. Since *foot* in Latin is "ped," such polyps are known as pedunculated polyps. More often, the polyp is spread over a relatively large area of the vocal fold. Such polyps are known as sessile polyps, stemming from the Latin word *sessilis* meaning low-lying.

Although the genesis of polyps is not completely understood, most clinicians believe they are the result of vocal abuse. Frequently, this abuse may be a one-time occurrence—much like a blister that develops after a couch potato rakes 3 acres of leaves. By contrast, nodules are thought to develop over time.

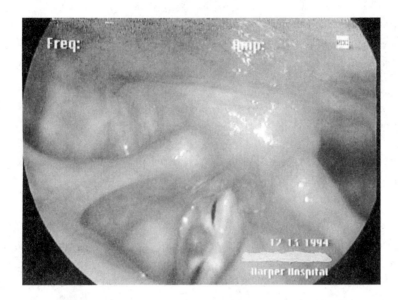

Figure 12–3. A unilateral, hemorrhagic polyp on the middle one third of a 47-year-old high school gym teacher. (From Dworkin, J. P., & Meleca, R. J., [1996], *Vocal pathologies: Diagnosis, treatment and case studies* [Figure 3-9, p. 70]. San Diego: Singular Publishing Group. Used with permission.)

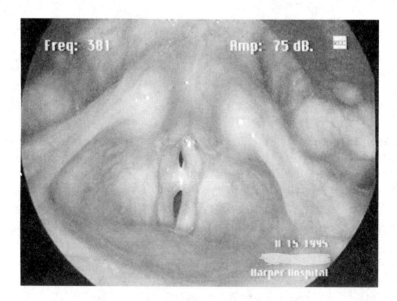

Figure 12–4. A sessile polyp in a 27-year-old salesman who admitted to intermittent vocal abusive behaviors. (From Dworkin, J. P., & Meleca, R. J., [1996], *Vocal pathologies: Diagnosis, treatment and case studies* [Figure 3-11, p. 71]. San Diego: Singular Publishing Group. Used with permission.)

Given what was stated previously about the genesis and location of nodules, where along the length of the vocal fold would you expect most polyps to develop?

A relatively hard nodule on one vocal fold tends to cause the creation of a nodule on the other fold. On the other hand, a soft, pliable polyp on one vocal fold does not tend to irritate the other fold. For this reason, polyps tend to occur on only one vocal fold (i.e., unilaterally). Since they may impede full adduction of the vocal folds during phonation, the voice tends to be breathy or hoarse. Their tendency to occur on only one vocal fold means that the two vocal folds may be substantially different in mass. In such cases, the two vocal folds may vibrate at different rates, causing a double voice **(diplophonia).**

As with nodules, polyps are most typically treated by SLPs whose goal it is to identify causative behaviors, such as yelling or excessive throat clearing, and help the patient eliminate them. However, unlike nodules, some "long-standing" polyps that do not respond to voice therapy may be surgically removed.

Contact Ulcers

Unlike nodules and polyps, contact ulcers—and the granulomas that frequently develop at sites of ulceration—do not appear on the membranous portion of the vocal fold. Instead, they arise further back, on the vocal processes of the arytenoids (see Figure 12–5). Contact ulcers can arise from a number of fairly disparate causes:

1. excessive slamming together of the arytenoid cartilages during the production of inappropriately low pitch;

2. frequent, nonproductive coughing and throat clearing;

3. gastric reflux resulting in acidic irritation of the membrane overlying the arytenoids (known as gastro-esophageal reflux disease or GERD); and

4. intubation trauma that can occur during surgery under general anesthesia.

Speech-language pathologists work with patients who present with the first two causative agents, since these are habit patterns amenable to therapeutic intervention. They might also be called upon to work with patients whose contact ulcers resulted from gastro-esophageal reflux disease (GERD) or intubation trauma. In the latter situations, the role of the SLP is to help patients adjust to the resultant hoarseness in a way that does not exacerbate the problem and hence prolong the recovery process. For patients with GERD, the primary treatment involves appropriate dietary changes and the

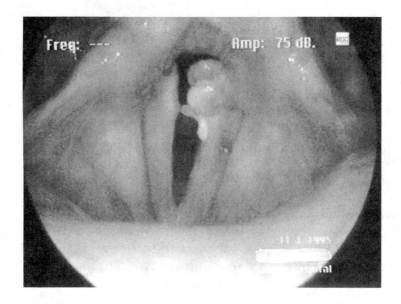

Figure 12-5. A contact granuloma on the left arytenoid cartilage, owing to agressive phonatory behaviors and chronic gastro-esophageal reflux disease (GERD) in a middle-aged industrial plant foreman. (From Dworkin, J. P., & Meleca, R. J., [1996], *Vocal pathologies: Diagnosis, treatment and case studies* [Figure 3-14, p. 75]. San Diego: Singular Publishing Group. Used with permission.)

CD-ROM

Gastro-Esophageal Reflux Disease	
CD-ROM segment Ch.12.01.	An ear, nose, and throat physician (ENT) uses rigid laryngoscopy to view the anatomic structures of the larynx. As noted previously, the subject presented with GERD. You will see that the posterior portion of each vocal fold is red (erythematous) as a result of irritation by stomach acid.
CD-ROM segment Ch.12.05.	Laryngeal compression during simulated weight-lifting maneuvers (viewed with a flexible scope). Using the larynx in this fashion can be abusive, if employed routinely. These compressions are followed by examples of coughing.

judicious use of antacids and/or beta-blockers, whereas intubation trauma is best treated with a "tincture of time," coupled with vocal use that is not hyperfunctional.

Papillomas

The human papilloma virus (HPV) causes warts, which can occur on any skin or mucous membrane surface. Most are easily treated and are not life-threatening. However, when they occur on the vocal folds, they can grow so large as to compromise the airway, making breathing difficult (see Figure 12–6). Children presenting with laryngeal papillomas are thought to contract the human papilloma virus (HPV) at birth from genital warts in the mother.

Fortunately, this condition is relatively uncommon. The incidence of laryngeal papillomas in the United States is approximately 7 cases per million people per year. It is also fortunate that the body develops some immunity to warts, and they usually go away without treatment. However, surgical removal is necessary in the case of papillomas whose size threatens the airway. Moreover, such growths tend to recur, necessitating repeated surgical procedures. Repeated surgery increases the likelihood of significant scar tissue formation that can adversely affect the vibratory activity of the vocal folds. In addition to postoperative voice therapy, an important role served by the SLP is detecting dysphonia in undiagnosed children and making an appropriate medical referral. Children with papillomas may go undetected for some time because some professionals may assume incorrectly that the child's hoarse-

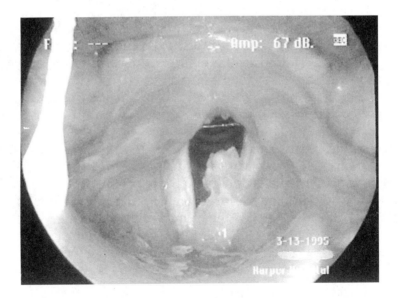

Figure 12–6. As you might imagine, this 28-year-old female suffered severe dysphonia as a result of her laryngeal papilloma. (From Dworkin, J. P., & Meleca, R. J., [1996], *Vocal pathologies: Diagnosis, treatment and case studies* [Figure 3-20, p. 84]. San Diego: Singular Publishing Group. Used with permission.)

ness is due to vocal nodules. This mistake is as understandable as it is inexcusable because the vast majority of children with a hoarse voice have vocal nodules, not papillomas.

Carcinoma

Cancer of the larynx affects approximately 11,000 new patients each year and constitutes approximately 10% of patients seen for voice problems by ENT physicians. Approximately 75% are found on the vocal folds, although they may appear above or below the folds. Unlike polyps and nodules, whose genesis tends to be from acute or chronic physical trauma, respectively, laryngeal cancer frequently arises from exposure to inhaled smoke that may occur over years. When physicians describe the smoking habits of a patient, they might say that "Mr. Jones is a 30 pack-year smoker" indicating that he smoked the *equivalent* of one pack of cigarettes per day for 30 years. Thus, someone who smoked 3 packs a day for 10 years would also be described as a 30 pack-year smoker.

For a reason that is not well understood, coincident smoking and alcohol consumption dramatically increases the chance of developing laryngeal cancer. That is, there appears to be an additive effect when drinking and smoking coexist. It is not unusual to find that many patients with laryngeal cancer report a history of smoking and moderate to heavy drinking.

Whereas polyps and nodules represent benign tissue changes that are localized to the outermost area of the vocal folds known as the "cover," squamous cell carcinomas are malignant tissue changes that arise in the squamous (flattened) cells found in the epithelial portion of the "cover." These malignant growths can invade the muscle or "body" of the vocal fold (see Figure 12–7). In addition, like other forms of cancer, laryngeal carcinomas may migrate (**metastasize**) to other locations within the body, thereby increasing the threat to life.

Patients with extensive laryngeal carcinomas may be candidates for complete removal of the larynx because of the life-threatening nature of cancer. With new advances in cancer treatment, only around 15–20% of laryngeal cancer patients now undergo total laryngectomy. For those who must undergo this radical procedure, it is the responsibility of the SLP to provide preoperative and postoperative counseling, coupled with postoperative therapy intended to optimize the communication abilities of the laryngectomized patient. We will return to this important topic after discussing the evaluation process.

THE VOICE EVALUATION

In Chapter 11, we mentioned that children born with cleft lip, cleft palate, or both should be evaluated and treated by a team of specialists with particular

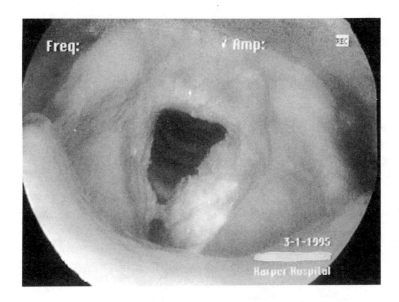

Figure 12–7. This patients presents with bilateral carcinoma of the vocal folds. Note the gross destruction of both folds. (From Dworkin, J. P., & Meleca, R. J., [1996], *Vocal pathologies: Diagnosis, treatment and case studies* [Figure 3-26, p. 92]. San Diego: Singular Publishing Group. Used with permission.)

expertise in this clinical area. While voice disorders typically do not negatively affect as many important functions as oral-facial clefts, voice problems are best managed by the joint efforts of a team. The core elements of such a team are the ENT and the SLP. In the ideal situation, which is most often realized in hospital settings, the ENT and the SLP evaluate the patient together. More often, patients are referred to the SLP by the ENT, a primary care physician, a school nurse, or the patients themselves. In all but the first case, it is incumbent upon the SLP to ensure that a trusted ENT is involved in the evaluation and treatment planning. This is particularly true since some laryngeal pathologies can be life-threatening.

A multiplicity of factors can cause and/or maintain a voice problem. Therefore, the evaluation must be far-reaching in scope. A thorough voice evaluation involves an extensive interview to obtain as much information as possible concerning the patient and his or her perceptions regarding the problem. It is also useful to include other family members in this part of the evaluation. Following the interview, the clinician conducts both a perceptual assessment and an instrumental evaluation of the voice.

Patient Interview

The interview is intended to provide extensive information concerning the patient and the problem. In addition to gathering basic demographic data, such as age and gender, it is important to explore thoroughly with patients their health history, professional and social activities, family milieu, dietary habits, use of stimulants, and level of concern regarding the voice problem. While it is not possible to discuss each of these factors in detail, an example may help you understand why an SLP must develop considerable interviewing skill.

Ms. Ima Patient was self-referred for what she described as a "frightening voice." She indicated that when speaking with people, she frequently is asked whether she is choking. She said it frequently feels as if someone is strangling her while speaking. The interview revealed that this condition began following the death of Ms. Patient's sister 6 months before and had been getting progressively worse ever since. She noted that her voice improved when she sang or spoke at a higher than normal pitch level and that it was worse when she spoke on the phone. Ms. Patient denied ever having experienced anything like this in the past, and her husband confirmed that report. Further discussion revealed that the family physician had examined the larynx with a laryngeal mirror and reportedly found "nothing wrong." After considerable probing, the husband reluctantly mentioned that his wife had been referred to a psychiatrist by her family physician approximately 2 months ago. However, that referral was rejected, and Ms. Patient became tearful when this topic was broached.

At first glance, it might appear that Ms. Patient's voice disorder is due to a psychological problem. However, you may have identified one or more of a number of clues in the preceding paragraph that suggest otherwise. Do you know what they are?

First of all, the descriptive terms of "choking" and "strangling" indicate the possibility of a neurologic disorder known as spasmodic dysphonia. As you know from our earlier discussion, it is not unusual for this condition to manifest itself following an emotional trauma, and it is easy to see why it frequently is thought to be a psychiatric disorder. Such a misdiagnosis may appear to be substantiated by a cursory examination of the larynx, because special equipment is necessary to uncover the laryngeal behaviors characterizing this condition. This equipment is rarely available to the family physician but is routinely used by ENT physicians. This is another example of why SLPs need to establish and maintain a close working relationship with an astute ENT.

Perceptual Assessment

During the interview, the patient may describe their voice problem using a number of terms. The characteristics that a patient reports are known as *symptoms.* The nine primary symptoms are hoarseness, fatigue, breathiness, reduced pitch range, lack of voice (aphonia), pitch breaks or inappropriately high pitch, strain/strangle, tremor, and lump in the throat (globus). Voice characteristics that can be observed or tested by a clinician are known as *signs*. Some symptoms, such as "high pitch" and "hoarseness" are also signs, whereas some, such as "something in my throat" and "fatigue," are not. The task of the SLP in the perceptual assessment part of the evaluation is to use listening skills to identify the presence and magnitude of the signs of a voice problem. Specifically, SLPs make judgments regarding pitch, loudness, and quality during a variety of tasks. A high-quality tape recording is routinely made of the patient, using a standard speech sample. While that sample varies across clinicians, it frequently includes the patient's name, the recording date, sustained vowel phonations, counting, reading, singing, spontaneous conversation, and pitch and loudness glissandos (a rapid sliding up and down a range).

 CD-ROM

Rising and Falling Glissando

CD-ROM segment Ch.12.06 shows rising pitch (rising glissando) during production of "hey" (viewed with a rigid scope). CD-ROM segment Ch.12.08 shows rising and falling glissando, including the falsetto register (viewed with a flexible scope).

Voice Quality

The literature pertaining to abnormalities of voice is replete with a variety of descriptive terms. Despite this extensive vocabulary, we can quite adequately describe voice quality disorders with three terms: breathy, hoarse, and harsh.

If you were to speak without allowing the vocal folds to vibrate, you would be whispering. That is, the source of sound would not be a rich set of harmonics, known as a laryngeal spectrum, but would be frictional noise created as air rushed through the glottis (the space between the vocal folds.) If, however, you were to allow the vocal folds to vibrate, but kept them from touching one another during vibration, your voice would be *breathy*. That is, your speech would be characterized by a spectrum of tones (voice) superimposed on a noise spectrum (whisper).

Now assume, for the moment, that you had a large growth on the medial aspect (inner surface) of your vocal folds. It should be apparent that the presence of such a growth would make it difficult to close the glottis completely. Since such a growth would cause an undesirable quality in the voice (breathiness), there is a natural tendency to increase vocal fold tension in an effort to eliminate that quality by forcing the vocal folds together. In fact, what happens as a consequence is that untoward vocal fold tension is introduced without the desired result of eliminating the breathiness. This combination of vocal fold tension (harshness), coupled with breathiness, is what we perceive as *hoarseness*.

An individual who does not manifest any irregularity of the medial margin of the vocal folds, and hence no breathiness, but does phonate with inappropriate vocal fold tension produces a tense voice that we describe as *harshness*. One previously mentioned clinical condition characterized by such tension and consequent voice quality is known as muscle tension dysphonia (MTD).

Hypertensive laryngeal function is often accompanied by pharyngeal (throat) muscle tension. The combination results in an amplification of high-frequency components that cause the speech—and hence the person—to appear strident. Given the inappropriate amount of tension in the vocal folds, it should be fairly easy to appreciate that such speakers run the risk of traumatizing the folds and causing the development of tissue changes in the vocal folds.

In judging the pitch, loudness, and quality of a patient's speech, clinicians use scales for grading the parameters of interest. One of the more commonly used scales is called equal-appearing-interval scaling. Most such scales use 5, 6, or 7 steps between polar opposites, such as high and low pitch, or between normal and severely impaired along a continuum such as hoarseness. For example, a 6-point scale regarding hoarseness might use the following assignments:

1 = normal voice quality

2 = mild hoarseness

3 = mild-to-moderate hoarseness

4 = moderate hoarseness

5 = moderate-to-severe hoarseness

6 = severe hoarseness

The phrase "equal-appearing" indicates that the clinician feels confident in stating that the psychophysical distance between mild and moderate is equal to the perceptual "distance" from moderate to severe. Assuming that this confidence is justified, *and it may not be,* the data collected utilizing this type of scale can be analyzed using relatively powerful statistics, known as parametric statistics.

Instrumental Evaluation

A voice evaluation that does not include instrumental assessment is considered a screening procedure. Instrumental data are an important way of confirming and extending information obtained by listening to the voice. They are also an extremely valuable means of documenting change, should the patient be enrolled in voice therapy.

Among a wide variety of instruments currently in use, two are of such particular value that we will mention them here. The first has already been mentioned: endoscopy. As you know already, this instrument enables the clinician to visualize the vocal folds and surrounding area. What we have not yet mentioned in this chapter is the technique known as *stroboscopy*.

 CD-ROM

Breathy Phonation

CD-ROM segment Ch.12.09 shows breathy phonation observed in real time and using stroboscopy to reveal the presence of a good mucosal wave (viewed with a rigid scope).

A stroboscope is a device that causes a light to pulsate at a particular frequency. If a light is turned on briefly every second, and a propeller is rotating once a second, it will appear as if the propeller is standing still. If the light is turned on briefly every 1.1 seconds, it will appear as if the propeller is rotating slowly. If the light is turned on briefly every 0.9 seconds, it will appear as if the propeller is slowly rotating backwards. That is the concept underlying laryngeal stroboscopy. A microphone is applied to the patient's neck, the purpose of which is to measure the fundamental frequency of that individual's voice. That signal is then used to drive the endoscope's light source. For example, let us assume that a male patient is phonating at 100 Hz (Hertz). A 100 Hz fundamental frequency admittedly is quite low, but it makes the math easier to follow. A fundamental frequency of 100 Hz means that the vocal folds move through an entire opening and closing cycle once every 1/100 of a second or every 10 milliseconds. A stroboscope will illuminate the vocal folds every 10.2 milliseconds, thereby creating the impression that the vocal folds are moving slowly. This slow-motion technique enables clinicians to examine closely the movement characteristics of the vocal folds, thereby enabling them to detect abnormalities that would otherwise go unnoticed.

Another instrument in wide use today is known as the *VisiPitch*. This instrument provides objective data regarding a number of acoustic parameters, not all of which will be mentioned here. With this machine, the clinician can obtain information regarding a patient's fundamental frequency and phonatory range, measured in Hertz (Hz). It is also possible to record voice intensity in decibels (dB) while the patient performs a number of tasks. In addition, this instrument can be used to determine the relative amount of spectral noise in the speech signal. Finally, it is used to determine instability in fundamental frequency while the patient attempts to maintain a constant tone for 2 seconds. This pitch instability is called *jitter*. The human larynx is not a perfect machine, and so we would expect some instability in a person's pitch, even when he or she was trying to produce a steady tone. However, extensive research on normal subjects and patients with voice disorders has shown that voices that are heard as normal do not manifest pitch instability, or jitter, that exceeds 1% of the person's fundamental frequency. That is, we would not expect moment-to-moment changes in fundamental frequency to exceed an average of 1 Hz in a male subject with a 100 Hz fundamental or 2 Hz in a female subject with a 200 Hz fundamental. Jitter values exceeding about 1% are associated with voices that are judged to be hoarse.

Disposition

Once the voice evaluation is complete, it is incumbent upon the SLP to make recommendations regarding referrals and the need for treatment, if any. Among all the patients seen by an SLP, some of the most challenging can be those individuals who have laryngeal cancer, and for whom the medical treatment involves surgical removal of the larynx **(laryngectomy).** These patients do not need to be treated for a voice problem. They need assistance adapting to the absence of voice.

LARYNGECTOMY

The larynx sits at the top of the trachea, or windpipe, and serves as a protective valve as well as a sound generator. Surgical removal of the larynx requires that the trachea be redirected to an opening on the front of the neck, known as a tracheal **stoma** (Figure 12–8). This causes alteration in a number of functions, some of which were discussed in Chapter 11. For example, because the cleansing action of the nose is eliminated by this redirection of the breath stream, **laryngectomees** (people who have had a laryngectomy) routinely wear some protective device over the stoma to ensure that foreign matter does not enter the lungs. This device may be a simple gauze pad or it may be a plastic valvular device that serves as an airway protector at the same time it facilitates phonation in a way that is described in the following sections.

It should take little imagination to appreciate how potentially devastating it would be to lose the ability to phonate. Those of you who have had a bad case of laryngitis have surely experienced short-term frustration in being unable to communicate verbally, but how would you feel if you thought that inability would be total and would be forever? Now try to understand the

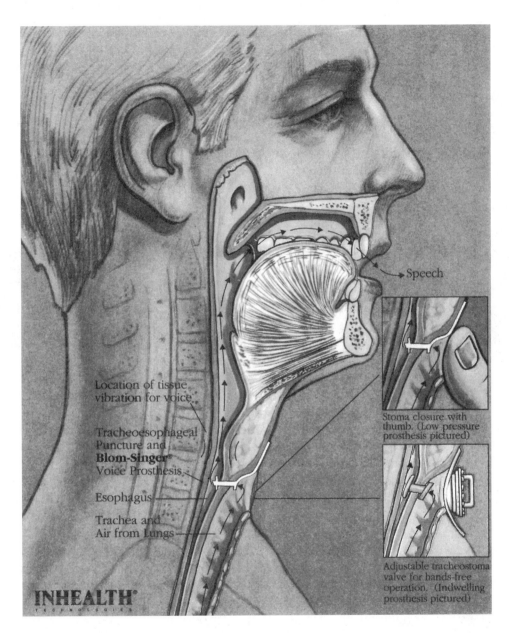

Figure 12–8. Illustration of the tracheo-esophageal puncture (TEP) surgical reconstruction technique following total laryngectomy. Note the position of the silicone prosthesis in the surgically created tunnel between the trachea and esophagus. Collars on both the esophageal and tracheal sides of the prosthesis ensure stable fit of the appliance. (From Dworkin, J. P., & Meleca, R. J., [1996], *Vocal pathologies: Diagnosis, treatment and case studies* [Figure 5-8, p. 145]. San Diego: Singular Publishing Group. Reprinted from *inhealth Technology* publication. Used with permission.)

impact of knowing that your sense of smell and taste will be compromised, your daily hygiene routine will be increased, showering will require special precautions to protect your airway, and swimming will no longer be possible.

If you are able to comprehend the emotionality associated with losing one's larynx, you can readily see why SLPs play such an important role in the counseling of patients both before and after surgery. We also play a major role in ensuring that these individuals do, in fact, regain the ability to communicate verbally. We do so by working with patients to help them adopt one, or more, of the following options.

Artificial Larynx

 CD-ROM

Artificial Larynx

CD-ROM segment Ch.12.10 is a short demonstration of an artificial larynx.

In anticipation of laryngectomy surgery, an SLP may work with patients to familiarize them with two types of artificial larynx they may choose to use after surgery. One of these involves a hand-held, battery-activated diaphragm that creates a sound source that, when held up to the air, actually sounds pretty obnoxious. However, when held against the neck, it produces a spectrum of tones in the throat that can be modulated by the articulators to produce intelligible speech.

In the immediate postoperative period, the throat area is quite tender. This is particularly true if the patient has undergone radiation therapy. As a consequence, a different type of artificial larynx is frequently recommended right after surgery. The principle difference is that the sound generated by the device is presented directly to the mouth by means of a small tube (catheter), thereby making it available for articulatory modulation.

Some laryngectomees are quite pleased with these mechanical devices and choose not to explore other options. On the other hand, many patients dislike the artificial, mechanical quality of voice and the "hassle" of dealing with a device that can be misplaced or lost.

Esophageal Speech

One such option is to force air down into the esophagus and then release the impounded air pressure in such a way as to cause vibration in the walls of the esophagus. Either you, or someone you know, is undoubtedly able to "speak on a burp." That is, in essence, **esophageal speech.** The primary difference involves the mechanism whereby the air is captured.

Instead of consuming enough carbonated beverage to create an air source, esophageal speakers actively force (inject) air down the esophagus past an area variously known as the **neoglottis,** the **pseudoglottis,** or the **pharyngeal-esophageal (PE) segment.** When the impounded air is released, it passes by the PE segment and draws the walls of the esophagus into vibration, much like air passing through the (true) glottis causes vibration of the vocal folds.

Since the esophageal walls are much larger in mass that the true vocal folds, esophageal speech is quite low-pitched. In addition, because there is little voluntary control of the muscles in the area of the pseudoglottis, pitch variability is quite limited.

The amount of air typically impounded for one esophageal utterance is only about 80 cubic centimerers, as opposed to a potential lung volume (vital capacity) of well over 2,000 cubic centimeters in both men and women. As such, utterance length is markedly limited, as is the ability to alter the force with which the impounded air escapes. Therefore, loudness variability is severely restricted. These latter constraints lead many laryngectomees to consider a third option for voice production.

Tracheoesophageal Speech

In tracheoesophageal speech, air is routed from the lungs into the esophagus via a tracheoesophageal speech prosthesis (see Figure 12–8). This is possible because patients undergo an additional surgery to create a small opening (fistula) between the trachea and esophagus. This operation is known as a tracheoesophageal puncture (TEP).[1]

Once the area has healed, a prosthesis similar to that shown in Figure 12–8 can be inserted. To force air from the trachea into the esophagus, the laryngectomee must either cover the hole (stoma) on the front of his or her throat with a finger or be fitted with a tracheostomal valve. Such a valve automatically shuts as exhaled lung pressure increases in anticipation of speech onset. The volume and pressure of shunted air available for vibration of the neoglottis is limited only by the respiratory capabilities of the individual. It is for this reason that TEP speakers manifest longer phrase length and greater pitch and loudness variability than esophageal speakers. Not all laryngectomized individuals are candidates for tracheoesophageal speech. However, when appropriate, most clinicians agree that TEP speakers achieve the most natural speech with the least therapy.

[1] Depending upon the surgeon, TEP may be performed at the time of laryngectomy or it may be performed as a secondary procedure.

Whichever speaking method is adopted by a patient, the SLP plays a critical role in the rehabilitation of these individuals. In the process, our principal reward is in knowing that we have helped our patients resume their rightful place in a society that relies heavily on the spoken word as a basis for human interaction.

SUMMARY

Voice disorders arise from changes in the structure and function of the larynx and result from a variety of causes. Abuse results in the formation of new tissue that changes the vibratory pattern and interferes with vocal fold closure. Neurological disorders may paralyze muscles of the larynx so that the vocal folds cannot be closed for phonation or fully opened for breathing. Cancer of the larynx frequently requires that the vocal folds be removed and an alternative sound source for speech must be developed. Psychological disorders may cause voice disorders, but there is no physical basis for the problems with phonation. Primary perceptual characteristics of voice disorders are breathiness, harshness, and hoarseness. Perceptual analysis of these signs, direct visualization of the vocal folds by nasendoscopy, the results of a medical evaluation, and a comprehensive case history provide the information necessary to diagnosis the disorder and to develop a program of treatment of voice disorders. Treatment depends on the type and severity of the disorder and requires the collaboration of the speech-language pathologist (SLP) and other health care professionals. In cases of abuse, therapy focuses on reducing the abusive phonation pattern. Paralysis may require medical intervention to provide improved vocal fold closure before therapy provided by a SLP. Psychologically based disorders may necessitate referral to other health care professionals for counseling. The ultimate goal of intervention is improved phonation for speech production.

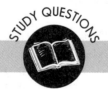

STUDY QUESTIONS

1. In this chapter, we noted that the presence of vocal nodules adversely affects voice *quality*. What effect on *pitch* would you expect from their presence?

2. A question for you, if you are a smoker: Why?

3. What are the essential differences between a polyp and a nodule?

4 What is meant by the terms "signs" and "symptoms"?

5 Name three different alternatives individuals have for producing oral speech following surgical removal of the larynx.

REFERENCES

Boone, D. R., & McFarlane, S. C. (1994). *The voice and voice therapy.* Englewood Cliffs, NJ: Prentice-Hall.

Case, J. L. (1996). *Clinical management of voice disorders.* Austin, TX: Pro-Ed.

Dworkin, J. P., & Meleca, R. J. (1997). *Vocal pathologies: Diagnosis, treatment, and case studies.* San Diego: Singular Publishing Group.

SUGGESTED READINGS

Brown, W. S., Vinson, B. P., & Crary, M. A. (1996). *Organic voice disorders: Assessment and treatment.* San Diego: Singular Publishing Group.

Dworkin, J. P., & Meleca, R. J. (1997). *Vocal pathologies: Diagnosis, treatment, and case studies.* San Diego: Singular Publishing Group.

Colton, R., & Casper, J. K. (1996). *Understanding voice problems: A physiological perspective for diagnosis and treatment.* Baltimore: Williams & Wilkins.

GLOSSARY

Abduction: Vocal fold movement away from each other.

Adduction: Vocal fold movement toward each other.

Aphonia: Loss of voice.

Atrophy: Withering or wasting away of tissues or organs.

Diplophonia: A "two toned" voice resulting from simultaneous vibration of two structures with differing vibratory frequencies.

Dysphonia: Disturbed phonation.

Dyspnea: Difficult or labored breathing; a shortness of breath.

Dystonia: Disturbed muscle tone.

Edema: Accumulation of an excessive amount of fluid in cells, tissues, or serous cavities; usually results in a swelling of the tissues.

Erythematous: Relating to or marked by erythema, redness or inflammation of the skin.

Esophageal speech: Alaryngeal speech in which the air supply for phonation originates in the upper portion of the esophagus, with the pharyngoesophageal segment functioning as a neoglottis.

Extrinsic laryngeal muscles: Muscles originating or acting from outside of the part where located or acting.

Glottis: usually used in our field to refer to the space between the true vocal folds.

Hyperfunction: Excessive forcing and straining, usually at the level of the vocal folds, but which may occur at various points along the vocal tract.

Hypofunction, vocal: Reduced vocal capacity resulting from prolonged overuse, muscle fatigue, tissue irritation, or general laryngeal or specific problems relating to the opening and closing of the glottis, characterized by air loss and sometimes hoarseness and pitch breaks.

Laryngectomee: One who has undergone a laryngectomy, which is surgical removal of part or all of the larynx.

Metastasize: To spread or invade by metastasis, said usually of a cancer.

Myopathy: An abnormal condition or disease of muscle.

Neoglottis: Vibratory segment or area that functions for vocal phonation in the absence of the glottis following surgical removal of the larynx. *See* Pseudoglottis.

Paramedian: Near the middle line.

Pharyngeal-esophageal (PE) segment: Pharyngoesophageal junction; another name for the neoglottis.

Pseudoglottis: Vibratory segment or area that functions for vocal phonation in the absence of the glottis; neoglottis.

Stoma: A small opening, such as the mouth; an artificial opening between cavities or canals, or between such and the surface of the body.

Unilateral: Pertaining to or restricted to one side of the body.

13

Fluency Disorders

Ronald B. Gillam

LEARNING OBJECTIVES

1 To understand and describe the primary behaviors of stuttering: word repetition, syllable repetition, sound repetition, prolongation, and block.

---

2 To differentiate between primary stuttering behaviors and secondary stuttering behaviors.

---

3 To learn what causes stuttering.

---

4 To learn about the factors that contribute to chronic stuttering.

---

5 To know the assessment procedures that are used in most stuttering evaluations.

---

6 To differentiate between the two primary types of treatment for stuttering: stuttering modification and fluency shaping.

---

7 To understand how the treatment of children who are beginning to stutter differs from the treatment of adolescents and adults who are chronic stutterers.

INTRODUCTION

Imagine yourself sitting in a restaurant. You overhear the man at the table next to you trying to order dinner. The man says, "I'll have, um, the, uh, spa, spa, spa (long pause) spaghetti (audible breath) and m-----meatballs." During the long pause after the third "spa," you can't help but notice that his lips are protruding and quivering. Then, when he says "meatballs," he holds the /m/ for about a second and his eyelids flutter a little before he gets the rest of the word out. The waitress looks surprised, smiles in an embarrassed sort of way, and hurries off. If you're like many other people, you might think he looks and sounds foolish, that he probably isn't very smart, and that he probably experiences social and vocational difficulties. You might laugh at him a little, or you might feel sorry for him.

If this person is like many other stutterers, you may have formed the wrong impressions. He may be a software developer, an architect, a real estate agent, or a college professor. He probably has a wife, children, and a number of close friends. It is likely that he had some speech therapy that has helped him lessen his stuttering even though he still stutters in some speaking contexts. He might not be terribly bothered by his stuttering anymore. In fact, he might live a happy, productive, and fulfilled life because he has refused to let the fact that he stutters interfere with his social, educational, and vocational choices.

This chapter reviews some of the more important findings about stuttering in children and adults and summarizes best practices in assessing and treating individuals who stutter. We will begin with a discussion of fluency, normal disfluency, and stuttering. Then we will examine what is currently known about the development of stuttering in children and the factors that contribute to continued stuttering in adolescents and adults. Finally, we will look into the ways speech-language pathologists (SLPs) assess and treat stuttering.

 CD-ROM

Overview of the CD-ROM Segments for Chapter 13

The CD-ROM that accompanies this book contains six short video segments of an adult who stutters. The first two segments demonstrate types of stuttering. Later you will use these segments to practice identifying stuttering. The other segments depict stuttering therapy. There are two segments that show an approach to therapy called "stuttering modification" and two segments that demonstrate an approach to therapy called "fluency shaping." You should watch all the segments before you read the remainder of this chapter. That way, you will have an idea about what stuttering looks like and how it can be changed.

Segments

Ch.13.01.   The individual is talking to a speech-language pathologist about one of his early speech therapy experiences. He is not employing any strategies to reduce or modify his stuttering.

Ch.13.02.   The individual reads a short passage from an article without using any strategies to reduce or modify his stuttering.

Ch.13.03.   The speech-language pathologist teaches the stutterer to "cancel" moments of stuttering. This is part of a technique called "speech modification."

Ch.13.04.   The stutterer practices a speech modification strategy called "pull-outs." This technique is also one of several intervention strategies that are referred to as "speech modification" approaches.

Ch.13.05.   The speech-language pathologist teaches the individual how to use a fluency shaping strategy that involves letting out a short breath before saying the first sound, slowing down the rate of speech, and saying sounds gently.

Ch.13.06.   The stutterer practices fluency shaping controls while reading a short passage about stuttering.

THE NATURE OF FLUENT SPEECH

Most children and adults speak with relatively little effort. Their speech is produced at a rate that makes it easy for listeners to perceive what they are saying, and their words flow together evenly. The term **fluency** is used to describe speech that is easy, rapid, rhythmical, and evenly flowing.

Speakers do not speak in a perfectly fluent manner all the time. Sometimes they repeat phrases (*My paper, my paper* is right here), words (*My, my* paper is right here), syllables (My *pa, pa*per is right here), or individual phonemes (*M, m, my* paper is right here). They may prolong some sounds a little longer than usual (*M---y* paper is right here). Sometimes they interject fillers (My paper is, *um,* right here), pause in unusual places (My [pause] paper is right here), or revise their sentences (*My paper, that paper I wrote last week* is right here). The term **disfluency** is used to describe speech that is marked by repetitions, interjections, pauses, and revisions like the ones just listed. Listen carefully to a friend during a phone conversation or to your professors as they lecture. You might be surprised at the number of disfluencies you hear. It is normal for speakers to produce disfluencies some of the time.

There are some individuals who have an unusual number of disfluencies or disfluencies that are physically tense. These disfluencies interfere with their ability to communicate effectively and may cause the speakers to have negative emotional reactions to their own speech. These individuals have a condition called **stuttering,** which is the most common form of fluency impairment. Stuttering is not the only type of fluency disorder. Some individuals speak disfluently as a result of neurological disease or brain injury. Other individuals have a condition called **cluttering,** which is characterized by very rapid bursts of dysrhythmic, unintelligible speech.

WHAT IS STUTTERING?

Guitar (1998) has proposed a three-part definition of stuttering. First, stuttering is characterized by an unusually high frequency or duration of repetitions, prolongations, and/or blockages (tense moments when voicing and/or the flow of air is interrupted) that interrupt the flow of speech. Second, these interruptions are often combined with excessive mental and physical effort to resume talking. Stutterers sometimes report that they lose their train of thought when they concentrate too much on ways to avoid stuttering, and they often tighten their speech musculature and push harder in order to escape from moments of stuttering. Ironically, avoidance and escape behaviors that are meant to decrease speech disfluencies often have the opposite effect; they actually make stuttering worse. Third, most stutterers have negative perceptions of their communication abilities due to their inability to say what they want to say when they want to say it. Some stutters develop unusually low self-esteem because they internalize the negative reactions of others.

Primary Stuttering Behaviors

There are primary and secondary stuttering behaviors. The **primary stuttering behaviors,** sometimes referred to as "core behaviors," are the disfluencies that were mentioned earlier (i.e., repetitions, prolongations, and blocks). It is not unusual for normal speakers to repeat phrases or whole words, to interject fillers like "uh" and "um," or to pause to collect their thoughts before continuing. People who stutter tend to have somewhat different kinds of disfluencies. They may produce three or four rapid repetitions of sounds at the beginning of words or even within words (*baseb,b,b,ball*). They also produce *prolongations* in which they hold out or "prolong" a sound for an unusually long period of time. For example, say the word *van*, but keep saying just the /v/ out loud for 2 or 3 seconds before you move into the "-an." That's a prolongation.

There is one more kind of disfluency, commonly called a *block,* that is rarely seen in the speech of people who do not stutter. Blocks are silent prolongations. Stutterers sometimes feel like they become stuck as they are producing sounds. When this happens, they hold the articulators in place to say the sound, but the articulators are so tense they do not allow any sound to come out for an unusually long time (1 or 2 seconds). Imagine you are going to say the word *car.* Put the back of your tongue up against the posterior (back) part of your hard palate and hold it there tightly. At the same time, push with your diaphragm so that your breath is trying to get out. It can't because your tongue is "blocking" the air from being released. Keep pushing your breath against your tongue for a few seconds, then release the tongue so that you say the word *car* with a hard /k/. The breath should come tumbling out all at once, and the word should be pronounced a little louder than usual. That is what it feels like to have a controlled (voluntary) block. Imagine how frustrating it might be if that often happened when you did not want it to. Do you think you might begin to feel frustrated and anxious about your speech?

Secondary Stuttering Behaviors

Secondary stuttering behaviors are counterproductive adaptations stutterers make as they try to get through primary stuttering behaviors or avoid them altogether. There are many different kinds of secondary stuttering behaviors. We have seen stutterers blink their eyes, open their jaws, purse their lips, change words, insert "uh" right before a word that they anticipate stuttering on, flap their arms, and even, in one case, stamp the floor with the left foot then the right foot in succession. Unfortunately, as these compensations become more and more automatic, they also become less and less successful as ways to escape or avoid stuttering. Soon, the secondary behaviors are as distracting, or in some cases even more distracting, than the primary stuttering behaviors.

 CD-ROM

Identify Primary and Secondary Stuttering Behaviors

Watch CD-ROM segments Ch.13.01 and Ch.13.02 again. Look for repetitions, prolongations, and blocks. Are there instances of stuttering in which the individual combined repetitions and blocks? What secondary behaviors can you identify?

Incidence and Prevalence of Stuttering

How common is stuttering? There are two ways to answer this question. You could consider the percentage of individuals who stutter at any given point in time. This percentage is referred to as the **prevalence** of stuttering. You might also want to consider the percentage of the population that has stuttered at any point during their lives. This percentage is called the **incidence** of stuttering. After an extensive review of the literature, Bloodstein (1995) concluded that approximately 1% of the population stutter at the present moment (the prevalence of stuttering), and that approximately 5% of the population report that they have stuttered for a period of 6 months or more at some point in their lives (the incidence of stuttering). If you could round up all these people, you would probably find that most of them are males. Across all ages of stutterers, there are approximately three male stutterers to every female stutterer.

INDIVIDUALS WHO STUTTER

Individual Variability

Not all individuals stutter in the same manner or with the same frequency. Mild stutterers have fleeting disfluencies, and these may occur only in the most stressful of speaking contexts. Typically, the duration of disfluencies averages less than 3 seconds, but in some cases an instance of disfluency can be much longer, even as long as 30 seconds. In addition, these disfluencies may occur in as many as 20% of the words that are spoken. Most individuals who stutter fall between those extremes, and the severity of their stuttering may change somewhat over time. For example, some stutterers report they experience periods of time when they are relatively fluent and other periods when they are disfluent.

Despite the considerable degree of individual variation among and within stutterers, there are some generalizations that apply to many individuals who stutter. Stuttering tends to be worse when speakers put the most pressure on themselves to be fluent. This often happens when there is critical content that must be communicated in one or two words (saying one's name, ordering in a restaurant), when speaking to authority figures (e.g., professors, parents, bosses), or when something needs to be said in a hurry.

Some types of speech tend to induce fluency. Most stutterers are completely fluent when they sing, when they are engaged in choral reading (as often happens during church services), or when they talk to babies or animals. It is not yet known exactly why these situations induce fluency in stutterers. It is interesting to note that none of these situations requires the speaker to convey critical new information to a listener. Also, in singing and choral reading, speech is not only slow, but the syllables tend to be linked together more smoothly. As we will discuss in more detail later, some therapy approaches are based on the fact that slower rate and smooth transitions between syllables and words induce fluency in most stutterers.

Differences Between Individuals Who Do and Do Not Stutter

There are a number of areas, apart from fluency, in which stutterers differ from nonstutterers. Individuals who stutter tend to have more negative concepts of themselves as speakers, and they have higher levels of concern about their speech. This seems reasonable because there are many instances in which stutterers know what they want to say, but they cannot say it in the fluent manner that they would like. In addition, some listeners form negative impressions about people who stutter. It is no wonder stutterers might feel less confident about their communication skills, and this might affect their self-concept in general.

There are also subtle differences in the language abilities of stutterers and nonstutterers. Language involves formulating what is going to be said and organizing the words and sentences that are needed to express one's thoughts. These functions are dynamically related to speech, which involves planning, initiating, and executing the motor movements that produce words and sentences. Difficulties formulating messages and organizing the words and sentences that best express those messages could affect speech production. For example, one might expect greater frequency of stuttering on words within long, grammatically complex sentences than on words within short, grammatically simple sentences. This is especially true for children who are in the process of learning language (Logan & Conture, 1995). In addition, adult stutterers are more likely to stutter on complex words that express the main idea or that are critical to the communication context. Clearly, stuttering tends to increase in relation to the complexity and importance of the information that is being expressed.

Results from some studies suggest there are differences in the motor systems of stutterers that interfere with their ability to react rapidly. Rapid motor responses are tested by presenting a cue (a visual picture or an auditory sound) and asking individuals to respond as quickly as they can by saying a word, producing a vowel sound, closing their lips, or just tapping a finger. In all of these response conditions, stutterers tend to have slower response times than nonstutterers. Studies of speech samples reveal similar findings. Even when they are not stuttering, individuals who stutter sometimes have slower voice onset times (the time between the release of a consonant at the beginning of the vowel as in the syllable /pa/), longer vowel durations, and slower transitions from one sound to the next. The implications of these findings are that stutterers have less efficient motor systems, and these differences may contribute to the development and/or the continuation of stuttering.

Finally, stutterers appear to use their brains a little differently than nonstutterers. Recall from Chapter 9 (Speech Science) that the left hemisphere is usually dominant for speech and language functions. Individuals who stutter present more right hemisphere activity during speech than nonstutterers. For example, Fox and his colleagues (1996) compared positron emission tomography (PET) scans of stutterers and nonstutterers. Stutterers presented greater activation of speech motor and language-processing areas in the right hemisphere, more activation in the cerebellum (which is responsible for co-ordination and smooth muscle actions), and less activation in left hemisphere language-processing areas than nonstutterers. They also found that individuals who stuttered showed more left hemisphere activation during their fluent speech than they did during stuttered speech. Results like these suggest stutterers may be using the right hemisphere for functions that are better handled by the left hemisphere. The stutterers who participated in these studies were adults. With more research, we hope to learn more about brain functions in children who stutter.

Taken together, these results suggest that stuttering is related to emotional, conceptual, linguistic, and motor performance. Given the rapid advances that are occurring in brain imaging technology, it is likely there will be important discoveries about the systems and processes underlying stuttering in the near future.

THE CAUSE OF STUTTERING

Research has yet to reveal the exact cause of stuttering. Over the years, many theories have been advanced to explain stuttering. Some theories that seemed to be reasonable explanations of stuttering at one time have been shown to be false. We will discuss two of these myths about the cause of stuttering, then we will summarize current thinking about the reasons why people stutter.

Myth: Stuttering Is a Nervous Reaction

Many people assume wrongly that stuttering results from excessive nervousness. We have heard parents and well-meaning friends say things like, "Just relax, there's nothing to be nervous about." when someone is disfluent. Unfortunately, these are not helpful comments. Many studies have shown that individuals who stutter are not more anxious than nonstutterers in general. Nervous disorders and other psychiatric disabilities are not more common in people who stutter than they are in the general population. Finally, relaxation-based therapies have not been particularly helpful for stutterers. For example, stutterers may stutter even though they are completely relaxed. The results of these studies suggest that people who stutter are not generally more anxious or nervous than people who do not stutter. However, nobody doubts that increased levels of anxiety lead to increased disfluencies in individuals who stutter. The key point, however, is that stuttering is not the result of a nervous condition.

Myth: Stuttering Is Caused by Overly Sensitive Parents

In the 1940s, an influential researcher named Wendell Johnson theorized that stuttering was caused by parents who were unnecessarily concerned about normal disfluencies their children produced. That concern was relayed to the child, and the child then became concerned about these behaviors (the disfluencies) and tried to avoid them. This theory was the intellectual springboard for many studies of the parents and families of children who stutter. Some of the more consistent results relating to similarities and differences between the families of stuttering and nonstuttering children are summarized in Table 13–1. Most of the differences between the parents of children who do and do not stutter appear to be reactions to disfluency. Today, most researchers and clinicians agree that parent reactions do not cause stuttering. In fact, Wingate (1976) and other researchers have suggested that parent corrections may help some children stutter less. Nonetheless, it seems likely that a stressful home environment or continuous negative reactions to children's' disfluencies could play a role in the development of stuttering in children who are sensitive to negative comments from others.

Current Thinking About the Etiology of Stuttering

Current models of stuttering depict the disorder as arising from complex dynamic relationships between internal (neurological and cognitive) factors and external conditions. The internal factors include inherited traits, temperament, cognitive abilities, language knowledge, information-processing mechanisms (attention, perception, memory, and reasoning), and speech motor control. The external conditions include culture, parental expectations,

Table 13–1. Similarities and Differences Between Families of Stuttering and Nonstuttering Children

Similarities	Differences
1. Socioeconomic status and number of siblings.	1. Children who stutter are more likely to grow up in less harmonious, less sociable, and less close families.
2. Parent personalities and emotional adjustment.	2. Parents of children who stutter are more anxious about their children's speech development.
3. Parents' general attitudes about childrearing.	3. Parents of children who stutter are more likely to be overprotective.
4. Parents' speech style and rate of speech.	4. Parents of children who stutter sometimes criticize their children's disfluent speech.

childrearing practices, educational experiences, and relationships with siblings and peers. It is important to understand that the sets of factors that may prompt the development of stuttering in one person are not necessarily the same factors that prompt stuttering in someone else. The next section provides more information about the kinds of factors that influence the development of stuttering.

THE DEVELOPMENT OF STUTTERING

Early Stuttering

Recall that normal speech is not completely fluent. Given the difficult motor patterns that must be refined during speech development, it should not be surprising that the speech of preschool-age children is often marked by word and phrase repetitions, interjections, and pauses. These disfluencies can occur in as many as 7% of the words that children speak. Repetitions of the first word in sentences or phrases is the most common form of disfluency in young children.

For the majority of children, the amount of disfluency declines over time. Unfortunately, some children's disfluencies increase in frequency, and their speech contains more sound repetitions, prolongations, and blocks. Conture (1990) referred to these as **within-word disfluencies** and suggested that most children who stutter present three or more within-word disfluencies per 100 words. According to Conture, this proportion of within-word disfluencies rarely occurs in the speech of children who do not stutter. In addition, children who stutter evidence feelings of frustration about their speech, and they begin to develop secondary stuttering behaviors. Behaviors that indicate the beginning of stuttering are listed in Table 13–2.

It can take months for normal disfluencies to evolve into early stuttering. However, changes from normal disfluency to stuttering-like disfluency may occur quickly. Some parents have reported that their child's stuttering developed within a day or two. Rarely, parents will report that their child was relatively fluent one day and exhibited many stuttering-like behaviors the next.

Genetic Influences

Could stuttering be a trait that is inherited? In a review of genetic studies of stuttering, Felsenfeld (1997) concluded that approximately 15% of the first-degree relatives (fathers, mothers, sisters, brothers, sons, daughters) of stutterers were current or recovered stutterers themselves. That means the likelihood of stuttering is three times greater for a person who has a first-

Table 13–2. Indicators of Early Stuttering in Children

Early Stuttering Behaviors

1. An average of three or more sound repetitions, prolongations, or blocks per 100 words.

2. Twenty-five percent or more of the total disfluencies are prolongations or blocks.

3. Instances in which repetitions, prolongations, or blocks occur in adjacent sounds or syllables within a word.

4. Increases in the rate and irregularity of repetitions.

5. Signs of excess tension or struggle during moments of disfluency.

6. Secondary behaviors such as eye blinks, facial tics, or interjections immediately before or during disfluencies.

7. Feelings of frustration about disfluencies.

degree family member who stutters. Because relatives of stutterers are generally at greater risk for stuttering than relatives of nonstutterers, it is likely that some aspect of the disorder, perhaps something like a predisposition for stuttering, may be inherited. Researchers have yet to discover a gene that carries stuttering, and studies of stuttering in families have not revealed a clear line of genetic transmission. Other developmental and environmental factors must interact with a predisposition for stuttering in order for the disorder to develop.

Environmental Demands and the Capacity for Fluency

Starkweather (1987) has suggested that disfluencies are likely to occur in children's speech when there is an imbalance between the demands for fluency and the child's capacity to produce fluent speech. There are four interrelated mechanisms that contribute to the capacity for fluency: neural development that supports sensory-motor coordination, language development, conceptual development, and emotional development.

Recall from Chapter 9 (Speech Science) that the brain is comprised of millions of interconnected neurons. As brain cells proliferate and differentiate, they create neural networks, some of which support motor coordination. In a process known as **neural plasticity,** neural circuits organize and reorganize themselves in response to interactions with the environment. But the environment is not all that matters for brain organization. Inheritance probably plays an important role in the rate of development and the patterns of neural activation that occur. Slowed neurological development and/or less efficient patterns of neural activation could result in a diminished capacity for producing fluent speech. When this reduced capacity is combined with the child's perception of excessive environmental demands, disfluency is the likely result. For example, if two parents are in a hurry to go somewhere at the same moment their child is trying to tell them something, the child might feel undue pressure to talk faster than his motor speech capabilities will allow. A disparity between the child's desire to talk faster in order to please his parents (who are in a hurry at that moment) and his ability to talk fast, would be likely to result in disfluent speech.

Children tend to be disfluent when they are not sure what to say or when they must expend a great deal of mental energy in order to solve a conceptual problem. For example, a child may want to tell his parents about a recent experience. To do so, he needs to weave together a series of sentences that represent the multiple events that were involved and the sequence in which they occurred. The demands inherent in formulating and organizing the story might exceed the child's linguistic and conceptual capacities to do so. This creates a situation in which disfluency is quite likely.

Emotional constancy also contributes to fluency and disfluency. Some children are inherently more sensitive than others, and some children are more likely than others to be disfluent in response to emotional stress. Imagine a child with a sensitive temperament who spilled ice cream in the living room, even though he knew there was a household rule not to take food out of the kitchen. A parent might ask this child to explain why he took food into the living room when he knew he was not supposed to. The child who stutters, sensing that his parent is displeased, might not be able to produce fluent speech under this emotional circumstance.

The demand-capacities explanation of the development of stuttering accounts for the fact that some children who are raised in relatively high-demand environments do not stutter, while other children who are raised in what appear to be less demanding environments might. The nature of the environment is not the critical factor in and of itself. What matters most for the development of stuttering is the balance between children's perception of the demands that are present in their environment and their motoric, linguistic, cognitive, and emotional resources for meeting the demands they place on themselves. Even in an environment that most people would consider to be relatively undemanding, increased disfluencies would be expected to occur in children who have extreme motoric, cognitive, linguistic, and/or emotional restrictions on their ability to produce fluent speech.

The Influence of Learning

Recall that children's brains are relatively plastic, meaning that experiences excite individual neurons and influence connections between networks of neurons. For some children, demand and capacity imbalances that contribute to increased disfluency may occur in many circumstances with many different listeners. When multiple experiences occur over time, as might happen during repeated instances of disfluency, new neural groups that are related to disfluency can form, grow, and strengthen.

In some instances, children's disfluencies may be more physically tense than they are in other instances. Children remember many aspects of their experiences, especially the ones that are distinct in some way. Children would be likely to recall instances when a disfluency was particularly tense or when they had an increased emotional reaction to a disfluency. Brains are good at spotting similarities across situations. Over a relatively short period of time, children would be likely to recognize subtle similarities in speaking contexts that induced more emotion or more tense disfluencies. Recognizing these similarities could prompt children to anticipate difficulties in speaking contexts that share common characteristics. This kind of anticipation is likely to heighten muscle tension, which then increases the likelihood of tense disfluencies and struggle. In this way, disfluency and struggle in a few situations can lead to a pattern of disfluency and struggle in many situations.

Consider the earlier example of a child who wanted to tell his parents about an experience he had. His story was disfluent, partially because the linguistic and cognitive requirements of storytelling were too demanding given the child's level of development. If this happened a few times, the child might begin to associate storytelling with disfluency. This association contributes to anticipation, which leads to heightened levels of neurological activity and increased muscle tension, which increases the likelihood of tense disfluencies. It is not long before tense disfluencies and negative emotional reactions become associated with storytelling in many contexts. Our brains work so efficiently that patterns of behavior, even undesirable patterns like stuttering, can strengthen and stabilize rather quickly.

FACTORS THAT CONTRIBUTE TO CHRONIC STUTTERING

Fortunately, stuttering resolves in 60 to 80% of the individuals who stutter during childhood. The resolution of stuttering often occurs before adolescence. The resolution of stuttering is probably related to growth spurts in developmental domains such as speech motor control, language, cognition, and temperament. Rapid developments in these domains could increase the capacity for fluency, thereby leading to a sudden reduction in stuttering. Such growth spurts can shift demands and capacities for fluency into greater balance. This new balance results in greater fluency, which begins to break down neurological and behavioral patterns of disfluency.

Unfortunately, many children continue to stutter into adolescence and adulthood. The term **chronic stuttering** is often used to refer to these individuals. The following section summarizes some of the factors that contribute to chronic stuttering.

Contributing Factor: Negative Feelings and Attitudes

Stutterers often report they are frustrated and embarrassed by their inability to say what they want to say in the way they want to say it. Adolescents and adults often feel their stuttering is out of their own control, like it is something that happens to them rather than something that they do. Some stutterers may also feel self-conscious about their speech. They may have been teased by classmates as children or laughed at as they struggled to get a word out. People sometimes avoid the person who stutterers because they have negative preconceptions of stutterers as being less intelligent or excessively nervous. They may be unsure about how to respond when the person is disfluent. They may wonder whether they should look away or finish the word for the stutterer. Unfortunately, avoiding talking to stutterers, looking away when they stutter, and finishing their stuttered words can contribute to stutterers' embarrassment about their stuttering.

Contributing Factor: Avoidance

Individuals who stutter sometimes avoid stuttering by changing the words they plan to say as they talk. For example, a stutterer we know tended to stutter more on words that contained the voiceless -th sound /θ/. Once, when he was making arrangements for a date, he told his friend, "I'll pick you up at six, uh, make that half past six." This was a way to avoid saying the word, *six-thirty.*

Another way to keep from stuttering is to avoid speaking situations that tend to exacerbate stuttering. Some stutterers simply refuse to answer the telephone, introduce themselves, ask questions, or speak in front of groups of people. Unfortunately, avoidance of any type adds to feelings that stuttering is controlling the individual rather than the other way around. In therapy, it is difficult to make changes in the speech pattern of someone who consistently avoids talking. As we will discuss later, an important aspect of therapy involves getting the person who stutters to deal constructively with his fear of stuttering by facing his stuttering head-on.

Contributing Factor: Difficulties With Speech Motor Control

Some stutterers evidence unusual patterns of breathing, vocalizing, and speaking even when they are not stuttering. They may tense the muscles in their chest, neck, larynx, jaw and/or face before they start to talk, and they may maintain excess tension in these areas while they are speaking. Some individuals who stutter have inadequate breath support for speech because they inhale too little air or exhale too much air before speaking. There are reports of stutterers whose rate of speech is very uneven. They speed up excessively when they think they are going to be fluent and slow down excessively when they anticipate stuttering. Overly tense musculature, breathing that is too shallow or too deep, and uneven rates of speech create a system that is conducive to stuttering.

The next section concerns the clinical management of stuttering. We begin by examining methods that are commonly used to assess stuttering. Then, we discuss the two principal approaches to treating stuttering known as speech modification and fluency shaping and the ways these approaches are applied to beginning stutterers and chronic stutterers.

ASSESSMENT OF STUTTERING

Evaluations of individuals who are excessively disfluent are designed to determine if the person is a stutterer, to describe the patterns of disfluency that are exhibited, and to determine what therapy procedures to use. It is critical for clinicians to remember that their primary concern is to serve the needs of the client. Clinicians should always ask individuals and/or their family members what they want to learn from an evaluation. Then, clinicians should do their best to collect the information necessary to respond to the individual's and his or her family's concerns.

Cultural Considerations

It is more and more common for clinicians to assess and treat clients and families who are members of ethnic and cultural groups that differ from their own. When this occurs, clinicians need to be sensitive to cultural issues that can affect childrearing practices, conceptions about disabilities, and interaction patterns. Clinicians will want to find out as much as possible about the cultural values and norms that affect communication. Clinicians should never assume that the communication traditions and patterns from one culture are more *correct* than those from another culture. Careful observation and family interviews are necessary for all evaluations. These assessment strategies are especially critical when the clinician is conducting an assessment of a child or an adult from a different cultural group.

Assessment Procedures and the Information They Yield

We have characterized stuttering as a dynamic interaction between internal processes and environmental conditions. Table 13–3 lists the procedures that are typically used to evaluate the internal and external factors that may contribute to stuttering.

Table 13–3. Assessment Procedures That Provide Information About Factors That Contribute to the Development and/or Continuation of Stuttering

Factor	Assessment Procedure
Internal Processes	
Genetic influences	Case history, family interview
Language ability	Language testing, language sample analysis
Temperament	Interviews, questionnaires, and observations
Cognitive ability	Screening and/or observation
Attitudes	Questionnaires
Avoidance	Speech sample
Speech motor control	Speech sample
External Conditions	
Culture	Interviews and observations
Parent attitudes and childrearing practices	Parent interviews
Family interactions	Family interviews, observations
Educational experiences	Teacher interviews, observations

Interviews and Case History

Evaluations should begin with a thorough case history. When assessing children, most of the history information is collected from parents. When assessing adults, history information is collected from the client. The clinician should always ask questions about other family members who stutter, changes in the rate and nature of disfluency over time, and perceptions about the person's fluency at the time of the evaluation. It is also a good idea for clinicians to interview family members and teachers of preschool-age and school-age children about their perceptions of the individual's speech and their reactions to disfluencies. The case history should reveal information about environmental conditions, reactions to disfluency, the consistency of disfluency behaviors across situations, and changes in disfluencies over time.

Speech Samples

Stuttering evaluations should include the collection and analysis of speech samples from a variety of speaking contexts including dialogue, monologue, and oral reading. Some clinicians use a commercially available test for collecting and analyzing speech samples called the *Stuttering Severity Instrument-3* (Riley, 1994), which is often abbreviated as the SSI. To administer the SSI (*Stuttering Severity Instrument-3*), examiners obtain speech samples in reading and conversation contexts. Reading passages are provided, and the conversation sample is obtained while the patient and the examiner converse about familiar topics such as school, jobs, recent holidays, favorite TV shows, or current movies. The SSI can be used to make judgments of stuttering severity. We use it to augment information we obtain from patient interviews, speech samples, and other speech and language tests.

Measures of Stuttering

At minimum, clinicians measure the frequency of certain types of stuttering. To do this, we select 4- or 5-minute segments of conversation and reading that seem to be representative of the individual's fluency and disfluency in those situations. We transcribe (write out) what the individual says, using conventional spelling, until we have 50 utterances. To measure the frequency of stuttering, we count the number of words that would have been spoken if there were no disfluencies. Then we count the number of words that contain within-word disfluencies (sound and syllable repetitions, prolongations, and blocks). The frequency of stuttering is simply the total number of words containing within-word disfluencies divided by the total number of words. This calculation yields a proportion. To convert the proportion to a percentage, simply multiply the proportion by 100. For example, in a sample with 400 total words, we counted 18 words that contained within-word disfluencies. Dividing 18 by 400 and then multiplying by 100, the frequency of stuttering was 4.5 within-word disfluencies per 100 words. Note that this value is higher (worse) than the frequency of disfluencies common for stuttering (refer to Table 13–2). This doesn't mean that the individual who was assessed was definitely a stutterer. The correct interpretation of this data is that the individual presented one indicator of stuttering-like behavior.

We also describe the kinds of disfluencies that are present. Figure 13–1 can be used for this purpose. We make a tic mark in the number box corresponding to each type of disfluency we observe. Then, we total the number of disfluencies. To calculate the percentage of each disfluency type, simply divide the number of disfluencies of each type by the total number of disfluencies and multiply that proportion by 100. This enables the evaluator to determine the relative percentage of types of disfluencies. Recall that prolongations and blocks often comprise 25% or more of the total disfluencies of children and adults who stutter.

Consistency and Adaptation

Some clinicians ask individuals who stutter to read a short passage over and over again. There are two patterns that stutterers are likely to exhibit. First, some stutterers tend to stutter on the same words in the same way each time. This is known as **consistency.** For example, across repeated readings, some

Description	Number	Percentage
Typical (Between-Word) Disfluencies		
Phrase repetitions		
Word repetitions		
Interjections		
Subtotal		
Atypical (Within-Word) Disfluencies		
Word repetitions		
Syllable repetitions		
Sound repetitions		
Prolongations		
Blocks		
Subtotal		
Total		

Figure 13–1. Types of disfluencies.

Frequency and Types of Disfluencies

Watch CD-ROM segments Ch.13.01 and Ch.13.02 again. This time, use Figure 13–1 to calculate the frequency of disfluencies. Does this stutterer present more or less than 3 within-word disfluencies per 100 words? Also, calculate the percentage of each type of disfluency. Are 25% or more of the moments of stuttering prolongations or blocks?

stutterers will have prolongations or block on the same words over and over. It is not unusual to find that 50 to 75% of the words that were stuttered in one reading were also stuttered in the previous reading.

As stutterers read the same passage over and over, they also tend to stutter less on successive readings. This effect is called **adaptation.** There is often a greater reduction the first two times a passage is repeated, after which the percentage of adaptation decreases. Some clinicians believe stutterers who have greater adaptation effects tend to improve more during therapy. However, a number of studies have failed to find much support for that idea.

Screening

As with every evaluation, the clinician needs to ensure that hearing sensitivity is within normal limits and that the structure and function of the oral mechanism are adequate to support speech. This means that, at minimum, the client should receive a hearing screening and a oral mechanism screening. We also make informal judgments about the individual's voice quality. When we evaluate children, we make informal judgments about the development of their articulation skills and the development of their language.

Feelings and Attitudes

We mentioned earlier that negative feelings and attitudes about communication contribute to the continuation of stuttering and can interfere with success in therapy. There are a number of scales that can be administered to assess attitudes and feelings related to stuttering. Many of these scales are available in the books that appear on the list of suggested readings at the end of the chapter. Clinicians usually administer these scales to get a sense of the extent to which negative attitudes and feelings contribute to stuttering behaviors. This can be useful information for planning treatment because different treatment approaches address feelings and emotions to different degrees.

Diagnosis and Recommendations

Clinicians should hold a feedback conference with the individual and/or the family after the assessment data have been analyzed. Clinicians should begin the feedback conference with a review of the assessment questions. The clinician should describe the characteristics of the individual's disfluencies and should indicate whether a diagnosis of stuttering is warranted. Information that revealed excessive amounts of concern by the individual, his parents and/or his teachers; high rates of disfluency that varied little across situations; and a pattern of increasing struggle would be indicative of a serious situation that required immediate therapeutic attention. In these cases, the clinician should work with the individual and the family to devise a treatment plan that is well-suited to the client's abilities and needs.

TREATMENT

We noted earlier that stuttering resolves in 60 to 80% of the individuals who have the disorder. This probably occurs most often in children who have been stuttering for a relatively short period of time. Adults who receive treatment are not "cured" often, but it does happen. Unfortunately, we do not know how often it happens. The good news is that many children, adolescents, and adults who receive treatment become fluent to the point where they can communicate effectively in their environments.

There are two types of treatment for stuttering. **Stuttering modification procedures** help the stutterer change or modify his stuttering so that it is relaxed and easy. **Fluency shaping** procedures establish a fluent manner of speaking that replaces stuttering. Many clinicians combine aspects of stuttering modification and fluency shaping in their therapy. This section summarizes two well-known stuttering modification and fluency shaping approaches and describes one method for integrating stuttering modification and fluency shaping procedures.

Stuttering Modification Therapy

Stuttering modification therapy is used to teach the stutterer to change the way he stutters. Charles Van Riper is probably the best known proponent of stuttering modification therapy. His approach (Van Riper, 1973) to treatment is frequently referred to by the acronym MIDVAS, which stands for Motivation, Identification, Desensitization, Variation, Approximation, and Stabilization. Table 13–4 lists the phases in MIDVAS, their primary focus, and some of the procedures that are used. The primary goal of Van Riper's therapy is to help stutterers acquire a speech style they find to be acceptable.

Van Riper believed attitudes and feelings about stuttering play a critical role in the development of the disorder, in its continuation, and in its remediation. In fact, four of the six stages of the MIDVAS approach (Motivation, Identification, Desensitization, and Stabilization) relate primarily to the stutterer's ability to deal with his own stuttering and the consequences of his stuttering in a rational manner.

The hallmarks of Van Riper's approach are the modification procedures that are taught in the Approximation phase. Van Riper proposed a three-step sequence for teaching stutterers how to stutter in a relaxed, controlled manner. First, stutterers are taught to stop as soon as a stuttered word is completed, pause, then say the word again in an easy (though not necessarily fluent) manner. This is called a *cancellation*. When they have mastered cancellations, they are taught to ease their way out of repetitions, prolongations, and blocks. This strategy is called a *pull-out*. Finally, stutterers are taught to modify

Table 13–4. A Summary of Van Riper's Approach to Stuttering Modification Therapy

Phase	Focus	Primary Procedures
Motivation	Prepare the client emotionally and mentally for the steps that follow.	1. Client teaches clinician to stutter 2. Discuss client's inner feelings 3. Explain the course of therapy
Identification	Help the client understand and explain exactly what he does and how he feels when he stutters.	1. Client describes his stuttering in detail 2. Speech assignments in which the stutterer observes listener reactions
Desensitization	Reduce the client's fears, frustrations, and embarrassment about his stuttering	1. Freezing—extending a moment of stuttering 2. Pseudostuttering (fake stuttering) in public
Variation	Teach the client to change his stuttering patterns	1. Speech assignments in which the stutterer explores different ways of stuttering in public
Approximation	Teach the client new responses that reduce stuttering.	1. Cancellations 2. Pull-outs 3. Preparatory sets
Stabilization	Help the client become his own clinician.	1. Practice techniques on feared words in feared situations 2. Practice placing fake stuttering into fluent speech

their stuttering before it occurs. That is, when they anticipate stuttering on an upcoming sound or word, they form a *preparatory set* in which they ease their way into the word that they thought they would stutter on.

 CD-ROM

Comparing Cancellations and Pull-outs

CD-ROM segments Ch.13.03 and Ch.13.04 show a stutterer practicing cancellations and pull-outs. Notice the differences between the two procedures. In cancellations (segment Ch.13.03), stuttering is modified after a stuttered word is completed. In pull-outs (segment Ch.13.04), stuttering is modified within the moment of stuttering. What does this stutterer do to modify his stuttering?

Fluency Shaping Therapy

Fluency shaping therapy is used to teach a new speech style that is free of stuttering. There are many different fluency shaping procedures, but most involve slower rates of speech, relaxed breathing, easy initiation of sounds, and smoother transitions between words. For example, Neilson and Andrews (1992) described an intensive 3-week fluency shaping therapy program. During the first week, stutterers are taught a new way of speaking in group and individual sessions. Stutterers slow their rate of speech down to 50 syllables per minute by extending the duration of consonants and vowels. (Try this yourself; you will find that it is very difficult to continue this abnormally slow rate of speech for very long.) They also learn to use a relaxed breathing pattern before they phonate, to initiate voicing in a very gentle manner, to use soft articulatory contacts during speech, to use constant voicing between syllables, and to move smoothly from one word to the next. When these skills are mastered at one speaking rate, the stutterer is allowed to speed up in 10 syllables per minute intervals. Once the individual reaches a rate of 100 syllables per minute, Neilson and Andrews teach appropriate speaking styles that incorporate such aspects as phrasing, rhythm, loudness, body language, and eye contact. They also teach stutterers how to use slower and smoother speech when they anticipate stuttering. In this way, individuals who stutter learn their new speech style in small increments.

During the second and third weeks of intervention, stutterers engage in "transfer" activities in which they use their new speech style in a variety of speaking situations outside the clinic. These outside activities help stutterers generalize their new way of speaking to the kinds of speech situations they routinely encounter in their everyday lives. Difficult speaking situations such as giving a speech, introducing oneself to a stranger, giving on-the-street interviews, and calling a radio talk show are practiced during the third week of therapy. To institute a new speech style, Neilson and Andrews give their clients repeated and varied opportunities to use their fluent speech style in real speaking contexts.

 CD-ROM

Examples of Fluency Shaping

CD-ROM segment Ch.13.05 shows a stutterer learning a fluency shaping strategy. In segment Ch.13.06, he practices this speech style during oral reading. Compare the speech in segments Ch.13.01 and Ch.13.02 to the speech in segments Ch.13.05 and Ch.13.06. Do you notice a difference between rate of speech, the onset of phonation, and the transitions between words? Does the speech in segments Ch.13.05 and Ch.13.06 sound "natural" to you?

Integrating Stuttering Modification and Fluency Shaping Methods

Many speech-language pathologists (SLPs) combine stuttering modification and fluency shaping techniques in therapy. Stutterers are shown how to alter their speech style so they are more likely to be fluent, but they are also taught how to modify their speech when they encounter moments of stuttering. Like Van Riper, most clinicians also believe individuals who stutter need assistance with reducing their negative emotions about stuttering, their worries about listener reactions, and their tendencies to avoid stuttering.

Therapy for Children Who Stutter

Therapy for children between 3 and 8 years of age involves many of the basic concepts and procedures from stuttering modification and fluency shaping approaches. Most clinicians utilize fluency shaping approaches somewhat more than stuttering modification because young children may not be developmentally ready for the amount of self-awareness that is required for stuttering modification. We have heard clinicians use the term "turtle talk" to describe the slower and easier fluency shaping speech style. Often, clinicians teach "turtle talk" in a step-by-step fashion, starting with single words, then advancing to short repeated phrases (e.g., "I have a _____"), short imitated sentences, longer imitated sentences, and finally multiple connected sentences in conversations and storytelling.

Clinicians who work with young children involve families in the therapy process as much as possible. They make sure parents understand exactly what will be done in therapy, and they enlist parental support in the therapy process. Clinicians help parents increase factors that induce fluency (such as slower speech, positive comments, stress-free environment, and so on) and decrease factors that disrupt fluency at home (such as rapid rates of speech, excessive questions, pressure to respond rapidly, and so on). Clinicians also invite parents to attend treatment sessions with their children so they can learn the fluency shaping and stuttering modification techniques that their children are using. Parents' involvement in the intervention process and their commitment to helping their child become more fluent are critical factors in the child's success in reducing or eliminating her or his stuttering-like disfluencies.

SUMMARY

In summary, stuttering is best conceived of as the unfortunate outcome of an imbalance between internal processes (e.g., inherited traits, speech motor control, language development, cognitive development, and temperament) and external conditions (e.g., culture; parent, sibling, and peer interactions; and educational experiences). The relationship between these internal and external factors is dynamic, meaning that it varies from individual to individual, and it even varies within a single individual over time. After stuttering develops, there are factors that serve to exacerbate the problem. These factors include negative feelings and attitudes, methods for avoiding stuttering, and maladaptive speech motor control processes that affect respiration, phonation, and articulatory rate.

Some children inherit traits that can contribute to the development of stuttering. These traits could relate to delayed neurological maturation or the development of inefficient neurological networks. Subtle neurological deficiencies and delays could affect various aspects of development, including language, cognition, temperament, and speech motor control. Environmental demands that exceed children's capacities for dealing with the requirements of the moment can result in disfluency.

During assessment, clinicians evaluate the internal and external factors that contribute to stuttering, determine the need for therapy, and plan intervention. If therapy is provided, clinicians usually combine aspects of stuttering modification and fluency shaping approaches. When the person who is being treated is a child, it is critical to involve the parents in the treatment process.

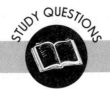

STUDY QUESTIONS

1 Give an example of the following primary behaviors of stuttering: word repetition, syllable repetition, sound repetition, prolongation, and block.

2 What is the incidence and prevalence of stuttering? What do differences between incidence and prevalence suggest about the likelihood of recovery from stuttering?

3 What is the difference between primary stuttering behaviors and secondary stuttering behaviors?

4 What are two myths about the etiology of stuttering?

5 Describe how the relationship between environmental conditions and individual capacities for fluency affect the development of stuttering.

6 What factors contribute to chronic stuttering?

7 What types of assessment procedures are used in most stuttering evaluations?

8 Why it is important to measure stutterers' attitudes and feelings about communication during an evaluation?

9 Describe cancellations, pull-outs, and preparatory sets.

10 What are the differences between stuttering modification and fluency shaping approaches to the treatment of stuttering?

REFERENCES

Bloodstein, O. (1995). *A handbook on stuttering* (5th ed.). San Diego: Singular Publishing Group.

Conture, E. G. (1990). *Stuttering* (2nd ed.). Englewood Cliffs, NJ: Prentice-Hall.

Felsenfeld, S. (1997). Epidemiology and genetics of stuttering. In R. F. Curlee & G. M. Siegel (Eds.), *Nature and treatment of stuttering: New directions* (2nd ed., pp. 3–23). Boston: Allyn & Bacon.

Fox, P. T., Ingham,, R., Ingham, J., et al. (1996). A PET study of the neural systems of stuttering. *Nature, 382,* 158–162.

Guitar, B. (1998). *Stuttering: An integrated approach to its nature and treatment* (2nd ed.). Baltimore, MD: Williams & Wilkins.

Logan, K., & Conture, E. (1995). Length, grammatical complexity, and rate differences in stuttered and fluent conversational utterances of children who stutter. *Journal of Fluency Disorders, 20,* 35–61.

Neilson, M., & Andrews, G. (1992). Intensive fluency training of chronic stutterers. In R. Curlee (Ed.), *Stuttering and related disorders of fluency* (pp. 139–165). New York: Thieme.

Riley, G. (1994). *The Stuttering Severity Instrument for Children and Adults* (3rd ed.). Austin, TX: Pro-Ed.

Starkweather, W. (1987). *Fluency and stuttering.* Englewood Cliffs, NJ: Prentice-Hall.

Van Riper, C. (1973). *The treatment of stuttering.* Englewood Cliffs, NJ: Prentice-Hall.

Wingate, M. (1976). *Stuttering theory and treatment.* New York: Irvington.

SUGGESTED READINGS

Andrews, G., Craig, A., Feyer, A., Hoddinot, S., Howie, P., & Neilson, M. (1983). Stuttering: A review of research findings and theories circa 1982. *Journal of Speech and Hearing Disorders, 48,* 226–246.

Andrews, G., Morris-Yeates, A., Howie, P., & Martin, N. (1991). Genetic factors in stuttering confirmed. *Archives of General Psychiatry, 48,* 1034–1035.

Bloodstein, O. (1993). *Stuttering: The search for a cause and cure.* Boston: Allyn & Bacon.

Curlee, R. F., & Siegel, G. M. (Eds.) (1997). *Nature and treatment of stuttering: New directions* (2nd ed.). Boston: Allyn & Bacon.

Guitar, B. (1998). *Stuttering: An integrated approach to its nature and treatment* (2nd ed.). Baltimore, MD: Williams & Wilkins.

Shapiro, D. (1999). *Stuttering intervention: A collaborative journey to fluency freedom.* Austin, TX: Pro-Ed.

GLOSSARY

Adaptation: The percentage of decrease in stuttering when a passage is read multiple times in succession. The percent of reduction is calculated for each repeated reading.

Chronic stuttering: Stuttering that continues into adulthood.

Cluttering: A fluency disorder that is characterized by very rapid bursts of disrhythmic, unintelligible speech.

Consistency: The percentage of stuttered words during repeated readings of the same passage.

Disfluency: The flow and ease of speech is disrupted by repetitions, interjections, pauses, and revisions.

Fluency: Speech that is easy, rapid, rhythmical, and evenly flowing.

Fluency shaping: A therapy approach in which the clinician teaches the stutterer a new way of talking that is designed to reduce the likelihood of stuttering.

Incidence: Lifetime risk. The percentage of individuals in a given population who report that they have, at one time or another, exhibited a particular disorder or condition.

Neural plasticity: The idea that neurological structures and pathways reorganize themselves and change over time in response to the kinds of experiences a person has.

Primary stuttering behaviors: Within-word disfluencies (i.e., repetitions, prolongations, and blocks) that are sometimes referred to as "core behaviors."

Prevalence: The percentage of individuals in a given population who present a particular disorder or condition at a particular point in time.

Secondary stuttering behaviors: Adaptations that stutterers make as they try to get through primary stuttering behaviors or to avoid them altogether. The most common secondary stuttering behaviors are eye blinks, lip pursing, arm movements, and head nods.

Stuttering: An unusual amount of tense, within-word disfluencies that interfere with the continuity of speech.

Stuttering modification procedures: A therapy approach in which the clinician teaches the client to alter the way he or she stutters.

Within-word disfluencies: Sound repetitions, prolongations, or blocks.

14

Dysarthria

Thomas P. Marquardt

1 To learn the major causes of cerebral palsy.

2 To understand differences between dysarthria in cerebral palsy and in adults.

3 To learn about diseases that cause dysarthria in adults.

4 To understand how dysarthria is identified and treated.

5 To learn about augmentative communication systems.

INTRODUCTION

Damage to central and/or peripheral nervous system pathways causes muscle dysfunction, that is, muscle weakness, incoordination, or paralysis. Speech disorders due to neuromuscular dysfunction are termed **dysarthria.** There are a number of different types of dysarthria; some affect a small part of the speech production apparatus, others the entire system. As a group, the dysarthrias involve all the major subcomponents of speech production: respiration, phonation, resonance, and articulation.

Dysarthria in children most commonly is associated with cerebral palsy; in adults it results from cerebrovascular or progressive neurological disease. Frequently the neuromuscular problems that underlie dysarthria cause difficulties in swallowing as well as in speech. In this chapter, we consider speech disorders in cerebral palsy and acquired dysarthria. Dysphagia, or disordered swallowing, is considered in Chapter 15.

 CD-ROM

Overview of the CD-ROM Segments in Chapter 14

The CD-ROM segments that accompany this chapter include two speakers with dysarthria. The first speaker (segment Ch.14.01) has an acquired dysarthria; the second speaker (segment Ch.14.02) has cerebral palsy. In segment Ch.14.03, the speaker with cerebral palsy demonstrates the use of an augmentative communication device.

CEREBRAL PALSY

Injury to the nervous system that occurs before, at the time of, or shortly after birth can cause cerebral palsy, a syndrome of deficits in visual, auditory, intellectual, and motor functions in the critical early development period for speech and language. At the center of the disorder is motor dysfunction. That is, the child's muscles are weak, paralyzed, and/or uncoordinated. Consider this description of cerebral palsy from the standpoint of developing speech and language. A child is born with vision, hearing, cognitive, and neuromuscular disorders. How might this affect speech and language learning?

The primary causes of cerebral palsy are anoxia, in which the brain has a restricted oxygen supply, and trauma, in which the brain is injured. Frequently, the causes are divided into three groups; *prenatal* (before birth), *perinatal* (at the time of birth), and *postnatal* (after birth). Disease or metabolic problems of the mother are prenatal causes of cerebral palsy. If the umbilical cord is wound around the neck causing strangulation, if there is a premature separation of the placenta, or if the birth process is delayed, the infant may be deprived of oxygen at the time of birth. The brain also may be damaged by trauma during the birth process or at a very early age due to falls or car accidents. Regardless of the cause, cerebral palsy is the result of nervous system damage, and it has an adverse effect on the development of speech and language skills.

Classification of Cerebral Palsy

There are several ways of classifying cerebral palsy: by the extremities affected (typography), by neuromuscular characteristics, and by severity of the disorder. We consider each of these classifications and then consider them together.

Orthopedic Classification

Orthopedic classification is based on the limbs affected. If one limb is involved, it is called *monoplegia*. If both legs are affected, it is termed *paraplegia*. Other terms are used when three limbs (*triplegia*) and four limbs (*quadriplegia*) are involved.

Neuromuscular Characteristics

Cerebral palsy also can be classified by underlying neuromuscular characteristics. Damage to the pyramidal tract and the associated extrapyramidal system yield a **spastic** type of cerebral palsy. Spasticity is characterized by an abnormal resistance to muscle lengthening and is produced by a hypersensitivity of muscle stretch reflexes. What this means is that when an attempt is made to stretch out the arm or to flex the leg, the muscles resist the movement. The **hypertonicity** is most prominent in antigravity muscles (muscles that allow us to stand, for example), which leads to a characteristic flexion pattern of the arms and extension pattern of the legs with inward rotation at the knees. The pattern includes arms that are bent upward and legs that are positioned like a scissors with the knees together but the feet spread apart. A feature of abnormal hypertonicity is chronic muscle shortening, which may be accompanied by muscle **atrophy** (wasting).

Involuntary movements characterized by a writhing and twisting motion typify **athetoid** cerebral palsy. In this case the primary damage is to the basal ganglia and associated components of the extrapyramidal tract (see Chapter 9 for a review of this tract). The involuntary movements progress from the body outward to the hands and feet, and the child may give the appearance of being in almost constant motion. The involuntary movements are superimposed on and interfere with voluntary purposeful movements. What this means is that when the child tries to reach for an item like a pencil or spoon, the arm may move back and forth and up and down repeatedly until the target is reached and then continue as the item is manipulated.

Ataxic cerebral palsy results from damage to the cerebellum. In ataxic cerebral palsy, the primary neuromuscular features are related not to increased or alternating muscle tone, but to a disturbance in movement coordination. Movements are characterized by errors in their speed, direction, and accuracy. When asked to carry out a rhythmic and precise motor activity like playing on a drum, the child has difficulty not only hitting the drum, but in maintaining the rhythm.

There are two other types of cerebral palsy that have been identified. **Rigid** cerebral palsy, with balanced hypertonicity and rigidity resulting from increased tone in muscles at both sides of a joint, and **tremor** cerebral palsy, characterized by rhythmic involuntary movements, are types that have a low frequency of occurrence and rarely occur alone.

Individuals with cerebral palsy infrequently have features of a single type of the disorder. Most often, spasticity occurs with athetosis or with ataxia. These types of cerebral palsy co-occur because multiple sites in the motor pathways have been damaged. Although one type of cerebral palsy may predominate, features of the other types of neuromuscular pathology are evident as well. Therefore, descriptions such as "primarily spastic" or "dominant athetosis" are often used as labels.

Severity

Severity ranges from mild to severe and is usually determined by an overall judgment of the level of impairment. This judgment is based on the degree of independence in communication, ambulation, and self-help skills. For example, clinicians ask themselves, "Is the child independent in self-help skills such as walking and feeding?" "What types of special equipment are required?" "Is speech understandable?" Table 14–1 lists the characteristics that

Table 14–1. Levels of Severity in Cerebral Palsy

Severity Level	Description
Mild	Self-help skills are adequate to care for personal needs, no significant speech problems, ambulates without appliances, no treatment necessary.
Moderate	Speech is impaired and special equipment may be needed for ambulation. Self-help skills are insufficient to meet daily care needs. Habilitation therapy is needed.
Severe	Poor prognosis for developing self-help skills, ambulation, and functional speech even with treatment and the use of adaptive equipment.

Source: Adapted from Rusk, H. (1977). *Rehabilitation medicine* (4th ed.). St. Louis, MO: Mosby.

are typically associated with mild, moderate, and severe forms of cerebral palsy.

A description of cerebral palsy for any individual is based on the three classification system components. Severe athetoid quadriplegia, mild spastic paraplegia, and moderate ataxic quadriplegia are typical diagnostic descriptions.

Motor Development in Children With Cerebral Palsy

Motor deficits are the focal point of a diagnosis of cerebral palsy, and delayed motor development is most frequently observed in children with the disorder. In general, children with cerebral palsy have developmental delays in sitting, standing, walking, and speech development related to the motor impairment. The basis of delayed motor development is twofold: impaired neuromuscular functioning and abnormal reflexes. We have already briefly discussed neuromuscular abnormalities in terms of type of cerebral palsy. These abnormalities have significant effects on motor development. Coupled with abnormal neuromuscular functioning is the lack of inhibition of primitive reflexes and the failure to develop the kinds of higher order reflexes that are seen in adults.

An infant's head movements elicit stereotypical patterns of limb movements. For example, movement of the head to the side elicits a pattern of arm and leg extension on the side to which the head is turned. This reflex, termed the asymmetrical tonic neck reflex, is expected to disappear by the time the infant is a year old. However, the reflex is not inhibited in cerebral palsy, and it interferes with the development of independent limb movement. Consider how difficult it would be to eat if, when your head turned to the right or left, your arm holding the spoon moved away from you. (See Table 14–2 for a brief review of some postural reflexes.)

Children with cerebral palsy often fail to develop higher level reflexes related to walking. For example, if you are shoved while standing, you adjust your posture by widening your stance and raising the arm in order to maintain balance. Children with cerebral palsy may not develop this righting reflex, making it more difficult for them to learn how to walk. Given the importance that reflexes have for development, is not surprising that children with cerebral palsy nearly always have delays in sitting, standing, walking, and speech development.

Speech and Language Development in Children With Cerebral Palsy

Speech disorders in cerebral palsy result from weakness and incoordination. All aspects of speech production are affected.

Table 14–2. Examples of Early Postural and Movement Reflexes

Reflex	Characteristics
Asymmetric tonic neck reflex	Turning the head to the side causes extension of the arm and leg on the side to which the head is turned and flexion of the limbs of the opposite side.
Symmetrical tonic neck reflex	Raising of the head results in extension of the arms and flexion of the legs. Legs are extended and arms are flexed when head is lowered.
Positive and negative supporting reactions	Contact of feet with ground causes simultaneous contraction of flexors and extensors of the legs and fixing of joints (positive); relaxation of the extensors of the legs occurs when the infant is lifted from the ground (negative).
Moro reflex	Adduction-extension reaction of the limbs with movement of the supporting surface, loud noise, or blowing on the face.
Neck righting reflex	Rotation of the head results in the rotation of the body as a whole to the side to which the head is turned.

Respiration

Respiratory activity is characterized by reduced vital capacity and impaired ability to generate and maintain relatively constant subglottal pressure (see Chapter 9 for a review of the relationship between respiration and speech). At least part of the reduced respiratory support for speech results from inefficient valving of the outgoing airstream at the glottis, velopharynx, and within the oral cavity by the lips and tongue.

Phonation

Laryngeal functions of children with cerebral palsy often are compromised by changing tonicity. Depending on the degree of vocal fold compression, this results in intermittent breathiness and a strangled harshness in voice quality as vocal fold tension decreases and increases. The tension may be so great that phonation does not occur at all even though the child appears to be trying to talk. Timing of respiratory and laryngeal activity also is disrupted. Expiration frequently begins before the vocal fold are closed, causing a loss of air. Errors in the production of the voiced-voiceless distinction in contrasts like /p/ and /b/ and /s/ and /z/ are frequent because of impaired timing in phonation onset.

Resonance

Resonance during speech production is disrupted in cerebral palsy. Netsell (1969) investigated aerodynamic aspects of speech production in cerebral palsy and found deviations of velopharyngeal functioning, including a gradual premature opening of the velopharynx during the production of syllables and a break of the velopharyngeal seal during nonnasal productions. These difficulties lead to hypernasality and nasal emission during speech production.

Articulation

Individuals with cerebral palsy frequently have significant articulation problems. The mandible may be hyperextended with the mouth open, making it difficult to round, protrude, or close the lips. The hyperextension of the jaw and abnormal tongue postures prevent precise shaping and constriction of the vocal tract for vowel and consonant production.

Prosody

Utterances in children with cerebral palsy may be limited to one or two words on each breath. Due to poor respiratory control, disrupted timing of respiratory and laryngeal functioning, and poor control of laryngeal tension, intonation and the ability to mark stressed words in an utterance are impaired.

The overall effect of neuromuscular impairment of the speech production components is to reduce the intelligibility of speech. Intelligibility may be so limited that words and phrases are not understandable unless the topic is known.

 CD-ROM

In CD-ROM segment Ch.14.01, an adult with cerebral palsy answers a series of questions. Can you understand his answers?

Speech Development

Speech sound development is delayed in children with cerebral palsy with the highest frequency of errors on fricatives and glides requiring tongue movement. Stops and nasals develop earlier than fricatives, and there are fewer errors on voiced consonants than on voiceless consonants. In general, the latest developing sounds in normal children, such as fricatives and affricates, are the most delayed in children with cerebral palsy.

The entire speech production system is affected in many cases of cerebral palsy due to reduced respiratory support and inefficient valving of the outgoing airstream at the glottis, velopharynx, and oral cavity. The developmental course of speech sounds follows what might be expected in normally developing children but at a reduced rate, with articulation errors continuing into adulthood. The melody of speech (prosody) also is affected and, in conjunction with speech sound errors, causes a reduction in speech intelligibility.

Language deficits also are a frequent concomitant of cerebral palsy. Reduced ability to explore the environment due to motor limitations, mental retardation, hearing loss, and perceptual deficits all work to limit the development of vocabulary, grammar, and discourse skills in children with cerebral palsy.

ACQUIRED DYSARTHRIA

Acquired dysarthria differs from cerebral palsy in several respects. In the case of acquired dysarthria, the adult developed speech and language before the onset of the disorder. Therefore, primitive reflexes do not contribute significantly to the speech deficits that are observed. In addition, adult patients usually present sensory problems related to the aging process.

Classification of Acquired Dysarthrias

Historically, acquired dysarthrias have been categorized by the causative disease process ("the dysarthria of multiple sclerosis") or the part of the body affected. However, with the seminal work of Darley, Aronson, and Brown (1975), a universal system of classification has been developed based primarily on the underlying dysfunction of muscle that characterizes the disorder. In many cases of acquired dysarthria, the disease progresses and speech becomes increasingly more difficult to understand. (See Table 14–3 for an overview of acquired dysarthrias.)

Flaccid Dysarthria

Interruption of normal input to the muscles from the peripheral nervous system causes muscle weakness and atrophy (wasting). Muscles that are cut off from their innervation due to peripheral nerve damage are flaccid. They are *hypotoned* (i.e., **hypotonicity,** reduced background electrical activity, results) and weak. Often, twitching of the muscle fibers associated with their wasting away **(atrophy)** occurs.

Table 14–3. Types and Characteristics of Acquired Dysarthria.

Type	Disease/Disorder Characteristics	Site of Lesion	Speech
Flaccid	Bulbar palsy Myasthenia gravis	Lower motor neuron	Audible inspiration, hypernasality, nasal emission, breathiness
Spastic	Pseudobulbar palsy	Upper motor neuron	Imprecise articulation slow rate, harsh voice quality
Ataxic	Cerebellar or Friedrich's ataxia	Cerebellum	Phoneme and syllable prolongation, slow rate, abnormal prosody
Hypokinetic	Parkinson's disease	Extrapyramidal system	Monoloudness, monopitch, reduced intensity, short rushes of speech
Hyperkinetic	Huntington's chorea Dystonia	Extrapyramidal system	Imprecise articulation, prolonged pauses, variable rate, impaired prosody
Mixed	Multiple sclerosis Amyotrophic lateral sclerosis	Multiple motor systems	Speech characteristics dependent on motor systems affected

The problem in flaccid dysarthria may be at the motoneuron cell bodies, at the peripheral nerve as it courses to the muscle, at the myoneural junction, or at the muscle fibers themselves. In other words, impulses from the central nervous system are interrupted as they course down to the muscle fibers.

Motoneurons can be injured by trauma, or they can deteriorate from degenerative disease. The myoneural junction is affected by a disorder called myasthenia gravis, in which neurotransmitter substances are depleted where the nerve endings synapse with muscle fibers. This requires longer than expected periods of time for the junction to restabilize. The individual may have almost normal muscle function following rest, but then will rapidly fatigue with prolonged motor activity. Hereditary conditions like muscular dystrophy cause the muscle fibers to deteriorate. In this progressive disorder, the muscles become weaker as the disease progresses. Depending on what parts of the motor unit (peripheral nerves and the muscle fibers they innervate) are affected, individuals with flaccid dysarthria demonstrate reduced muscle tone, with atrophy and weakness and reduced muscle reflexes.

The parts of the speech musculature affected by flaccid dysarthria depend on the underlying problem. If a single nerve, such as the hypoglossal nerve (cranial nerve XII, which innervates the tongue), is damaged on one side, then only the tongue on that side will be weak or paralyzed. If the brainstem is damaged on one side and involves several cranial nerves, then one side of the face, tongue, and palate will be impaired. In conditions like muscular dystrophy or myasthenia gravis, the entire speech production apparatus is affected.

The speech characteristics of flaccid dysarthria are due primarily to weakness. Speech rate is slow with breathy phonation, hypernasality, weak production of stops and fricatives, articulatory imprecision, and reduced phrase length. Reduced breath support due to respiratory weakness and air wastage at the glottis, velopharynx, and oral cavity cause phrases to be short, with monoloudess and monopitch.

Spastic Dysarthria

When the pyramidal and extrapyramidal tracts are damaged bilaterally at or near the cortical surface, impaired innervation to the muscles causes them to be weak, *hypertoned* (i.e., **hypertonicity,** too much background electrical activity), and **hyperreflexic** (exaggerated responses to reflex elicitation). When stretched, the muscles contract before releasing with continued extension **(spasticity).** This leads to the types of muscle spasms that are characteristic of spastic dysarthria. There may be some atrophy, but it is due to a lack of muscle use due to weakness.

All four limbs of the body are affected in spastic dysarthria as well as the trunk, head, and neck. In contrast to flaccid dysarthria, where muscles of a single speech structure may be completely paralyzed, the whole speech production musculature is affected in spastic dysarthria. Speech is characterized by articulatory imprecision, slow rate, short phrases, and a harsh voice quality. Prosody is affected with reduced loudness and pitch variation.

There are a variety of conditions that can lead to spastic dysarythria. Pseudobulbar palsy, for example, is caused by small strokes in the white fiber pathways beneath the surface of the brain. The individual typically is elderly, with both speech and swallowing problems.

Ataxic Dysarthria

The primary characteristics of ataxic dysarthria relate to coordination. In ataxic dysarthria, movements are inaccurate and dysrhythmic. However, in contrast to flaccid and spastic dysarthrias, reflexes are normal and there is only minimal weakness. Ataxic dysarthria results from damage to the cerebellum, which functions to coordinate the direction, extent, and timing of movements.

Like the other dysarthrias, ataxic dysarthria has a negative impact on speech production. In these cases, prosody tends to be monotonous and there are disruptions in stress patterns. Normally stressed syllables are sometimes unstressed and unstressed syllables are stressed. The rate of speech is usually slowed, and vowels, in particular, are increased in duration. The good news for individuals with ataxic dysarthria is that speech intelligibility frequently is only mildly affected. This is quite unlike the speech of individuals with flaccid and spastic dysarthrias, who may have marked difficulty in making themselves understood.

Hypokinetic Dysarthria

In hypokinetic dysarthria, the individual's muscles are hypertoned and rigid, resulting in reduced movement. Many people with hypokinetic dysarthria experience a resting tremor that disappears with voluntary movement. The hand may tremble rhythmically, but the tremor disappears when the person reaches for a spoon or other object. There may be difficulty starting and stopping movements. For example, when trying to move from a chair to another room, the individual begins getting up from the chair, stops, and then starts again to get to a standing posture. Small shuffling steps move him to the next room, but he has to put his hand on the table to stop so he can sit down. There is an apparent difficulty initiating, continuing, and terminating movements.

Parkinson's disease is the primary example of a disorder that results in hypokinetic dysarthria. Parkinson's disease is caused by a degeneration of dopamine-producing cells of the basal ganglia, which are three large nuclei that are deep within the cerebral hemispheres. The effect of this deficit is a balanced hypertonicity of the musculature and resting tremors of the head and limbs.

The speech movements of individuals with hypokinetic dysarthria are small, but their speech rate sometimes sounds fast. If fact, hypokinetic dysarthria is the only dysarthria in which accelerated movements and short rushes of speech characterize the disorder. Speech melody is flat with monoloudness, monopitch, and reduced intensity.

Hyperkinetic Dysarthria

When the basal ganglia of the extrapyramidal system are damaged, involuntary movements are a telltale sign. In Parkinson's disease, the involuntary movements disappear with movement. In other disorders such as Huntington's chorea and dystonia, however, the involuntary movements are superimposed on voluntary movements of the body. Depending on the underlying cause, the involuntary movements in hyperkenetic dysarthria may be slow or fast, rhythmic or dysrhythmic, involve the entire body, or be restricted to a single structure like the jaw.

Involuntary movements interfere with speech production. Articulation is imprecise in individuals with hyperkinetic dysarthria, and they often have breakdowns in the flow of speech, which sound like hesitations in unusual places. The person with hyperkinetic dysarthria often speaks with short phrases, and there are long pauses while he or she waits for the involuntary movement to subside. After the involuntary movements, the person continues with speech. The voice quality of these individuals may be breathy or strangled sounding depending on the state of the fluctuating tonicity of the laryngeal musculature and the degree of breath support.

Mixed Dysarthrias

Several disease processes affect more than one part of the motor system at the same time. Multiple sclerosis, a disease in which the myelin covering of axons is damaged, may affect the spinal cord, brainstem, cerebellum, cerebrum, or any combination of these structures. Another example of a disease that affects more than one part of the motor system is amyotrophic lateral sclerosis, which damages the upper motor neurons of the pyramidal tract as well as the peripheral motoneurons of the brainstem and spinal cord. How speech production is affected will depend on which systems are damaged and may vary from a barely detectable change in speech production in multiple sclerosis to completely unintelligible speech in advanced amyotrophic lateral sclerosis.

 CD-ROM

In CD-ROM segment Ch.14.03, an adult with mild mixed dysarthria talks about himself. Note that although his speech is intelligible, prosodic aspects of speech production are impaired.

ASSESSMENT OF INDIVIDUALS WITH DYSARTHRIA

When assessing an individual with dysarthria, the speech-language pathologist (SLP) needs to evaluate each subsystem of the speech production process—respiration, phonation, velopharyngeal function, and articulation—in order to determine the type and extent of dysarthria.

The Oral-Peripheral Examination

The anatomic and functional integrity of speech production structures is determined from completion of an oral-peripheral examination. What this entails is a careful examination of structures such as the tongue, jaw, and lips at rest and during nonspeech (rounding and spreading the lips, opening and closing the mouth) and speech (saying syllables rapidly) activities. A key element in the evaluation of the individual with dysarthria is the determination of speech intelligibility, because it serves as the index of dysarthria severity, progression of the disease, and effects of treatment.

In addition to the oral-peripheral examination, there are several evaluation protocols for dysarthria. The Frenchay dysarthria assessment (Enderby, 1983) is one such test. It includes tasks to assess reflex and voluntary activities of speech structures during nonspeech and speech activities. For example, in the evaluation of the tongue, the speech-language pathologist (SLP) asks the patient to move the tongue in side-to-side and in-and-out movements, to push the tongue against the inside of the cheek on both sides. The assessment findings may be used to assign the individual to a specific dysarthria group like hypokinetic or ataxic.

Intelligible speech requires a stable subglottal air pressure as a power source for vocal fold vibration and for additional sound sources in the upper airway. Respiratory dysfunction, except in the severest forms of neuromuscular disease, seldom is the basis for reduced intelligibility. Movements of air that are sufficient to support life are nearly always sufficient for producing short sequences of understandable speech.

Respiration should be assessed during nonspeech and speech-related tasks. Quiet respiration and respiration for speech are observed carefully for lack of coordination and signs of compensation for muscular weakness. One simple device to evaluate nonspeech respiration is to place a straw in a water-filled glass that has centimeter markings on the side (Hixon, Hawley, & Wilson, 1982). If bubbles can be blown in the water with the straw inserted 5 centimeters below the surface for 5 seconds, respiratory function is sufficient for speech.

Speech-language pathologists evaluate laryngeal function by making subjective judgments of voice quality. They ask patients to produce prolonged vowels during syllable production and during connected speech. The degree of hoarseness, harshness, breathiness, and fluctuations in voice quality are estimated during these activities and others in which the patient in instructed to increases loudness and pitch. See Chapter 12 for a discussion of additional activities that are used to assess voice production.

The SLP also looks for evidence of weakness and/or coordination of the velopharynx. These judgments should be based on physical examination of the mechanism at rest and during production of a prolonged vowel. Nasal emission of air is assessed during the articulation of syllables containing stops and consonants in connected speech. If the SLP hears nasal emission and hypernasality during speech production, there is probably abnormal function of the velopharynx due to weakness and/or incoordination.

Articulatory structures of the upper airway, including muscles of the tongue, jaw, and lips, should be assessed to determine if they are weak, atrophic, and/or uncoordinated. The SLP should look for reductions in strength, speed, range or motion, and coordination. The face is examined at rest and during rounding and retraction of the lips to assess facial weakness. The examiner may ask the individual to hold a tongue depressor between their lips. This is routinely performed on the left side and on the right sides to see if one side is weaker. Alternating lip rounding and retraction at maximum rates may reveal problems with speech and coordination. Similarly, the examiner evaluates jaw strength on each side by attempting to close the jaw after he asks the patient to hold the jaw open and assesses strength by testing the compression of a tongue depressor between the teeth on each side. Requesting maximum up-and-down movements of the jaw provide information on speed and coordination. The tongue is tested by evaluating function during protrusion and retraction, lateral movement, and rapid alternating movements. Based on these systematic observations, the clinician obtains an estimate of the functional integrity of each subcomponent of the speech production system.

The Speech Examination

Several aspects of speech production provide important information about the type and extent of dysarthria. The clinician requests that maximum rates of syllable production be generated using bilabial (/b/, /p/), lingualveolar (/k/, /g/), and linguavelar (/t/, /d/, /s/) consonants plus a vowel. If dysarthria is present, the number of syllables that can be produced is decreased compared to normal performance.

Speech samples serve as assessment vehicles to estimate articulatory precision, speech rate, prosodic patterning, and other perceptual features. Typically, a standard passage is read and a sample of conversational speech is obtained. The SLP listens to these samples for evidence of altered speech characteristics that are indicative of dysarthria. Behaviors that indicate dysarthria include slow rate, hypernasality, and harsh voice quality.

There are several measures of speech intelligibility administered to individuals who are suspected of having dysarthria. Perhaps the measure most often used is the *Assessment of the Intelligibility of Dysarthric Speech* (Yorkston & Beukelman, 1981). The patient reads or repeats words and phrases. These speech samples are recorded and are evaluated by a second listener to provide estimates of word and sentence intelligibility. In general, we expect sentences to be more intelligible than words, It is important to point out that the severity of impairment to any major component of the system may have major effects on speech intelligibility. For example, mild weakness of the entire speech production system may result in only mild reductions in intelligibility. Severe impairment in tongue or velopharyngeal functioning, even if the rest of the system is intact, may render speech almost entirely unintelligible

TREATMENT OF INDIVIDUALS WITH DYSARTHRIA

A team of professionals including physicians, SLPS, occupational therapists, audiologists, special educators, and physical therapists works to help the child develop functional independence. Drugs are prescribed to reduce spasticity and involuntary movement; bracing and special seating equipment are useful for preventing contractures and for facilitating sitting and walking; prescipive glasses and hearing aids may improve sensory functioning; specialized teaching is employed to deal with deficits in attention, memory, and learning; and counseling may help to reduce emotional lability.

Treatment for dysarthria may take several forms. Surgery and drugs are beneficial for some disorders in which dysarthria is an symptom. For example, individuals with Parkinson's disease benefit from the administration of dopamine. This drug is used to replace naturally produced dopamine, a substance that is required for brain metabolism. Patients with Parkinson's disease do not produce dopamine in sufficient quantities due to degeneration of cells in the basal ganglia. Other drugs can be prescribed that serve to reduce involuntary movements or spasticity. In some cases, improved motor performance has been brought about by surgical intervention that destroys a part of the thalamus or a portion of the globus pallidus. There also have been efforts to transfer fetal brain cells to patients with Parkinson's disease to replace those that have been destroyed. An early consideration in dysarthria, then, is the use of drugs and surgery to benefit motor performance.

Surgical and prosthetic management may be used to directly improve speech performance. In unilateral vocal fold paralysis, it may be beneficial to surgically move the fold to the midline so that it can be approximated by the noninvolved fold during phonation. An alternative is to fill the paralyzed vocal fold with teflon, effectively moving it to a closed position for better closure during approximation of the unparalyzed fold. For severe velopharyngeal inadequacy, a palatal lift or pharyngeal flap may reduce nasal emission and hypernasality, which results in improved speech intelligibility.

Postural supports are important for children with cerebral palsy and for adults with acquired dysarthrias because it is necessary to place the individual in a better position for speaking. These supports take the form of slings to hold up the arms and adapted wheelchairs for maintaining upright supported posture. For example, an adapted wheelchair in which the head is stabilized may restrict the eliciting of reflex patterns that interfere with voluntary arm movements.

Speech therapy is often geared toward improving speech intelligibility. In children with cerebral palsy, treatment may initially focus on the development of a stable respiratory pattern. For example, the child may be placed in a supine position (on his back) with the legs, arms, and neck flexed. Touching the skin with ice will cause the child to take several deep breaths. Attention is focused on the sensations associated with this pattern of rapid inhalation followed by prolonged expiration. As the child develops control over the respiratory pattern for speech, he is asked to phonate a prolonged vowel with expiration. When phonation is consistent, superimposing constrictions in the mouth, like closing the lips, results in the production of the voiced /b/ with a vowel. In general, treatment focuses the development of coordinated volitional control of the speech production system.

For adults, speech intelligibility can be improved by reductions in speech rate, increases in intensity, and exaggerated articulatory movements during speech production. A particularly effective program for Parkinson's disease (Ramig, Countryman, Thompson, & Horii, 1995), for example, focuses on increasing speech intensity with careful self-monitoring of intensity. This is followed by practice in talking louder in therapy sessions and in self-practice outside the clinic. Talking louder results in an increase in movement of the speech structures with greater articulatory precision. For individuals with good intelligibility, the focus of treatment may change to improving the naturalness of speech. Speech may be fully understandable, but calls attention to the speaker because of abnormal intonation or stress. Treatment focuses on feedback during speech production to focus on words that should be stressed and intonation patterns appropriate to the utterance.

What if intelligible speech was not an option? What if the neuromuscular condition was so severe that the child with cerebral palsy or the adult with acquired dysarthria cannot be understood, even by family members who knew him or her well? What can they do to communicate?

AUGMENTATIVE COMMUNICATION

We all augment our communication with facial expressions and gestures. If you were asked to communicate a message but could only use one word, you would probably use gestures or pantomime to convey the information. Augmentative communication refers to supplementing or augmenting speech using various techniques and aids. Sometimes the communication system we employ temporarily replaces speech. Examples of these systems include using writing or gestures in a particularly noisy environment. But in contrast to the unimpaired speaker who relies on augmentative communication only in particular situations, individuals with dysarthria or severe language impairments may need to use an augmentative communication system all the time.

Augmentative communication can take various forms. Some systems do not require any type of communication aid or device. Think for a moment that you need to convey three messages without speaking: *stop, yes,* and *I don't know.* How would you do it using gestures? The gestures you would probably come up with are the hand held palm forward in a vertical direction with an arm extended for *stop,* upward and downward movements of the head for *yes,* and a shrugging of the shoulders for *I don't know.* In this case, you needed no tool or device other than your own body to communicate. What if you were paralyzed except for movements of your left foot? How would you communicate in this situation? In all likelihood you would need some type of device to accomplish message transmission. A switch triggered by movements of your foot that activate and stop a cursor moving across a screen with printed words, however, would allow you to stop on the word you wanted to communicate. This is an example of an aided augmentative communication, because more than your own body was required to accomplish communication. The two systems also are different because one is nonelectronic (gestures) and the other is electronic (scanning system).

Based on this short description, it is apparent that augmentative systems are extremely diverse and depend on the capabilities of the communicator. They may be as basic as words or pictures on a board that the user employs to communicate everyday needs like requests for a drink or food, to technologically advanced systems based on speech synthesizers capable of storing hundreds of phrases and words.

 CD-ROM

The adult with cerebral palsy shown in CD-ROM segment Ch.14.01 uses an augmentive communication device to respond to questions. View segment Ch.14.01 again and compare the intelligibility of his responses using speech and the augmentative system.

Augmentative communication differs in several important respects from oral speech. Augmentative communication is slower. We might expect an unimpaired individual to produce approximately 150 words per minute while speaking. With an augmentative system, even when items are directly selected from a picture or word array or from a series of stored phrases on a speech synthesizer, communication will be slower. This is particularly true when a cursor must be used to scan across a field of possible options. If a communication board is used that requires a communication partner to view it, he must be positioned behind the user. Neither of the partners can see the other's face. If gestures are used, then the partner must interpret what the gestures convey; both communicators must know the code. Some environments may be difficult if a speech synthesizer is used, because the output may not be sufficient to overcome background noise.

For individuals with dysarthria due to cerebral palsy or acquired motor system damage, augmentative communication may be the primary means of conveying messages (see Figures 14–1 and 14–2). No system is ideal and frequently there are multiple options available. To help an individual decide

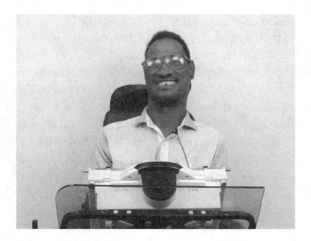

Figure 14–1. Adult male with cerebral palsy who uses an augmentative communication system.

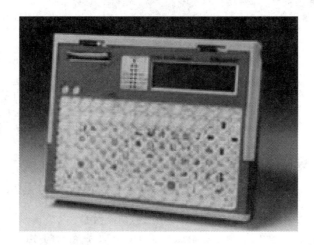

Figure 14–2. Liberator augmentative communication system. (Courtesy of Prentke-Romich Company)

which system to use, we need to assess intellectual, sensory, motor, and academic skills. Knowing which motor behaviors are available will help to decide whether a gestural system is possible or what size the keys on a keyboard need to be in order to access a word-based augmentative system. If the individual can read, words rather than pictures can be used on the communication device. The degree of cognitive functioning is important in determining whether a symbol system can be used as part of the display and whether the individual is capable of learning how to use the system.

An assessment of the person's communication needs is perhaps as important as his abilities. What and how meaning is conveyed by the augmentative communication user depends on his or her age and situation. An 8-year-old child with cerebral palsy may need to communicate in a classroom setting with his teacher and classmates, not only on academic topics such as mathematics and reading assignments, but on social events and activities outside the classroom. The needs of the adult with severe multiple sclerosis may be markedly different. The ability to communicate to meet everyday functional needs and to discuss family issues may be paramount.

The overriding goal is to develop an augmentative system within the capabilities of the user that meets communication needs with maximum efficiency. Few individuals with cerebral palsy are speechless or entirely unintelligible. The augmentative system may be the primary communication mode for some individuals; for others it serves to supplement speech only in difficult communication situations.

A period of training with the system is essential. For the child or adult who has had limited opportunity to communicate, this training may take the form of demonstrating turn-taking, initiation of communication, and question asking. In adults with acquired dysarthria and severely reduced intelligibility, it may focus on using the procedure of pointing to the first letter of each word verbalized to increase the probability that the communication partner can interpret the content of the intended message. In thinking about augmentative communication systems, it is always important to remember that speech is faster, more flexible, and more efficient. The initial focus of rehabilitation should be to maximize oral speech function and to augment or to substitute an alternative communication system only if necessary.

SUMMARY

Neuromuscular speech disorders result from damage to the motor systems of the central and/or peripheral nervous system. Speech is affected because muscles are weak, paralyzed, or uncoordinated. Although there are similarities between dysarthria in cerebral palsy compared to acquired nervous system damage, children with cerebral palsy demonstrate visual, auditory, and cognitive impairments that have a bearing on the development of speech and language abilities. This is because the injury or damage responsible for the cerebral palsy occurred near the time of birth. The assessment of dysarthria focuses on speech production, but may include language and cognitive assessment since deficits in these domains of communicative functioning also may be associated with the cause of the disorder. The purpose of drug, prosthetic, and behavioral intervention is to maximize the communication ability of individuals with dysarthria. Augmentative communication systems may have an important role in meeting this goal, particularly for the severely impaired individual.

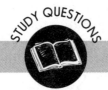

STUDY QUESTIONS

1 What neuromuscular disorders have involuntary movement? Why?

2 How does the assessment of dysarthria differ for an adult compared to a child?

3 What are the major causes of cerebral palsy?

4 What are two diseases that result in mixed dysarthria?

5 How is speech intelligibility assessed?

6 How does augmentative communication differ from oral speech production?

REFERENCES

Darley, F., Aronson, A., & Brown, J. (1975). *Motor speech disorders.* St. Louis, MO: W. B. Saunders.

Enderby, P. (1983). *Frenchay dysarthria assessment.* Austin, TX: Pro-Ed.

Hixon, T. J., Hawley, J. L., & Wilson, K. J. (1982). An around-the-house device for the clinical determination of respiratory driving pressure: A note on making the simple even simpler. *Journal of Speech and Hearing Disorders, 47,* 413–415.

Netsell, R. (1969). Evaluation of velopharyngeal function in dysarthria. *Journal of Speech and Hearing Disorders, 34,* 113–122.

Ramig, L., Countryman, S., Thompson, L., & Horii, L. (1995). A comparison of two intensive speech treatments for Parkinson disease. *Journal of Speech and Hearing Research, 39,* 1232–1251.

Rusk, H. (1977). *Rehabilitation medicine* (4th ed.). St. Louis, MO: Mosby.

Yorkston, K., & Beukelman, D. (1981). *Assessment of intelligibility of dysarthric speech.* Austin, TX: Pro-Ed.

SUGGESTED READINGS

Blackstone, S. (1986). *Augmentative communication: An introduction.* Rockville, MD: American Speech-Language-Hearing Association.

Brookshire, R. (1997). *Introduction to neurogenic communication disorders* (5th ed.). St. Louis, MO: Mosby.

Love, R. (1992). *Childhood motor speech disability.* New York: Macmillan.

McDonald, E. (Ed.). (1987). *Treating cerebral palsy.* Austin, TX: Pro-Ed.

GLOSSARY

Ataxia (ataxic): Neuromuscular disorder characterized by errors in the direction, force, and timing of movements due to cerebellar damage.

Athetosis (athetoid): Congenital neuromuscular disorder characterized by writhing involuntary movement caused by extrapyramidal tract damage.

Atrophy: Muscle wasting.

Dysarthria: Neuromuscular speech disorder.

Hyper-/Hypotonicity: Abnormally increased (hyper-) or decreased (hypo-) background activity of a muscle due to nervous system damage.

Hyper-/Hyporeflexia: Abnormally increased (hyper-) or decreased (hypo-) reflexes due to nervous system damage.

Rigidity (rigid): Balanced hypertonicity that results in resistance to movement.

Spasticity (spastic): Abnormal muscle tone, primarily in antigravity muscles, due to upper motor neuron damage.

Tremor: Rhythmic involuntary movements due to basal ganglia disease/damage.

15

Dysphagia

Dena Granof

1 To learn the normal processes involved in feeding and swallowing.

2 To understand the causes of swallowing disorders.

3 To learn clinical and instrumental procedures for evaluating dysphagia.

4 To learn the speech-language pathologist's (SLPs) role in assessing and treating swallowing disorders in children and adults.

INTRODUCTION

Dysphagia (dis-fa-ja) is a difficulty in swallowing or an inability to swallow. A swallowing problem affects a person's ability to eat, which serves two primary purposes: (1) nutrition and hydration and (2) pleasure. To remain healthy, to recover from illness or trauma, or to grow, both of these functions must be achieved in a safe and efficient manner. When patients have dysphagia, they are unable to consume enough food or liquid safely and efficiently. Food plays an important role in all cultures and families and is a significant part of our social interactions. Dysphagia also impairs a person's ability to participate in social gatherings or events.

CD-ROM

> **Overview of CD-ROM Segments for Chapter 15**
>
> Normal (CD-ROM segment Ch.15.01) and disordered (CD-ROM segment Ch.15.02) swallowing are shown during modified barium swallow (MBS) studies. Barium swallow studies allow viewing of the bolus as it is moved from the mouth through the pharynx to the esophagus.

Examples of Dysphagia

The following two case studies illustrate what happens when a person has dysphagia (see Figure 15–1 for a view of the anatomical structures involved in the swallowing process). Ms. T is a 73-year-old woman who recently had a stroke affecting the left side of the brain. The brain damage caused by the stroke impairs the function of the muscles of the face, mouth, larynx, and pharynx. Because of this muscle dysfunction, Ms. T has trouble chewing and moving the food around in her mouth. When she attempts to swallow or move the food from the mouth to the stomach, the weakness of her muscles makes it difficult for her to push the food into the pharynx and then into the esophagus so it can continue on to the stomach. Some food remains in the part of the mouth that is now paralyzed and no longer has sensation. After every two or three bites, Ms. T coughs because food is going toward the tracheal airway and lungs instead of the stomach.

When the food enters the airway it is called **aspiration.** Aspiration may occur because the weak and/or paralyzed pharyngeal and laryngeal muscles cannot control the food. Ms. T is only able to eat and drink small amounts at a time. She may not be a "safe" eater since the impaired muscle function may allow food to enter the lungs and cause possible aspiration or choking. Ms. T's nutrition, hydration, safety, and eating pleasure are negatively affected by the symptoms of her stroke.

The second case study is an example of dysphagia in a child. Rebecca is 4 years old and has spastic cerebral palsy. She uses a wheelchair with supports for her head and trunk. She is able to say one word at a time, but due to severe dysarthria, her speech is not very understandable. Rebecca drinks small sips of thickened liquids out of a special cup and eats food that is of a puree or

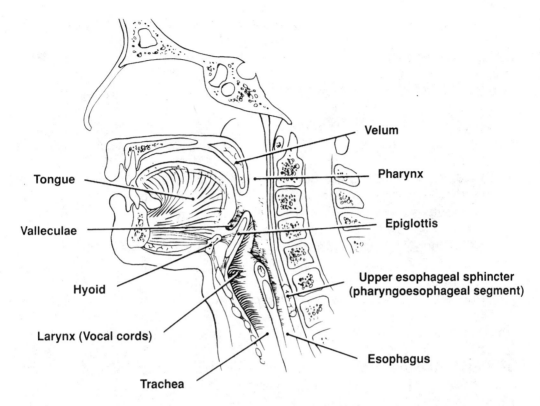

Figure 15–1. Anatomical structures involved with swallowing. (From Cherney, L. R. [1994]. *Clinical management of dysphagia in children and adults* [Figure 1-5, p. 6]. Gaithersburg, MD: Aspen Publishers. Reprinted with permission.)

pudding consistency. Because of abnormal muscle tone and slow movement, it takes over an hour for Rebecca to finish a meal. She frequently coughs and chokes toward the end of her meals. Rebecca has been diagnosed with dysphagia because she is not able to eat enough food to maintain good nutrition for growth or to drink an adequate amount of liquid. Her coughing indicates that some food may be going down her airway.

Role of the Speech-Language Pathologist

For both Ms. T and Rebecca, the speech-language pathologist (SLP) will be an integral part of the dysphagia team that assesses and treats their swallowing problems. Speech-language pathologists (SLPs) have been involved with swallowing since the 1930s when they treated the feeding problems of children who had cerebral palsy (Miller & Groher, 1993). Over the past 25 years, there has been an expansion of the practice of speech-language pathology into medical settings such as hospitals and nursing homes. Additionally, more multidisabled children are being served in the public schools. According to the 1995 American Speech-Language and Hearing Association Omnibus Survey (American Speech-Language-Hearing Association [ASHA], 1995), approximately 52% of practicing SLPs are involved in the management of dysphagia.

There are several reasons that SLPs are a key part of a dysphagia team. Communication and swallowing problems frequently occur together. A study by Martin and Corlew (1990) surveyed 115 patients at a veteran's administration medical center. Of these patients, 81% had swallowing problems and 87% of those with swallowing problems also had communication disorders. Similar results were reported in a Rehabilitation Institute of Chicago study (Cherney, 1994) of 973 consecutive referrals to the Department of Communicative Disorders. This study found that 307 or 31.55% of these patients had dysphagia.

Communication and swallowing problems often co-occur because these two functions share some common structures and functions. Historically, SLPs have been trained to understand the structure and function of the oral mechanism, pharynx, and larynx and to apply this knowledge to the assessment and treatment of speech disorders. These same structures and functions are an important part of the swallowing process; thus, it is more efficient to have one professional managing these overlapping areas. In 1987, the Ad Hoc Committee on Dysphagia Report (ASHA, 1987) set out guidelines regarding the role of the SLP in the area of dysphagia. The report clearly states that dysphagia should be included in the scope of practice and that the SLP should be involved in the evaluation and treatment of dysphagia with or without the presence of a communication disorder.

STAGES OF SWALLOWING

Before examining the reasons for dysphagia and what techniques or skills the SLP uses to evaluate swallowing problems, it is important to understand

 CD-ROM

A Normal Swallow

CD-ROM segment Ch.15.01 is a modified barium study (MBS) of a normal swallow. Note the rapid movement of fluid from the mouth through the pharynx to the esophagus.

the normal swallow. The process of swallowing is viewed in terms of different stages. These include an anticipatory stage, oral stage, pharyngeal stage, and esophageal stage.

The Anticipatory Stage

The anticipatory stage of swallowing occurs before the food actually reaches the mouth. Sensory information about what is going to be eaten is provided through vision and smell. These senses allow the person the opportunity to prepare to eat. They help the person "get ready" for the food by understanding what is on the plate and whether it is a desirable thing to eat.

The Oral Stage

The oral stage marks the actual beginning of events that lead up to the swallow. There are two parts to this stage, and both are under voluntary control. In the preparatory part of the oral stage, a **bolus** (food after it has been chewed and mixed with saliva) is being readied for a safe swallow. Figure 15–2A shows the position of the bolus during the oral stage. Once the food enters the mouth, a labial or lip seal is needed to prevent the food from falling out, and there needs to be an open nasal airway for breathing. The pharynx and larynx are at rest. At the same time, the buccal or cheek musculature prevents the food from falling into lateral sulci, which are the spaces between the cheek and the mandible. The bolus is masticated (chewed) and manipulated by the tongue and jaw in a rotary lateral movement. Sensory input about the taste, texture, temperature, and size of the bolus determines the amount of oral motor movement and strength that is needed. During this process, the back of the tongue is usually elevated to keep the bolus in the oral cavity.

The second part of the oral stage, sometimes called the transport phase, begins when the tongue pushes the bolus against the palate, moving it in a posterior or backward direction towards the pharynx. The size and consistency of the bolus affect the amount of lingual strength that is necessary to complete this movement. The oral stage of the swallow is completed when the bolus passes the anterior faucial arches and enters the pharyngeal area. It is at this point that the pharyngeal stage of the swallow is triggered.

The Pharyngeal Stage

The pharyngeal stage (see Figure 15–2B) begins with the triggering of the pharyngeal swallow. The two purposes of the pharyngeal stage are to protect the airway and to direct the bolus toward the stomach. The pharyngeal

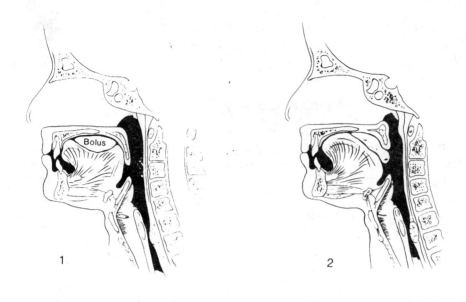

Oral Phase

A

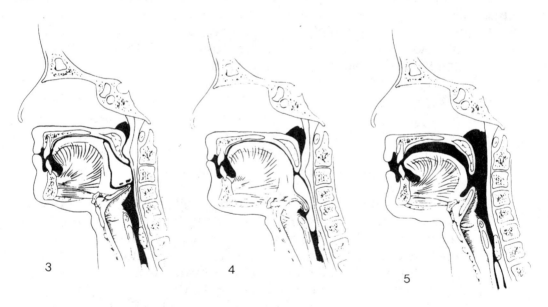

Pharyngeal Phase   Esophageal Phase

B

Figure 15–2. Stages of swallowing: **A.** Oral stage (parts 1 and 2). **B.** Pharyngeal phase (parts 3 and 4) and Esophageal phase (part 5). (From Cherney, L. R. [1994]. *Clinical management of dysphagia in children and adults* [Figure 1-7, pp. 8-9]. Gaithersburg, MD: Aspen Publishers. Reprinted with permission.)

swallow motor pattern is initiated by sensory information sent from the mouth and oropharynx to the brainstem. According to Logemann (1998), there is a sensory recognition center in the medulla (lower brainstem) that interprets this incoming sensory information. The recognition center in the medulla sends the information to the nucleus ambiguous (also in the medulla), which initiates the pharyngeal swallow.

A number of simultaneous physiological events occur as a result of the swallow. The velum elevates and contracts to close off the velopharynx so food cannot enter the nasal cavity. The larynx and hyoid bone move upward and forward. There is closure of the larynx to prevent food from entering the airway beginning at the level of the vocal folds and moving superiorly or upward to the false vocal folds and then the aryepiglottic folds. As the larynx elevates and moves forward, the epiglottis comes over the larynx to provide additional airway protection.

When the swallow is triggered, there is initiation of pharyngeal **peristalsis.** The bolus is transported through the pharynx toward the esophagus by the contraction of the muscles of the superior, medial, and inferior pharyngeal constrictors. These muscles are on the back part of the pharyngeal wall. The upper esophageal sphincter, which is on top of the esophagus, relaxes or opens with the upward and forward movement of the larynx. This allows the food to enter the esophagus.

The Esophageal Stage

The esophageal stage (see Figure 15–2B) begins with the lowering and backward movement of the larynx and resumption of breathing. The upper esophageal sphincter contracts to prevent food from re-entering the pharynx. The bolus moves through the esophagus to the stomach in a series of peristaltic waves.

DYSPHAGIA IN ADULTS

Swallowing requires both cognitive and motor skills. Cognitively, a person must be able to recognize the need to eat and decide what to eat. From the description of the different stages of swallowing, it can be seen that the normal swallow requires an intact motor system. Swallowing is a process of finely coordinated, sequential muscular movements. When there is an illness or injury that affects either the cognitive or the motor skills, there is a high risk for dysphagia. Following is information on some of the most common etiologies of dysphagia in adults and the resultant swallowing problems.

Cortical Stroke

Left Hemisphere Cerebrovascular Accident (CVA)

Persons who suffer cerebrovascular accidents (CVAs), or strokes, to the left hemisphere often have an oral stage difficulty due to weakened or paralyzed facial musculature including labial, lingual, and mandibular function. There may be a delay in initiating the pharyngeal swallow, which could cause the bolus to be aspirated.

Right Hemisphere Cerebrovascular Accident (CVA)

Individuals who suffer right hemisphere strokes often have oral stage difficulties due to reduction in labial, lingual, and mandibular strength. They also have a delayed pharyngeal swallow, which could cause aspiration. There is a reduction in pharyngeal peristalsis, which contributes to food getting "stuck" in the throat. Cognitive deficits including impulsivity, errors in judgment, and attention difficulties may compound these muscular difficulties.

Brainstem Stroke

Individuals who have brainstem CVAs (cerebrovascular accidents) often have oral stage difficulties due to reduced labial, lingual, and mandibular sensation and strength. These persons also have a delayed or absent pharyngeal swallow, causing incomplete laryngeal elevation and closure and reduced upper esophageal sphincter opening. This may result in possible aspiration and an inability for the bolus to enter the esophagus.

Traumatic Brain Injury

Dysphagia symptoms due to traumatic brain injury vary according to the location and severity of the injury, but problems usually exist at each stage of the swallow. Cognitive deficits in orientation, memory, judgment, attention, and reasoning may affect the ability to choose foods, control the rate of eating, and maintain attention to the task of eating. Common oral stage problems include reduced tongue control, abnormal reflexes, and difficulty with chewing. There may be a delayed or absent pharyngeal swallow, reduced pharyngeal peristalsis and aspiration.

Dementia

Dementia causes cognitive deficits such as reduced attention, reasoning, judgment, and poor orientation skills. These deficits can significantly affect the initiation of the eating process. There may be an overall reduction in oral awareness, resulting in slow oral preparatory movements. Food may be held in the mouth for an extended period of time and not recognized as something to be swallowed. As a result, there is often a delayed pharyngeal swallow. Since dementia is frequently a part of a neurological disease, the muscular deficits of that disease serve to compound the problems of dementia and cause swallowing dysfunction in all of the stages.

Neuromuscular Disease

Multiple sclerosis (MS), amyotrophic lateral sclerosis (ALS), Parkinson's disease, myasthenia gravis, and muscular dystrophy (MD) are progressive neuromuscular diseases that cause changes in strength, rate, and efficiency of muscular movements. As these diseases progress or get worse, muscular movements frequently become weak and uncoordinated. This causes difficulty at all stages of the swallow.

 CD-ROM

A Comparison of Normal and Abnormal Swallows

View the normal swallow in CD-ROM segment Ch.15.01 again. Now view segment Ch.15.02 that shows a modified barium swallow (MBS) from a stroke patient. Note that the muscles that control swallowing are weak, the time required for the liquid to pass from the mouth to the esophagus is slow, and there is a significant amount of liquid left in the pharyngeal area.

MANAGEMENT OF ADULT DYSPHAGIA

Assessment and treatment of adult dysphagia requires a team approach. The speech-language pathologist is one part of a dysphagia team that can include occupational and physical therapists, nurses, nutritionists, and a variety of medical doctors such as radiologists, neurologists, gastroenterologists, or pulmonologists. The patient and family are also an integral part of this team. The dysphagia assessment is comprised of a number of procedures, including review of the patient's history, a bedside examination, and an instrumental examination. Based on the results of the assessment, the team meets and decides on a treatment plan.

The following case study will be used to illustrate assessment procedures, decision making, and formulation of a treatment plan. Tim, a 17 year old, was involved in a motorcycle accident. He was thrown off his motorcycle while driving around a curve too quickly and sustained a traumatic brain injury (TBI). He was taken by ambulance to the nearest trauma center where he remained unresponsive (in a "coma") for 72 hours. During this period of time he was nourished through **intravenous (IV)** solutions. Upon awakening, Tim was confused and disoriented; he did not know where he was, how he got there, or the day or time. One side of his body, including his face and neck, had reduced muscle movement and strength. The neurologist assigned to his case requested a dysphagia evaluation. The purpose of the evaluation was to determine if Tim could begin eating orally again. To make that decision, a number of questions needed to be answered. They included: (1) Are the muscles in Tim's tongue, lips, and jaw able to adequately prepare a bolus? (2) Do the pharyngeal and laryngeal muscles have enough strength and movement to elevate the larynx to close off the airway and direct the bolus to the esophagus? (3) Is Tim aware of the food on his plate and can he feed himself? (4) Can Tim eat safely (without aspiration) and maintain adequate nutrition?

Review of History Prior to the Accident

Upon receiving the referral for a dysphagia evaluation, the SLP needs to collect relevant feeding, behavioral, and medical information. The SLP needs to know if the patient had swallowing problems prior to the illness or accident. Information about any preexisting illness or trauma is also important. Additionally, the SLP needs to find out what medications, if any, the patient had been taking. This information can be ascertained from both a review of the medical chart and an interview with the patient's family.

Tim was a healthy young man with no history of illness or trauma. Prior to the accident, he had no swallowing or eating problems. In middle school, he had been diagnosed with a mild learning disability and had been on medication to improve his attention.

Current Medical Status

The next step in a dysphagia evaluation is to review the patient's current medical condition. The dysphagia team, including the SLP, needs to know if the patient is medically stable, the respiratory status, what medications have been prescribed, and the current level of cognitive functioning. The team also needs to know how the patient is currently receiving nutrition. The patient may be eating orally, receiving nutrients through an intravenous tube (like Tim), being fed through a tube placed in the nose that goes to the stomach (**nasogastric** or NG tube), or by a tube surgically placed directly into the stomach (**gastric** or G-tube). The way in which the dysphagia assessment is structured will depend on the answers to these questions. It is more complicated to perform a dysphagia assessment when there are respiratory or cardiac problems. Some medications that are given to patients after traumatic brain injury (TBI) cause drowsiness, and knowledge of this effect will allow the evaluation to be scheduled at an optimal time. If a patient is disoriented and confused, he or she may not understand the instructions of the SLP or even comprehend that food is something to be eaten. If the patient is not currently receiving oral nutrition, there are safety considerations related to the use of food in the assessment. This information is gathered from the medical chart, by consulting with the nurses and doctors on the dysphagia team, and by observing the patient.

Tim was medically stable; however, he was being given a medication to control seizures, which are common after TBI. This medication made him very sleepy. He could not maintain adequate alertness for more that 10 minutes at a time. He was also confused and did not understand why he was in the hospital or why he was unable to get out of bed and walk. He could not remember any of his therapists, nurses, or doctors, even though they were each in his room several times a day. He had not eaten orally in the 3 days since his accident.

Noninstrumental Clinical Exam (NICE) or Bedside Clinical Assessment (BCA)

This is the point in the assessment process that the SLP sits down with the patient and assesses his or her ability to take food off the plate, prepare the bolus, and safely swallow. The cognitive and motor skills necessary to perform these actions are evaluated. The examination procedures are influenced by the information gathered by the review of the patient's medical history and the patient's current medical status.

In Tim's case, we know he may have a short attention span and have difficulty following directions. Given his medical history, we expect he will have some motor difficulty with chewing and swallowing. We also know he has not eaten food for 3 days.

First, the SLP observes the patient's level of alertness, ability to follow directions, and any other behaviors that might interfere with the ability to attend to the feeding process. This is followed by an examination of the structure of the oral anatomy. The SLP examines the lips, tongue, cheeks, jaw, palate, and teeth, noting any abnormalities such as scarring or asymmetry.

During the oral-motor examination, the SLP will observe the patient's ability to perform the motor movements necessary for a safe and adequate swallow to occur. Based on the SLP's review of the patient's current medical status, food may or may not be used to assess these skills. The SLP observes (1) lip closure and lip strength, (2) jaw and cheek movement and strength, (3) lingual ability to move the food around in the mouth for both bolus preparation and the transporting of the bolus to the posterior of the oral cavity, and (4) initiation of the pharyngeal swallow. Once the bolus moves into the pharyngeal area, it can no longer be observed.

As was discussed previously, a safe swallow occurs when the larynx moves upward and forward while opening the upper esophageal sphincter that is at the top of the esophagus. This allows the food to go toward the stomach. The pharyngeal constrictor muscles propel the bolus through the pharynx to the esophagus. Because this cannot be directly observed, there are several "signs" that help the SLP to understand what is happening to the bolus after it moves through the oral cavity. These include (1) watching the neck along with placement of two fingers under the chin to determine if there is upward and forward laryngeal movement; (2) listening for coughing, which could mean that the bolus or part of the bolus is going down the "wrong way" toward the lungs; (3) and listening for a "gurgly" sound after swallowing, which might indicate that part of the bolus is on the vocal folds.

Pharyngeal stage problems cannot be diagnosed by the bedside clinical assessment. However, an indication of possible pharyngeal stage deficits can be ascertained through the information provided by this evaluation. Weak and uncoordinated oral motor movements may indicate the presence of poor pharyngeal stage movements. The initiation of the swallow may be delayed, which could cause possible aspiration. Laryngeal movement may be judged to be inadequate, which could cause incomplete protection of the airway. The patient may cough after the swallow or complain that it feels as if food is stuck in his or her throat. Or, the patient may have a diagnosis such as dementia or a stroke in which pharyngeal stage problems are common. When pharyngeal stage problems are suspected, an additional assessment procedure is performed.

Observation of Tim's oral structures indicated good dentition, but asymmetry in both the tongue and cheeks. This was evidenced by a "droop" on the right side of his face and tongue, which could mean reduced or absent muscular movement. Food was used as a part of Tim's bedside clinical assessment, but he had to be constantly reminded that he needed to put the spoon in his mouth and chew and swallow. Chewing was slow and labored. He had trouble making a bolus with crackers and could not use his tongue to efficiently move the bolus to the back of his mouth. He had much better control and ease of movement with the chocolate pudding. The initiation of the swallow appeared delayed, and Tim coughed for several minutes after each of the four bites. It appeared Tim had possible pharyngeal stage deficits. Therefore, he was referred for an instrumental assessment.

Instrumental Assessment of Dysphagia

An instrumental assessment is used to get a better understanding of pharyngeal stage functioning. The most commonly used instrumental procedure is referred to as **a modified barium swallow (MBS).** This procedure is a fluoroscopic image that is recorded on videotape. The SLP and a radiologist perform this procedure together. The patient is brought into the room where X-rays are taken. The patient sits in a special chair that can be positioned for optimal eating. The SLP places barium-coated food in the patient's mouth, and the radiologist takes a moving picture or fluoroscopy of the patient chewing and swallowing. Pharyngeal stage functioning can be visualized, and any abnormalities in structure or function can be identified on the video X-ray image. If the patient aspirates, this can also be seen on the video. Use of the modified barium swallow (MBS) allows the dysphagia team to understand the cause of the dysphagia and to make recommendations for treatment. It also provides key information as to whether the patient is able to eat safely.

Another commonly used instrumental procedure is **videoendoscopy.** A flexible scope in inserted through the nose and positioned just above the epiglottis. The patient is then given food that has been mixed with dye. As the patient eats, the pharyngeal structures and functions are observed through the scope. As with the MBS, videoendoscopy provides information about the adequacy and safety of the swallow.

Based on the results of Tim's bedside clinical assessment, he was referred for a modified barium swallow study. He was given three consistencies of food: thin liquid barium, pudding-like barium, and a cookie coated with barium. The video study showed that Tim had a delayed swallow and weak pharyngeal constrictor muscles. The delayed swallow caused a small amount of the thin liquid to be aspirated before the swallow was initiated. Pieces of the cookie got "stuck" in his throat, and it took several extra swallows to clear all the food from the pharyngeal area. This situation was due to the weak pharyngeal muscles.

Treatment Planning

The entire dysphagia team reviews all of the information that has been gathered about the patient and writes a treatment plan that will allow the patient to be well nourished and safe. This plan usually address a number of different aspects of the eating and swallowing process (Table 15–1).

Once a dysphagia treatment plan has been formulated, the team determines the procedures for carrying out the recommendations. The entire dysphagia team works together to ensure that the patient remains safe and well nourished. Dysphagia assessment and treatment is an ongoing process.

Table 15–1. Typical Aspects of a Treatment Plan for Dysphagia

Aspect	Questions
Positioning	What is the best position for the patient while eating? Does the patient need any special head or neck support? How long should the patient remain upright after eating?
Environmental Modifications	Does the patient need a quiet room to eat in? What kind of reminders or cues does the patient need to put the food in his or her mouth and remember to chew and swallow?
Adaptive Feeding Equipment	Does the patient need a nonslip bowl, a spoon with a special handle, or a cup with a spout?
Bolus Modifications	What consistency of food is easiest and safest for the patient to eat? Is it thin or thickened liquids or finely chopped or pudding-like food? Does the patient do better with hot or cold foods? How much food should be given for each swallow?
Swallowing Techniques	Can the patient be taught any compensatory strategies to avoid aspiration? Does the patient need instructions for safe swallowing such as multiple swallows for each bolus or alternating liquid and solid foods?

Patients continually change and improve, and the treatment plan needs to reflect these changes as they occur.

Tim had many of the dysphagia symptoms that are common after TBI, and his treatment plan reflected the presence of these symptoms. Tim's treatment plan contained four important elements that were directed toward his current level of swallowing: (1) *Positioning*—Tim needed to be positioned upright in his wheelchair. This aided him in the use of his weakened muscles and helped direct the food toward the esophagus and reduced the risk of aspiration. (2) *Cueing*—Tim had another person sitting with him during the meal to remind him to chew and swallow each bite of food before putting another bite in his mouth. Tim tended to stuff too much in at one time, which is a safety concern. Tim also needed to be reminded that there was food on his plate and that he needed to eat it. (3) *Bolus modifications*—the results of the dysphagia assessment showed that Tim had difficulty with thin liquids because of his delayed swallow and with foods that needed to be chewed because of his weak pharyngeal constrictor muscles. The dysphagia team recommended that Tim's diet consist of thickened liquids and foods with a pudding consistency. This allowed Tim to eat safely and obtain adequate nutrition. (4) *Swallowing strategies*—during the MBS, it was observed that it took Tim several swallows to clear the pharyngeal area of food. Based on this finding, it was recommended that, after every three or four bites, Tim be directed to take two or three "dry swallows." As Tim continued to improve in both his cognitive and motor skills, the dysphagia plan was revised to meet his changing skills.

DYSPHAGIA IN CHILDREN

The focus of pediatric dysphagia is different from that of adult dysphagia. Adult dysphagia deals with the treatment and assessment of swallowing after an injury or the onset of an illness. These patients had normal swallowing abilities that were impaired as a result of the illness or injury. In cases of pediatric dysphagia, the SLP is treating children who have yet to acquire normal eating skills. These children have a medical condition, genetic disorder, or illness that has been present since birth or shortly after birth and therefore prevents the development of normal swallowing skills. The goal of dysphagia assessment and treatment with children is to aid in the development of skills needed to keep the child safe and well nourished. At the same time, the dysphagia team develops a plan to ensure that the child will stay well nourished while these skills are being developed. Children may be referred for a dysphagia evaluation based on a number of different referral criteria or etiologies. Following are two of the most common etiologies, prematurity and cerebral palsy, and the resultant swallowing problems.

Prematurity

The ability to suck and swallow develops prenatally. Swallowing is thought to begin somewhere between 12 and 17 weeks gestation. It is known that the fetal swallow aids in controlling the amount of amniotic fluid. However, sucking is not firmly established until 30–34 weeks gestation. Along with the development of sucking, there are primitive reflexes that help the newborn to establish a functional eating pattern. These reflexes also develop during the last 4 to 8 weeks of gestation. For this reason, a premature baby may not have the ability to suck milk from a nipple. Weak facial muscles and underdeveloped lungs can also contribute to this difficulty. The full-term normal infant uses a rhythmic suck/swallow/breathe pattern to take in nutrition. The premature baby may exhibit an uncoordinated suck and swallow, a weak suck, or breathing disruptions during feeding.

Cerebral Palsy

Children with cerebral palsy have a wide range of feeding problems. The type and severity of the feeding problem depends on the degree of motor deficit. There are several different kinds of cerebral palsy, and each has a different movement pattern. Typically, there is an increase in muscle tone and a decrease in the range of movement.

Cognitive deficits can also result in problems that affect all stages of the swallow. With cognitive deficits, the child may not understand what food is or that it needs to be put in the mouth to be eaten. There may be a reduction in lip closure, lingual control, or jaw control. Bolus formation is often poor, and increased time may be required for oral transit. Children with cognitive deficits may have inadequate velopharyngeal closure, which causes a delay in the pharyngeal swallow. Laryngeal elevation and pharyngeal peristalsis may also be affected by the abnormal tone and muscle strength. The child with cerebral palsy is often a slow, inefficient eater who is at high risk for aspiration.

Pediatric Dysphagia Evaluation

The assessment procedures for children are similar to those for adults. The SLP reviews past medical history and current medical status, performs a non-instrumental clinical examination, and then, if warranted, proceeds to do an instrumental examination. For children, each step has a different focus or different questions to be answered. The following is a review of each of the assessment procedures with the key changes that are needed for the pediatric population.

Review of Medical and Feeding History and Current Feeding Methods

Because the focus of pediatric dysphagia is on children who are having difficulty acquiring normal eating skills, it is crucial to understand any underlying medical conditions and how these conditions may contribute to current feeding problems. Therefore, to understand why a child has not developed normal eating and swallowing skills, information must be gathered about the child's prenatal history, birth history, early feeding problems, preferred positioning, preferred textures, types of utensils, respiratory status, use of alternative feeding methods, medications, seizures, and signs of distress during eating.

Bedside Clinical Assessment

The bedside assessment provides information about a child's current eating status. The examination includes information about the child's level of alertness, muscle tone, movement patterns, respiratory status, and structure and function of the face and mouth. As with adults, the beside clinical assessment leads to a determination of whether it is safe to use food as a part of the swallowing assessment. If food can be used, sucking or chewing is observed. The SLP looks for lip, tongue, and jaw movements, along with any changes in respiratory function. With children, the way in which the lips and tongue are used to get the food off the spoon is also noted, along with the kind of motor movement that is used for chewing. If a baby is being evaluated, the rate and strength of sucking is assessed, along with the suck/swallow/breathe sequence. Any additional behaviors such as nasopharyngeal reflux, lethargy, coughing, choking, gagging, or arching of the back are noted. As with adults, if the results of the noninstrumental clinical examination (NICE) indicate possible pharyngeal stage problems, then an instrumental assessment is completed.

Instrumental Assessment

Currently, the modified barium swallow procedure (MBS) is used to a much greater degree than videoendoscopy with the pediatric population. When doing an MBS with children, additional procedures include (1) conducting the MBS in the child's current seating system; (2) using food textures that are similar to what the child currently eats; and (3) using the child's own utensils—bottle, special cup, spoon, and so on.

Pediatric Treatment Planning

Based on the information gained from the review of the child's medical and feeding history, NICE, and MBS, the dysphagia team formulates a treatment plan designed to address two major goals. The first goal is a way for the child to meet current nutritional needs while remaining safe so that the child can grow and remain healthy. The second goal is focused on techniques or strategies that will improve both oral-motor and pharyngeal-stage functioning. This second goal is also directed toward "normalizing" the child's eating and swallowing skills.

SUMMARY

Swallowing includes a series of overlapping stages that prepare food and move it through the pharynx and esophagus to the stomach. Swallowing disorders frequently occur with speech disorders and fall within the professional province of a speech-language pathologist (SLP). Clinical and instrumental procedures are use to identify the stage of swallowing affected and to develop strategies that allow the individual to maintain nutrition and hydration.

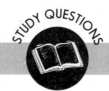

STUDY QUESTIONS

1 What are the stages of swallowing?

2 What are three disorders that cause dysphagia?

3 What is the speech-language pathologist's (SLPs) role in assessing and treating swallowing disorders?

4 How are swallowing problems different in children compared to adults?

5 What happens when food or fluid enters the trachea?

REFERENCES

American Speech-Language-Hearing Association. (1987). *Ad hoc committee on dysphagia report.* Rockville, MD: American Speech-Language-Hearing Association.

American Speech-Language-Hearing Association. (1995). *Omnibus survey results; 1995 edition.* Rockville, MD: American Speech-Language-Hearing Association.

Cherney, L. (1994). *Clinical management of dysphagia in adults and children* (2nd ed.). Gaithersburg, MD: Aspen.

Logemann, J. A. (1998). *Evaluation and treatment of swallowing disorders* (2nd ed.). Austin, TX: Pro-Ed.

Martin, B., & Corlew, M. (1990). The incidence of communication disorders in dysphagic patients. *Journal of Speech and Hearing Disorders, 55,* 28–32.

Miller, R. M., & Groher, M. E. (1993). Speech-language pathology and dysphagia: A brief historical perspective. *Dysphagia, 8,* 180–184.

SUGGESTED READINGS

Arvedson, J. C., & Brodsky, L. (1993). *Pediatric swallowing and feeding.* San Diego: Singular Publishing Group.

Logemann, J. A. (1998). *Evaluation and treatment of swallowing disorders* (2nd ed.). Austin, TX: Pro-Ed.

Perlman, A. L., & Schulze-Delrieu, K. (1997). *Deglutition and its disorders.* San Diego: Singular Publishing Group.

Rosenthal, S. R., Sheppard, J. J., & Lotze, M. (1995). *Dysphagia and the child with developmental disabilities.* San Diego: Singular Publishing Group.

Aspiration: The presence of food or liquid in the airway below the level of the true vocal folds.

Bolus: A term used to describe food after it has been chewed and mixed with saliva.

Dysphagia: Difficulty in swallowing or an inability to swallow.

Gastric tube: A feeding tube that is placed directly into the stomach through an incision in the skin.

Intravenous (IV): A needle that is placed into a vein through which liquid nutrition or medication can be given.

Modified barium swallow (MBS): A moving X-ray picture of a swallow.

Nasogastric tube: A feeding tube that goes through the nose then the pharynx and into the stomach.

Videoendoscopy: The insertion of a flexible scope through the nose to look at the anatomy of the pharynx and to observe the pharynx and larynx before and after swallowing.

LANGUAGE AND LANGUAGE DISORDERS

16

Language Science

Ronald B. Gillam and Lisa M. Bedore

LEARNING OBJECTIVES

1 To understand how our biology contributes to language development.

2 To learn about information processing mechanisms that support language development and use.

3 To be able to define what is meant by the term, *universal grammar.*

4 To differentiate between functionalist and nativist theories of language.

5 To understand how biology, psychology, and specialized linguistic knowledge interact to support language development and use.

INTRODUCTION

We use the term *language science* to refer to research about the biological, psychological, and linguistic bases of language development and use. We explained in Chapter 2 that heredity, learning mechanisms, experience, and prior knowledge combine to influence language development and use. This chapter examines some of the evidence that supports the role these factors play in language development. The section entitled, "The Biological Basis of Language," summarizes the role of heredity and biology. The following two sections explore learning mechanisms. The section entitled, "The Psychological Bases of Language," primarily concerns information processing mechanisms that support language learning. The section entitled, "The Linguistic Bases of Language," concerns the representation of linguistic knowledge that underlies language development and use. This is important information for speech-language pathologists (SLPs) and audiologists because a complete understanding of the factors that support language development should be the basis for everything that is done in language assessment and intervention.

THE BIOLOGICAL BASIS OF LANGUAGE

Humans appear to have a special ability to learn language easily and quickly. There are a number of indications that our ability to learn our first language so effortlessly is related to our biology. This section explores three of these indications in some detail: (1) the fact that some language functions are localized in certain areas of the brain, (2) the fact that complex language appears to be unique to humans, and (3) the fact that some language disorders are hereditary. Our primary point in this section is that human biology is well adapted for learning and using language, especially when other important social and intellectual supports are available. What this means is that biology is important, but it is not sufficient, in and of itself, to account for language development. What really matters is the interaction between biology and other factors such as socialization, psychological learning mechanisms, and prior knowledge.

Brain Localization

Recent advances in brain-imaging techniques have made it possible for researchers to investigate the parts of the brain that are involved in various activities. This new information, together with years of studies of the speech and language behaviors that change after brain damage, suggests that certain parts of our brains are specialized for language.

In most people, language functions are lateralized to the left hemisphere. There are three areas in the left hemisphere that are especially important for language: Broca's area, Wernicke's area, and the arcuate fasciculus (Figure 16–1). **Broca's area** is located in the left hemisphere at the lower part of the frontal lobe. It is close to the part of the motor strip that controls the tongue

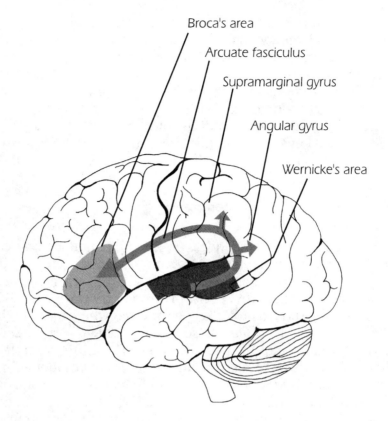

Figure 16–1. A lateral view of the left side of the brain showing Broca's and Wernicke's areas and the arcuate fasciculus. (From Webster, D. B. [1999], *Neuroscience of communication* [Figure 11-1, p. 322]. San Diego: Singular Publishing Group.)

and lips. Broca's area is responsible for planning speech and for some aspects of grammar. **Wernicke's area** is located at the posterior two-thirds of the left temporal lobe. This area is responsible for language comprehension and for many semantic functions. The **arcuate fasciculus** is a band of fibers that connects Broca's area and Wernicke's area.

When you are listening to someone, you process their words in Wernicke's area. As you think of a response, the representation of the words and meanings you want to express travel from Wernicke's area, through the arcuate fasciculus, to Broca's area. There, the brain programs motor commands for producing the words and sentences.

These areas are not as specialized for language in young children as they are in adults. Recall from Chapter 9 (Speech Science) that the brain is comprised of millions of interconnected neurons. Infants have fewer connections between neurons than adults do. As brain cells proliferate and differentiate, they organize themselves into neural networks. Some of these networks (e.g.,

Wernicke's area, Broca's area, and the arcuate fasciculus) support language comprehension and production. It is likely that we are genetically predisposed for establishing certain patterns of neural development and certain areas of localization. We probably also inherit factors that influence the speed at which new connections form in the brain. There are many instances in which the parents of children who have language delays and disorders report that they had language learning difficulties themselves. It is possible that slower neurological development and/or less efficient patterns of neural activation of language centers could be inherited.

Species Specificity

When considering whether language is biologically motivated, we can ask, Is language unique to humans? If so, it would suggest there may be something special about our biology that makes language learning and use possible.

There is no doubt that many species of animals communicate. Bees dance and ants touch antennas to indicate to each other where food can be found. Many wild animals produce different sounds for danger warnings, for searching for a mate, or to signal their return home. These are examples of communication, but they are not necessarily examples of language. Recall from Chapter 2 that human language is intentional (we plan for someone to understand our message) and conventionalized across speakers (people who speak the same language understand what the conventions of that language are). The animal communication that we just mentioned seems to fit these requirements. However, language is also symbolic (sounds and words represent objects, ideas, and feelings) and productive (words can be combined in unique ways). Natural communication between animals does not seem to meet these requirements. Animals in the wild do not seem to use sequences of conventionalized sounds to represent objects and ideas, and there is no evidence of productivity in animal communication. Further, their communication systems may have something like words, but, as yet, there is no evidence of communications that have a syntax in which word-like units are sequenced in conventional ways.

Recently, there have been interesting attempts to teach human language to animals. Probably the most famous experiments involve teaching American Sign Language to chimpanzees. These animals seem to be able to learn signs (albeit very slowly and with a great deal of effort), and some have put signs together in creative ways. Pepperberg (1996) reported on an African Gray parrot that puts items into categories, exhibits an understanding of concepts such as same/different, and creates new utterances it has not been specifically taught. Clearly, species other than humans are capable of learning and using simple language-like behaviors.

Yet, there are real differences in the degree to which linguistic-like abilities are demonstrated by humans and other species. Most humans acquire language easily. Children learn the language that surrounds them within a few years with no special training. Other species learn language very slowly, and only with special help. No animals have yet to produce anything like complex sentences or stories, and they do not tend to use languages that humans teach them in creative or functional ways. What this seems to suggest is that there are certain ecological and evolutionary pressures that result in complex language. These pressures are not completely unique to human beings. However, we appear to be the only species that has access to the right combination of biological, social, and intellectual supports for rapid and effortless language learning.

Hereditary Influences on Language Disorders

As noted in Chapter 2, there are a group of children who have unusual difficulty learning language despite adequate hearing, vision, intelligence, and social experiences. These children have a condition known as **specific language impairment (SLI).** There have been a number of recent studies of the family members of children with SLI (specific language impairment). It is clear that the immediate relatives of children with SLI have a higher rate of language difficulties than is encountered in the general population.

There have also been studies of identical (monozygotic) and fraternal (dizygotic) twins who have SLI. Identical twins share all their genes. Fraternal twins share only 50% of their genes, just like any siblings. If there are strong hereditary factors in language development, there should be many instances in which both identical twins present specific language impairment and fewer instances in which both fraternal twins have impaired language. Studies of SLI in identical and fraternal twins have found nearly twice as many identical twin pairs with SLI as fraternal twin pairs with SLI (Tomblin & Buckwalter, 1994). Family and twin studies of children with SLI demonstrate that some aspects of language development are genetically determined.

In summary, some aspects of our biology prepare us to learn and use language, especially when other important social and intellectual supports are available. Three lines of evidence supporting the importance of biology were discussed. There are special areas of our brains that handle many of our language processes, and these areas are in the same location in the left hemisphere for most individuals, regardless of the language they speak. Studies have indicated that nonhuman species can learn simplified languages, but it seems to be the case that human beings are the only species that learn *complex* language easily and well. While there does appear to be an inheritance factor in language impairment, as is the case with any genetic trait, not every member of a family will inherit a language disorder.

Adequate biological support for language may be important, but biology is not the only factor that is critical for language development. Biology matters, but it is only important with respect to the way it interacts with other factors such as socialization, psychological learning mechanisms, and prior knowledge.

THE PSYCHOLOGICAL BASES OF LANGUAGE

The extent to which general cognitive mechanisms support language development is often debated. Recall from Chapter 2 that some scholars believe language learning requires the same sorts of psychological processes that are involved in many other kinds of learning. Other scholars believe language acquisition requires additional mental mechanisms that are specialized for language learning. Nearly everyone agrees, however, that language is an important aspect of information processing and that language learning makes some use of the mind's information processing system.

Information Processing

Information processing usually refers to the means by which mental representations are derived from environmental stimulation (information) and modified mentally to influence knowledge and actions (processing). The information processing functions that are thought to play a critical role in language development and use are attention, perception, and memory.

Imagine a young child who is sitting in his living room. This child has not yet learned the words *pet* or *kitty*. His mother is sitting in a chair watching television. The family's pet cat walks into the room. As it does, both the child and the mother look at it. His mother says, "There's the kitty. Let's pet the kitty." She picks up the cat, takes it to where the child is sitting, and moves the child's hand across the cat's back. As she does so she says, "Pet the kitty. Yes, you're petting the kitty."

To learn the words *pet* and *kitty*, this child must attend to the sounds his mother said and to what is happening in the room. He then constructs mental representations (mental images) of the sequences of sounds that he heard and searches his memory to determine whether he has heard any of those sequences before. If he has, he needs to remember what those sequences meant and apply them to the current situation. If the words are new to him, as they are in this example, he must hold the sound sequences in mind while he tries to figure out what they might mean.

In this example, the child must figure out something about the sound sequences in the words *pet* and *kitty* (phonology), their meaning (semantics), their relation to other words that were spoken (syntax and morphology), and their use with respect to the context they were spoken in (pragmatics). If the child is a good language learner, he will figure out that *pet* refers to an

Table 16–1. Basic Assumptions of Information Processing Approaches to Cognition

1. Mental representations are the physical embodiment of information.
2. Mental processes transform representations.
3. Information processing has stages and substages.
4. Transmission of information takes time.
5. The nature and efficiency of information processing varies according to the amount and types of information.

Source: Based on Massaro and Cowan (1993).

action and *kitty* refers to the object that the action is performed on. He will also figure out that the action is stated before the object in the sentence. It is likely that he will store in memory whatever he can deduce about *pet* and *kitty* so that this information will be available to him the next time he hears these words. Later, when his brother says, "Where's the kitty?" the child will activate his newfound language knowledge of *kitty* when he recognizes similarities between the sounds that were just spoken and the sounds that comprised the word *kitty* that he learned earlier. Given this scenario, it should be clear that success in language learning and use might depend heavily on attention, perception, and memory processes.

According to Massaro and Cowan (1993), there are three important assumptions in information processing explanations of cognition. First, information processing approaches assume that the mind processes mental representations, which are bits of knowledge. Most information processing theorists believe these bits of knowledge are the product of communication between neurons. Recall from Chapter 9 (Speech Science) that the brain is comprised of literally billions of neurons that communicate with each other via electrical impulses. These impulses are carried from one cell body to another by the axons and dendrites. Neurons have activation levels that correspond roughly to the firing rate on the axon or to the degree of depolarization on the dendrite. Neurons interact by driving up or driving down the activation levels of other neurons. All this electrical activity results in mental images, which are representations of visual, auditory, and haptic (touch) experiences.

The smallest unit of mental representation is called a **proposition.** You know that *a* is a letter of the alphabet. That is a proposition. You put many propositions together to form a network. If we asked you to think of as many words as you can that start with the letter *a,* you would answer our question by activating a network. Two types of proposition networks that play important roles in language development are called **schemas,** which represent large concepts (you are developing a schema of "life in college"), and **scripts,** which represent sequences of events (you have a script for what usually happens when you go to a fast-food restaurant).

The second important assumption in information processing accounts of cognition is that the brain processes information in different ways. Sometimes processing occurs in a **serial** manner. When this happens, it is done one step at a time. For example, you could perceive the sounds in one word, then think of their sequence, then think of their meaning. Most of the time, though, processing occurs in a **parallel** manner. In parallel processing, the brain completes multiple processing functions all at once. For example, upon hearing a new word, the brains of skilled language learners figure out something about its phonology, its morphology, its meaning, and its syntactic relationship to the other words in the sentence all at same time.

The third important assumption in information processing theories is that individuals have different **capacities** for mental activities. Most researchers think of capacity as the amount of information that can be processed in a given period of time. Our capacity for processing information is related to the amount of prior knowledge we have about something, the speed at which we activate that knowledge, and the way we have organized our knowledge into networks. If you already know a great deal about a subject and you have organized what you know in an efficient and logical manner, you should be able to process more new information than someone who knows less about that topic.

Attention

You are probably thinking about various things right now. Hopefully, you are trying to understand what information processing is and what it has to do with language development and use. We suspect there are plenty of other things for you to think about too. What other chapters or articles do you need to read for your other classes? How is your sick friend feeling? What is that noise that you just heard? What's the weather like outside? These other concerns may drift in and out of your mind as you read. The extent to which individuals are mindful of different sensations or thoughts is known as **attention.** We will discuss the goals and manifestations of attention, and we will explain how attention relates to language development, language disorders, language assessment, and language intervention.

There are two important goals of attention. When you want to do something well, you devote more of your mental energies to it. So, increased attention can increase the accuracy of an activity. For example, children will learn new words faster when they are mindful of what others are saying and when they are actively engaged in the interaction. That is why children do not learn much language from watching television. They tend to be much less engaged while they are watching television than when they are interacting with people. Increased attention also helps you perform a mental activity faster. We respond more quickly when we expect something to happen. For example, you pick up the phone faster when you are expecting a call, or you raise your hand faster when you are expecting a question.

LaBerg (1995) explains that there are three manifestations of attention—selection, preparation, and maintenance—that result in increased speed and accuracy of mental functions. First, we use **selective attention** to determine what we want to be mindful of. At some moments we may be mindful of the words we are reading on the page. At another moment, we may become mindful of voices around us. Sometimes it is good to select new information to be mindful of (i.e., to shift attention). For example, if a car was approaching right when you were about to cross the street, it might be to your benefit to shift your attention to a honking sound. At other times, shifting attention is detrimental to performance. To learn something new, like a new word, it helps to be thinking about the way it was said, the actions that were occurring while it was said, and the other words that were said with it. Shifting your attention to the sound of a dog barking outside right after hearing a new word would not be helpful for learning the meaning of the word.

We explained before that expectation leads to increased speed and accuracy of performance. Sometimes, we decide to attend to something before it actually happens. LaBerg (1995) refers to this phenomenon as **preparatory attention** or expectation. Imagine you are listening to a lecture, and your professor asks a question. A student who was anticipating the question would be more likely to give a coherent answer if she was called on and would be less likely to stumble over her words than a student who was not anticipating the question.

Finally, **maintenance of attention** refers to the length of time that we are mindful of something without shifting our attention to other matters. Maintaining attention means selecting something to attend to and holding that selection. We are also talking about increasing states of mindfulness. Some children continually shift their attention from what their teacher is saying to their growling stomach, to a bug crawling on the window outside their classroom, to the noise of an airplane flying overhead, and then back to the teacher. They do not maintain their attention selections, and they are not thinking about anything intensely. Children who do not maintain their attention adequately are not likely to learn as much about the lesson that is being presented as children who are thinking carefully about what the teacher is saying without shifting their attentional energies very often.

Attention is important for language development and language disorders. Children learn language faster when they are actively engaged in interactions with others, that is, when they selectively attend to the words that are being said and the context they are being said in, and when they maintain their attention on the critical aspects of the interaction for longer periods of time. It should not be surprising that some children with language disorders have attention problems. Some of these children shift their attention too often. As a result, they may not maintain their attention on an interaction long enough to profit from the experience. Problems with attention are especially prevalent in children with neurological problems such as cerebral palsy, children who have had brain injuries, and children with a condition known as attention deficit disorder (ADD).

Perception

The detection of a sound is a sensation. When audiologists administer pure tone hearing tests, they are measuring sensation (i.e., the person's knowledge that they heard *something*). **Perception** refers to the ability to recognize *what* is seen and heard, and to interpret it as meaningful. There is a great deal of information about visual perception, but we will focus on auditory perception (especially speech perception) because it is most closely related to communication.

Try saying the following sentence out loud, "Don't forget to buy some milk at the store." Listen as you say it. Did you pause between each word? If you are like most speakers, you did not. Now, imagine saying this sentence to someone who does not know English. The person essentially hears the equivalent of, "Don'tforgettobuysomemilkatthestore." How could a listener who did not know English well decide whether the words in the middle were, "for geto" or "forget to"? Now, have a couple of friends say this same sentence. Did they say it exactly like you did, with the same rate, volume, speed, and intonation patterns? Did they even say the sounds exactly like you said them? Probably not. Yet, 99 out of 100 listeners would probably say that you all spoke the same sentence. Speech perception involves two difficult tasks: (1) deciding what words have been said and (2) being able to interpret words that have been spoken in a number of different ways.

Perception involves the ability to analyze features of speech. Think back to our discussion of speech sounds in Chapter 2. We said phonemes could be differentiated by their place of articulation (the point where the vocal track was closed or constricted during production), their manner of production (the way the vocal track was closed or constricted), and their voicing (whether the vocal folds were vibrating or not during production). A number of experiments have shown that listeners tend to confuse phonemes that share many features. For example, if we asked you to listen to the sounds [b], [p], and [s] played with lots of background noise, you would tend to confuse [b] and [p]. You would rarely say that a [b] sounded like an [s]. That is because [b] and [p] share the features of place of articulation and manner of articulation, but [s] is produced at a different place in the mouth and in a different manner (it is a fricative but [b] and [p] are stops). One important aspect of speech perception is the ability to recognize features of the sounds that are spoken.

Some sounds, like [b] and [p], differ in only one dimension (voicing). Yet, speakers are remarkably good at deciding when a sound is [b]-like and when it is [p]-like. The ability to perceive sounds as belonging to distinct categories is called **categorical perception**, and this is another critical aspect of speech perception. The categorical perception of [b] and [p] has been studied in some detail. Recall that these sounds differ only in voicing, with [b] being voiced and [p] being unvoiced. Think of the words *bat* and *pat*. How can you tell them apart? One sound, [b] has a voice onset time that is shorter (the vocal folds are vibrating when the lips are opened). The other sound, [p], has a longer voice onset time (there is an interval of time between the point that the lips are opened and the point at which the vocal folds start to vibrate for the production of the vowel).

Not all speakers produce [b] and [p] with exactly the same voice onset times. At what point does a [b] become a [p]? Researchers have used computer-generated speech to answer this question (see Remez, 1994, for a review of this literature). At a voice onset time of 10 milliseconds, nearly everyone agrees that the sound is a [b]. At the voice onset time of 45 milliseconds, nearly everyone agrees that the sound is a [p]. There is a switch in the perception of [b] to the perception of [p] at around 25 milliseconds, and this is the same point for nearly all speakers of English.

Very young infants categorize [p] and [b] at almost the exact same voice onset point as adults do. This finding suggests that our hearing system and our language systems are very much in tune with each other. It appears that the kinds of differentiation between sounds that our ears are able to make are the kinds of differentiation that matter in speech.

Speech is not only perceived according to its features and categories. We also use context cues during speech perception. We do not always hear everything someone is saying. Sometimes, there are interfering sounds in the environment. For example, imagine that you are talking with your friend outside and a car honks as it passes. You might hear your friend say something like, "I had lots of homework last night so I couldn't (honk) out with them." The general context provided by the words that you were able to hear makes it possible for you to interpret this sentence even though you might not have heard each word. In fact, most people would guess that the missing word was "go." Listeners can do this quite easily because our general knowledge of semantics and syntax contributes to our interpretation of perceptual features. When higher level language concepts influence perception, it is called **top-down processing.**

Some children and adults with language disorders have perceptual difficulties. Children with perception problems appear to process information slowly or incompletely. Difficulties processing rapidly incoming information or incomplete mental representations of sounds could interfere with feature detection and categorical perception, which could then interfere with language development. There are also a number of adult patients who have difficulty recognizing speech even though they can recognize nonspeech sounds, and they can produce sounds. Adult patients with speech perception problems usually have brain lesions in their left temporal lobes. When perception influences higher level language and thought, it is called **bottom-up processing.**

Memory

Figure 16–2 depicts the dynamic relationships between sensory memory, long-term memory, working memory, and central executive functions. This

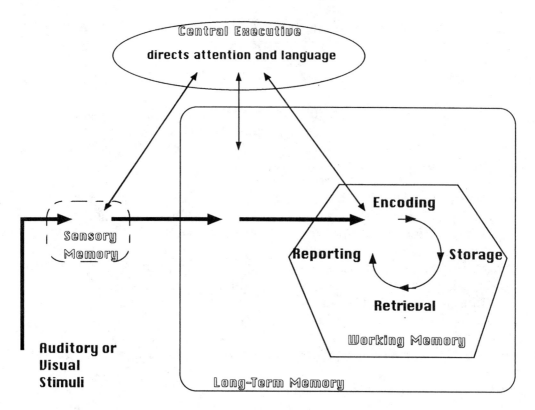

Figure 16-2. A simple model of memory.

model shares many concepts in common with Cowan's (1995) basic model of information processing. While this model does not represent all aspects of memory, it does include many of the mechanisms and relationships that are important for understanding the role that memory plays in language development and language disorders.

There are three memory systems: sensory memory, long-term memory, and working memory. **Sensory memory** is a very brief afterimage that is active for less than a second after hearing a sound or seeing a picture. Visual and auditory afterimages in sensory memory tend to decay quickly (within a few hundred milliseconds). The sensory memory box in Figure 16–2 has gaps to represent the fleeting nature of sensory memories. The heavy line in Figure 16–2 represents the path that a stimulus takes through the auditory system. Notice that this line is broken within the sensory memory box. That is because some traces fade away before they enter our working memory.

There is evidence that some information gets into our **long-term memory** even though we may never consciously think about it. We will not consider unconscious memories further, because it is unlikely they play an important role in language learning. Most of the information that makes it into long-term memory does so through conscious encoding and storage processes that are necessary for retrieving and reporting that information minutes, hours, days, or even years later. The memory processes necessary for storage and retrieval primarily occur within a memory system called **working memory.**

Working memory is often described as the storage and processing functions within long-term memory that are active at a given moment. Working memory is not seen as a distinctly different kind of memory. Rather, it is the portion of long-term memory that is busy processing information. This processing involves simultaneously encoding information, storing it, retrieving related information that has already been stored, and/or reporting it. Learners represent information in their minds **(encoding),** hold it for immediate or later use **(storage),** access the information when they need it **(retrieval),** and communicate what they have remembered **(reporting).** The connections between these phases represent interdependencies among encoding, storage, retrieval, and reporting. For example, the way information is initially encoded affects the way it is stored, the kinds of cues that will necessary for retrieval at a later time, and the amount of information that will be available for reporting.

Figure 16–2 also shows a central executive mechanism that acts with respect to the learner's motivation and goals to direct attention and language knowledge. More effective learners are those who are more alert, process more information, have higher levels of language development, and have more conceptual understanding about a particular topic. They will encode, store, retrieve, and report information more completely and more efficiently than learners who are less motivated, who are less alert, who process information slowly, who have less complex language abilities, and/or who know less about the subject at hand.

Finally, the memory model depicted in Figure 16–2 assumes a general memory capacity that limits the amount of encoding, storage, retrieval, and reporting that can be accomplished at any given time. This general capacity is thought to result from the dynamic relationships between information processing functions, language abilities, and knowledge. The capacity limitations that are often discussed in relationship to language impairment are understood in this model to be a combination of attention processes, perceptual processes, speed of activation, phonological, lexical, syntactic, and discursive language knowledge, and general knowledge of the topic at hand. Some children may have deficiencies in one or two of these areas, while others may have deficiencies in nearly all of these areas.

Functionalist Approaches to Language Acquisition

Like information processing theorists, **functionalists** believe there is no need to hypothesize that children need innate linguistic knowledge in order to learn the language that surrounds them. Functionalists suggest that because humans are well adapted to learn language, we typically acquire the words and grammar of our native language(s) quickly and efficiently with the general learning mechanisms available to us. Children learn language quickly because they are adept at attending to linguistic cues in the environment. By repeated exposure to the language models that children hear around them, children learn to associate grammatical structures and meaning. Children pick out the most salient and reliable information to them and use that to interpret language and build up their representation of language.

In this section we will introduce two functionalist models of language acquisition. One is called the **competition model** (Bates & MacWhinney, 1987; MacWhinney, 1987). This model will give you an idea of how learners come to attend to the most reliable **cues** to accurately interpret the language around them. We will also discuss connectionist modeling (e.g., Plunkett & Marchman, 1993). **Connectionism** focuses on the way associations are formed between sound and meaning. This will give you an idea of how children come to represent language in the mind from a functionalist perspective.

The Competition Model

The competition model was first proposed by Elizabeth Bates and Brian MacWhinney (Bates & MacWhinney, 1987; MacWhinney, 1987). This model focuses on two basic issues in development: (1) how language acquisition is similar across languages and (2) how language acquisition differs from one language to another. A basic assumption in this model is that learners mentally represent knowledge about words (i.e., Does a word function as a noun or verb, and how can it be used?). When listeners hear sentences, they activate their representation of the words and grammatical markers of the sentence. Different interpretations of a word (e.g., *fly* could be a noun or a verb) "compete" for activation strength. The activation with the most weight (i.e., the strongest representation) determines how the sentence will be interpreted.

Much of the work done to test this model seeks to determine how speakers use linguistic cues available in their native language to break the linguistic code. If we think about different languages, we can see they all have systematic ways of encoding ideas. English, for example, tends to use subject-verb-object (SVO) word order, but it has relatively few markers for verb tenses. If you have studied a language such as Spanish or Italian, you know these languages make greater use of grammatical cues and have freer word order than English. Learners of each of these languages may rely on a slightly different constellation of cues to figure out what is being said to them.

One important concept in the competition model concerns the use of cues to interpret sentences. We can think about the strength of cues and about the validity of cues. A cue is said to be strong if it is highly probable that a form and function go together. A cue is valid if it is reliable or consistently present in the input. Cue validity and strength are highly related. If a cue is regularly present in the input, then it is likely that it will lead to correct interpretation. When cues lead to correct interpretation of sentences, they increase in strength.

By observing how speakers interpret sentences, investigators can determine how cues are used. Some cues that have been hypothesized to be useful for speakers of different languages include word order and animacy (animate nouns can act on other objects). In one experiment, speakers of English or Italian were given small objects and asked to act out simple but ambiguous sentences such as, *The eraser the pig chases/La gamma il maialino bacia* or *Licks the cow the goat/Lecca la mucca la cabra.* Because these sentences are ambiguous due to the noun that is first mentioned (i.e., the eraser) or the way the words are ordered, we can see what speakers attend to as they attempt to interpret the sentences. Some children attend to word order more closely and make the eraser "chase" the pig; other children attend to animacy cues and make the pig the actor, since erasers cannot chase anything. Comparing the responses of the different language groups, it becomes apparent that the language they are learning influences children's response patterns. English speakers tend to focus on word order cues. If the eraser is the first noun in the sentence, then it is most likely to be interpreted as the actor or subject even though the animacy cues suggest that such as interpretation is not plausible. Italian speakers, on the other hand, tend to rely more on the animacy cues and act out the sentence as if the pig were the actor or subject. Each group's response pattern reflects the influence of their native language. English has a strong tendency to use subject-verb-object (SVO) sentences. In Italian, word order can vary so speakers rely more on the animacy cues. This gives us a feel for the way listeners develop biases based on their linguistic experience to interpret sentences.

We have just shown how cues in the language compete for activation in the minds of language learners. Language learners can activate different sorts of representations of the words and grammatical markers they hear. Potential interpretations of the grammatical roles and meanings of words "compete" with each other for activation strength. Different languages have different sorts of cues. As learners acquire a language, they tend to formulate activation patterns particular to the structural boundaries of the language being learned. In the next section, we summarize a somewhat different idea about the way mental representations of a language are formed and maintained. This theory, known as connectionism, is based on computer models of the mind.

Connectionism

Connectionism focuses on the way learners build up representations of phonological, semantic, and grammatical processes. Studies in connectionism have focused on patterns in the language and the means by which learners can mentally represent their meaning. Unlike investigators in other aspects of language, connectionists model language acquisition using computers and then evaluate whether the pattern of errors in the way the computer learns language resembles what is known about the way children learn language.

One basic assumption of connectionism is that symbolic processes are not the key to language acquisition. Rather, it assumes that language learning is an associative process in which the connections between two units (such as phonemes or words) become more or less strong. Because the language is systematically patterned, the network is able to reduplicate that which is observed in the environment. By changing the computer program to alter or specialize the network used to learn different behaviors, different kinds of learning can take place. Furthermore, like humans, connectionist networks can become more adept learners over time.

Connectionists have studied word learning, grammatical learning, and reading. One well-known example in the study of connectionist modeling demonstrated that learning the English past tense could be modeled. In several places, we have mentioned the learning of tense. Learning past tense in English is challenging because there are irregular forms that can be memorized and regular forms that are formed by adding -ed to the verb. In development, children start by using irregular forms and regular forms with relatively high levels of accuracy. As they become aware of the rule for past tense, they begin to make errors and overgeneralize. As they learn the rule, correct use of past tense forms increases. Plunkett and Marchman (1993) were able to show that a connectionist network could learn English past tense in much the same way that children learn this grammatical morpheme.

Information processing models, competition models, and connectionist models of the processes involved in learning are quite similar. They all assume that mental processes related to attention and activation influence the way language is coded, stored, retrieved, and used. The mechanisms by which this happens might be a little different, but the basic message of these theories is clear: there are a number of basic psychological processes that play important roles in language learning. It is possible (some would say it is likely) that there are also learning mechanisms that are specialized for the acquisition of language. We consider the evidence supporting the existence of specialized linguistic mechanisms in the next section of this chapter.

LINGUISTIC BASES OF LANGUAGE ACQUISITION

As we mentioned in Chapter 2, some scholars believe language is a special ability that humans are innately endowed with. The quickness and ease at which some children acquire their native language have led a number of scholars to argue that children are born with some sort of a **universal grammar (UG).** Proponents of this view are sometimes called **nativists.** UG (Universal Grammar) contains a basic design for grammar that permits a child to learn whichever language (or languages) he or she is exposed to. Innate learning mechanisms enable young language learners to crack the grammatical code of their language quickly and easily. In this section, we discuss the evidence for UG, explain what the content of UG is proposed to be, and describe two of the learning mechanisms that have been proposed within nativist accounts of language acquisition.

Before we talk about the content of UG, let's return for a moment to the evidence for innate language knowledge. Three main reasons that nativists believe humans have innate linguistic knowledge are (1) minimal input is needed to learn language, (2) learners rely on grammatical input and minimal correction or negative input, and (3) most children tend to learn language quickly. Let's talk about more about these. Imagine that you were reading and came to the following sentence: *The crenious iggle mons a fibberish ook under grue soll.* Could you begin to guess who did what to whom? If you are a (native) speaker of English, it is most likely you know that something *mons* something or someone. This ability to pick the verb out of a series of nonsense words illustrates how little exposure you need to begin to interpret an unfamiliar lexicon. You have only read this sentence once or twice. Yet, based on your knowledge of grammar, you can hypothesize the grammatical roles of these new words. Is it possible that children who are just learning language do something quite similar? Perhaps they can interpret the grammatical roles of unknown words based on some sort of innate knowledge of the way language works.

The second important point is that children learn based on input. It is interesting that children do not seem to benefit from negative input or correction from adult speakers. Young children produce many "errors" as they are learning to speak. Some that we touched on in Chapter 2 were frequent omissions of morphemes (e.g., *yesterday he jump*) and mispronunciations of words (i.e., /tot/ instead of *coat*). Occasionally, caregivers do correct children in exchanges such as the following:

Child: Mom I eated a sucker.
Mother: You ate a sucker? Say ate.
Child: Ate. I eated a good sucker.

As you see, this child does not appear to immediately benefit from adult corrections. Furthermore, studies have shown that only a small number of the errors that children produce are corrected in this way. This suggests that most children do not benefit from negative input. Rather, they adjust their linguistic system on the basis of the language that surrounds them.

The third factor that nativists have taken as evidence that language learning is innate is the speed with which children acquire language. Children are able to rapidly interpret new words (such as you did previously in the example of a nonsense sentence), and they learn as many as 5 to 10 new words each day. Knowledge of sentence structure helps children figure out meaning and semantic roles. Mechanisms such as bioprograms and maturation are thought to be the key elements in language acquisition.

Obviously, children are not born speaking. So, you may be wondering just what a universal grammar is. Universal grammar (UG) can be thought of as blueprint for languages. This means that languages will share common elements and will behave in systematic ways. If you have studied a foreign language, you know that many languages share the same kinds of words. Word types such as nouns, verbs, and words that mark grammatical relations such as articles, prepositions, and grammatical morphemes are commonly found in the world's languages. Languages behave in systematic ways that are not entirely dissimilar from one another.

If we look at the ways language is structured, we see that languages rely on internal structures. The ordering of elements within the parts of a sentence, such as the noun phrase or prepositional phrase, is illustrated in the syntactic trees illustrated in Figure 16–3. When we form questions based on

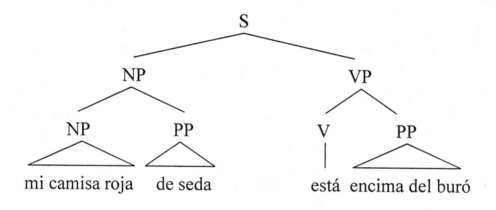

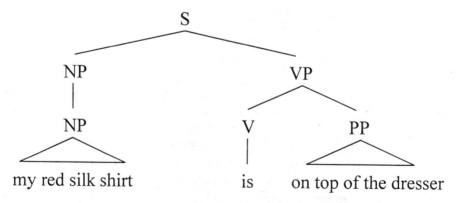

Figure 16–3. Syntactic trees that illustrate the way elements within a sentence are ordered.

these utterances we see that the elements of the sentence move together systemically. Thus, in English, it makes sense to say *Is my red silk shirt on top of the dresser?* but not *On top is my silk red dresser of the shirt.* Similarly, in Spanish, you can say *Está mi camisa roja de seda encima del buró?* but not *Está camisa mi roja encima de buró del seda.*

On the other hand, there are also systematic differences between languages. English is a language that requires the use of subjects. We cannot just say *went to the bus stop.* For this to be a complete utterance, we need to use a noun or pronoun to specify *who* went. Thus, we would say, *Joe went to the bus stop* or *She went to the bus stop.* Other languages do not have this rule, so subjects can be omitted. In Spanish, for example, the subject is not produced in a sentence such as *fui a la tienda ([I] went to the store),* but a subject might be included in a context where emphasis or clarification is needed such as **mi mamá** *fue a la tienda (**my mom** went to the store).*

Universal grammar (UG) also serves as a guide or blueprint for language acquisition. If we look at children acquiring languages such as English, German, or French, we see that learners of these languages make similar kinds of errors as they acquire their native language. For example, most children learning English do not start to use tense marked forms on a regular basis until they are around 3 years old. One current theory proposed by Wexler (1994) is that children go through a stage, called optional infinitive, during which they do not realize that tense marking on verbs is required. Because they think tense is not required, they use unmarked or infinitive forms. Thus, a 2-year-old English-learning child might say, *baby cry* instead of *baby cries* or *baby cried.* A child acquiring Spanish might say, *bebé llorar* (baby to cry) instead of the tensed forms *bebé llora* (baby cries) or *lloró* ([baby] cried). Although the rules for each of the languages are different, the error patterns are similar. Clearly, there are important similarities in the acquisition process that cross languages.

Nativists suggest there is some type of language acquisition mechanism or device that propels the language acquisition process. However, within this school of thought, there is ongoing debate over the nature of this mechanism. Some theorists support what is referred to as the principles and parameters approach (e.g., Hyams, 1986; Lust, 1999). They suggest that children have access to linguistic knowledge (i.e., grammatical principles) from the outset, but that they need input from the environment to determine what the parameters of the language should be. Proponents of this type of language acquisition device stress the importance of exposure to the native language. Sufficient exposure will trigger children to select the parameter that is appropriate to their native language. A common example used to illustrate this point is the use of subjects in sentences. As we mentioned previously, some languages like English require subjects; other languages like Italian or Spanish do not. Across languages, children start out using short sentences without subjects. When children start to use subjects, it is taken as an indication that the parameter for their language has been triggered. From this theoretical perspective, it would be expected that children would make consistent use of the structure in question once it was triggered.

In contrast, other theorists (e.g., Borer & Wexler, 1992) argue that some aspects of UG only become available to the child as he or she matures. Children start out with an incomplete version of UG that matures into a full adult version of UG. This process has been likened to a tadpole turning into a frog (Gleitman, 1981). The transition from the use of unmarked verb forms to marked verb forms, discussed as part of the optional infinitive hypothesis, is proposed to result from such a mechanism. Wexler (1999) suggests that children do not have access to the aspect of UG that guides verb marking until a certain level of maturation occurs. This explanation emphasizes the role of growth of the UG rather than the role of exposure to the language as a means of change in children's language use.

SUMMARY

Heredity, learning mechanisms, experience, and prior knowledge combine to influence language development and use. The best evidence is that there are biological, psychological, and linguistic mechanisms that are involved in dynamic relationships that influence language development and use.

Findings of brain localization, species specificity, and hereditary influences on language disorders suggest that some aspects of our biology prepare us to learn and use language.

There are also psychological mechanisms that contribute to language development and use. According to information processing theorists, children who attend more closely, who process information faster, who retain more of the information they process, and who retrieve that information efficiently when it is needed are well equipped to learn language. Theorists known as "functionalists" tend to agree with this perspective. The competition model suggests that different representations of the grammatical roles and meanings of words "compete" with each other for activation strength. The strength of the activations are consistent with the nature of word order, inflection, and meaning cues that are available in linguistic input. Connectionists are interested in creating computer models that learn language much the same way that children learn language. Connectionists assume that language learning involves association (connections) between two units of knowledge, and these theorists have been successful in creating computer programs that learn language much like children do.

It is also likely that innate learning mechanisms enable language learners to crack the grammatical code of their language quickly and easily. There may be some type of a language acquisition device that helps children learn language quickly and easily. On the other hand, it may be possible for children to reach the same levels of language knowledge simply by making multiple associations between language form and language meaning. These associations enable learners to build representations of phonological, semantic, and grammatical processes.

Finally, it is likely that some aspects of language learning, especially grammatical morphology and syntax, benefit from innate linguistic knowledge. We explained how this knowledge may consist of a universal grammar (UG). The UG may rely on input from the environment to drive development, or it may rely on internal maturational mechanisms to take effect. This is known as the nativist perspective.

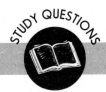

STUDY QUESTIONS

1 What are three types of evidence that humans are biologically endowed to learn language?

2 What are the differences among attention, perception, and memory? How might these processes contribute to language development?

3 Describe two functionalist theories of language development. How are they similar to information processing theories? How are they different?

4 What is a universal grammar?

5 What is the difference between functionalist and nativist theories of language?

6 Summarize how biological, psychological, and specialized linguistic mechanisms might interact to support language development and use.

REFERENCES

Bates, E., & MacWhinney, B. (1987). Competition, variation, and language learning. In B. MacWhinney (Ed.), *Mechanisms of language acquisition* (pp. 157–193). Hillsdale, NJ: Lawrence Earlbaum.

Borer, H., & Wexler, K. (1992). Bi-unique relations and the maturation of grammatical principles. *Natural Language and Linguistic Theory, 10,* 147–189.

Cowan, N. (1995). *Attention and memory: An integrated framework*. New York: Oxford University Press.

Gleitman, L. (1981). Maturational determinants of language growth. *Cognition, 10,* 103–114.

Hyams, N. (1986). *Language acquisition and the theory of parameters*. Dordrecht, The Netherlands: Reidel.

LaBerge, D. (1995). *Attentional processing: The brain's art of mindfulness*. Cambridge, MA: Harvard University Press.

Lust, B. (1999). Universal grammar: The strong continuity hypothesis in first language acquisition. In W. Ritchie & T. Bhatia (Eds.), *Handbook of child language acquisition* (pp. 111–145). San Diego: Academic Press.

MacWhinney, B. (1987). The competition model. In B. MacWhinney (Ed.), *Mechanisms of language acquisition* (pp. 249–308). Hillsdale, NJ: Lawrence Earlbaum.

Massaro, D. W., & Cowan, N. (1993). Information processing models: Microscopes of the mind. *Annual Review of Psychology, 44,* 383–425.

Pepperberg, I. M. (1996). Categorical class formation by an African Grey parrot (Psittacus erithacus). In T. R. Zentall & P. M Smeets (Eds.), *Stimulus class formation in humans and animals, Advances in Psychology, No. 117* (pp. 71–91). Amsterdam, Netherlands: Elsevier.

Plunkett, K., & Marchman, V. (1993). U-shaped learning and frequency effects in a multilayered perception: Implications for child language acquisition. *Cognition, 48,* 21–69.

Remez, R. E. (1994). A guide to research on the perception of speech. In M. A. Gernsbacher (Ed.), *Handbook of psycholinguistics* (pp. 145–172). San Diego: Academic Press.

Tomblin, J. B., & Buckwalter, P. R. (1994). Studies of genetics of specific language impairment. In R. V. Watkins & M. L. Rice (Eds.), *Specific language impairments in children* (pp. 17–34). Baltimore: Paul H. Brookes.

Wexler, K. (1994). Optional infinitives, head movement and the economy of derivations. In D. Lightfoot & N. Hornstein (Eds.), *Verb movement* (pp. 305–382). Cambridge, UK: Cambridge University Press.

Wexler, K. (1999). Maturation and growth of grammar. In W. C. Ritchie & T. K. Bhatia (Eds.), *Handbook of child language acquisition* (pp. 55–109. San Diego: Academic Press.

Webster, D. B. (1999), *Neuroscience of communication*. San Diego: Singular Publishing Group.

SUGGESTED READINGS

Cowan, N. (1995). *Attention and memory: An integrated framework*. New York: Oxford University Press.

Ericsson, K. A., & Kintsch, W. (1995). Long-term working memory. *Psychological Review, 102*(2), 211–245.

Gillam, R. B. (Ed.). (1998). *Memory and language impairment in children and adults: New perspectives*. Gaithersburg, MD: Aspen.

Just, M. A., & Carpenter, P. A. (1992). A capacity theory of comprehension: Individual differences in working memory. *Psychological Review, 99,* 122–149.

Karmiloff-Smith, A. (1992). *Beyond modularity: A developmental perspective on* cognitive science. Cambridge, MA: MIT Press

Pinker, S. (1994). *The language instinct: How the mind creates language.* New York: William Morrow.

Thelen, E., & Smith, L. B. (1994). *A dynamic systems approach to the development of cognition and action.* Cambridge, MA: MIT Press.

GLOSSARY

Arcuate fasciculus: A band of neural fibers that connects Broca's area and Wernicke's area.

Attention: The extent to which we are mindful of different sensations or thoughts.

Bottom-up processing: Lower-level perceptual information gleaned directly from the auditory or visual signal is used to comprehend meaning.

Broca's area: An area at the lower part of the frontal lobe in the left hemisphere that is primarily responsible for planning articulatory movements.

Capacity: The amount of information that can be processed at any given time.

Categorical perception: The ability to perceive sounds as belonging to different phoneme categories (e.g., the ability to differentiate between /p/ and /b/).

Competition model: Language-learning model that emphasizes the representation of linguistic structures in the mind and the role of psychological processes in the buildup of this process.

Connectionism: A computational approach to modeling human behavior.

Cues: Word or phoneme that causes the listener to key into a certain source.

Encoding: Mental representations of information that is seen and heard. Vi-sual information can be represented as mental pictures called icons. Speech is represented as sequences of sounds.

Functionalist: Theorists who posit that general learning mechanisms will account for language learning.

Information processing: The way the mind represents and manipulates auditory, visual, and haptic (touch) information from the environment. Information processing usually includes to attention, perception, memory, and reasoning functions.

Long-term memory: The processes involved in recalling information for minutes, days, months, or years at a time. Long-term memory has a large storage capacity and is not susceptible to outside interference.

Maintenance of attention: The length of time that an individual is mindful of something without shifting attention to other matters.

Nativist: The term for theorists who posit the presence of an innate language-learning device.

Parallel processing: A type of information processing in which two or more processing functions occur at once.

Perception: The ability to recognize and attribute meaning to what is seen or heard.

Preparatory attention: Anticipation and expectation can lead individuals to prepare themselves to attend to something before it actually happens.

Proposition: The smallest unit of knowledge. Propositions are combined to form a network of mental representations called schemas and scripts.

Reporting: The processes involved in telling about retrieved memories.

Retrieval: The processes involved in accessing memories that have been stored.

Schema: A network of propositions that represent all that is known about concepts such as "mathematics," "college life," or even "Christmas."

Script: A proposition network that represents the typical sequence of actions or spoken messages that are related to an event such as "church," "birthdays," or "eating at a fancy restaurant."

Selective attention: What an individual is mindful of at any given moment.

Sensory memory: An auditory or visual afterimage that lasts a few hundred milliseconds after hearing a spoken word or seeing a picture. These afterimages tend to decay quickly.

Serial processing: Information processing that occurs in sequential steps.

Specific language impairment (SLI): Unusual difficulties learning language despite normal environmental supports and the absence of hearing, vision, motor, or cognitive disorders.

Storage: The amount of information that is retained after it has been encoded.

Top-down processing: The use of higher level semantic and syntactic knowledge to inform the interpretation of the auditory and visual stimuli that are being perceived.

Universal grammar (UG): An innate blueprint that guides the acquisition of grammar.

Wernicke's area: An area of the left hemisphere located behind Broca's area. Wernicke's area plays an important role in language content and in language comprehension.

Working memory: Processing functions within long-term memory that are active at a given moment.

17

Language Disorders in Infants, Toddlers, and Preschoolers

Elizabeth D. Peña and Barbara L. Davis

LEARNING OBJECTIVES

1 To understand what a language disorder is.

2 To differentiate between language problems in the areas of language form, content, and use.

3 To become familiar with different service-delivery settings.

4 To have a basic understanding of the components of an assessment for young children.

5 To compare/contrast different intervention approaches.

INTRODUCTION

As noted in Chapter 2, there are many different kinds of children who have difficulty learning language. Recall that children who are born with Down syndrome (a genetic cause of mental retardation), severe hearing impairment (a sensory deficit), or fetal alcohol syndrome (difference in prenatal development caused by maternal alcohol use) are likely to have problems learning and using language. In addition, there are children who have problems acquiring language even though they do not present any type of obvious cause. This is usually referred to as a **developmental language disorder** or a **specific language impairment.**

Children with developmental language disorders may communicate differently from their peers. That is, their language may seem to be more like the language of children who are much younger. Decisions about clinical diagnosis and appropriate intervention strategies are often based on comparisons of the child's language abilities with children of the same age and/or

 CD-ROM

CD-ROM Summary

Volume 2 of the CD-ROM that accompanies this book contains four short video segments of two children (ages 3 and 5) with language impairment. All the segments provide examples of the kinds of language difficulties that are experienced by children with language impairments. The first segment (Ch.17.01) shows language form errors. The second (Ch.17.02) and third (Ch.17.03) segments provide examples of content-based expressive difficulties. Finally, the fourth segment (Ch.17.04) shows a 3-year-old child with limited language output who nevertheless demonstrates appropriate social interaction (pragmatics).

Segments

Ch.17.01   The 5-year-old girl is interacting with her clinician playing with a house and a set of figures. She is pretending to be an older boy who wants to drive. She makes tense agreement errors during this interaction.

Ch.17.02   In this video clip, you see a 3-year-old girl reading a book with the examiner. She responds to questions posed by the examiner.

Ch.17.03   This video clip shows the 5-year-old girl playing with a stuffed giraffe and a doctor's kit. She pretends to examine the giraffe. This segment shows her using nonspecific language in response to clinician questions.

Ch.17.04   In this example, the 3-year-old girl is playing with a dish and food set. She responds to contextualized requests nonverbally and uses some single-word utterances.

with children who have the same types of language differences. We explore these issues in detail in this chapter, but first, we define some important terms to help you understand preschool language disorders.

CHILDREN WITH DEVELOPMENTAL LANGUAGE DISORDERS

Definition of Language Disorder

According to the American Speech-Language and Hearing Association, "a language disorder is the impairment or deviant development of comprehension and/or use of a spoken, written, and/or other symbol system. The disorder may involve (1) the form of language (phonologic, morphologic, and syntactic systems), (2) the content of language (semantic system), and/or (3) the function of language in communication (pragmatic system) in any combination" (American Speech-Language-Hearing Association, 1982, p. 949).

Let's think about this definition. We can recognize errors in the form, content, and use areas of language. Form errors are reflected in ungrammatical sentences. For example, a child with language form errors might say something like, *The block falled down.* Utterances with content errors do not make sense. For example, a child might say, *The ball is on the table* when it is really under the table. Finally, use errors interfere with social appropriateness. Children with language use errors may interrupt people repeatedly, fail to contribute to conversations, or change the topic too often. We know typically developing children make the kinds of errors just described, and children who come from different cultural and linguistic backgrounds sometimes produce these same kinds of errors. So, errors alone are not a definite indicator of a disorder. How do we know when a language error indicates an impairment? What standard should language performance be compared to?

Parents and teachers become concerned about children's language development when it appears they are not expressing themselves as well as other children their same age. There are two ways to think about the concept of "same age." **Chronological age** refers to the amount of time that has elapsed since a child's birth. We typically use chronological age in years and months to determine a child's age and to compare him or her to other children of the "same age." This is done by subtracting the child's date of birth (expressed in years/months/days) from the date of assessment (also expressed in years/months/days) to obtain an age that is expressed in years-months-days. Days from 16–31 are rounded up to 1 month, and days from 1–15 are rounded down to 0 months so that the chronological age is expressed in years and months. Assume, for example, that you were collecting a language sample on August 21, 2000 (2000/8/21) from a boy who was born on December 9, 1995 (1995/12/9). This child would be 4 years, 9 months, and 16 days old the day you collected his language sample. Rounding the days up, we would say this child was 4 years, 10 months old, and we would write his chronological age as, 4;10 (years; months).

Developmental age refers to the typical chronological age at which a child can perform a skill in a given area, in this case, language. We determine developmental age by collecting samples of the child's language and comparing the child's content, form, and use of language to what we know about typical ranges of development. Children with language disorders nearly always present a pattern in which their developmental language age is lower than their chronological age. Recall from Chapter 2, however, that there is a great deal of individual variation in the rate of language development, making it impossible to pinpoint a specific age at which a particular aspect of language develops. Rather, we usually think about ranges of development. For example, a child who is 4 years old may only combine two words together into short, incomplete sentences (e.g., "want car"). Sentences like this would be typical for a child who is between 18 to 24 months old. In this example, it appears that the child's chronological age may be 2 years greater than his language developmental age.

Some clinicians consider comparisons between a child's chronological age and his or her language developmental age when they diagnose language disorder. In the past, it has been common for clinicians to use a 1-year difference between a child's chronological age and his or her language developmental age as a criterion for identifying a language disorder. There are two problems with this way of thinking. First, as we noted previously, it is nearly impossible to pinpoint a child's language developmental age. Second, a 1-year discrepancy between chronological and developmental age in a 2-year-old child is not quite the same as a 1-year discrepancy between chronological and developmental age in a 4-year-old child. For this reason, clinicians often base their decisions about the presence or absence of a language disorder on a variety of factors, including discrepancies between chronological age and developmental age.

Some clinicians use poor performance on formal tests as an indicator of disorder. They give language tests to compare a child's language ability to that of other children of the same chronological age and social/cultural background. The purpose of testing is to determine if a child's test score is significantly lower than the average score for children his age. If a child scores too low on one or more language tests, it is assumed he or she has a language disorder. This approach to diagnosis, known as the **neutralist approach,** does not account for social and cultural influences on language development or for the kinds of language expectations that exist in the child's everyday environments. Instead, it relies solely on comparisons between one child's performance and the average performance of other children of the same age. The word *neutralism* has been applied to this position because formal language tests are *neutral* on the importance of considering social norms and expectations in identification.

Fey (1986) defines a language disorder as "a significant deficit in the child's level of development of the form, content, or use of language" (p. 31).

He goes on to suggest that clinicians should take into account how language problems affect daily interaction with others. If a child's language problems are likely to result in negative social, psychological, educational, and vocational consequences, then Fey believes he or she should receive language intervention. Fey's approach to identifying children with language disorders is sometimes called the **normativist approach** because it values social norms and focuses on the functional consequences of problems with language.

A growing number of clinicians combine the neutralist and normativist approaches to identifying language disorder. Paul (1995) suggests that language impairment should be defined relative to both social expectations and performance on formal language tests. Speech-language pathologists who take this perspective consider the child's test scores in light of the social norms in the child's environment, parental or teacher expectations, and the child's functional communication at home, at daycare, or at preschool.

Types of Language Disorders

Language disorders are often categorized according their cause. Nelson (1998) classifies the factors that play a role in language disorders into central processing factors, peripheral factors, and environmental and emotional factors. Central processing factors are those that are thought to relate to the part of the brain that controls language and cognitive development. Types of disorders in this category include specific language impairment, mental retardation, central auditory processing disorder, autism, and acquired brain injury. Peripheral factors are those that directly cause impairment in the motor or sensory systems. Peripheral factors influence how language is perceived and processed. Hearing impairment, visual impairment, deaf-blindness, and other physical impairments are examples of the types of peripheral factors that are related to language disorders. These factors may contribute to language impairment, but the presence of these factors does not always cause language impairments. Environmental and emotional factors that do not have a physical cause can influence language development. Problematic environmental and emotional factors include neglect and abuse, behavioral problems, and emotional problems. Finally, some language problems may be a result of a combination of factors. Unfortunately, mixed factor causes often result in more severe disabilities that involve the cognitive, sensory, and motor systems.

Nelson's (1998) system for categorizing language disorders helps us classify children with language impairments and suggests possible causes for the disorder. This system is not perfect, however. In most cases, we can only speculate about the factor or factors that may have led to a language disorder originally. In addition, clinical categories of language disorders are not completely independent of each other. Many children with language impairments present language profiles that could fit into more than one category. For example, the language abilities of a child with mental retardation may be quite similar to the language abilities of a child who has been neglected or abused. Sometimes, the setting the child is observed in and the measures used during evaluation can influence how children with language impairment are identified. For example, children with language impairment may appear to fit a "central factor" diagnosis in a clinical setting based on formal language measures, while in a school setting, they may fit a "behavioral" factor diagnosis based on a combination of cognitive, language, and social-adaptive measures. The final problem with attempts to place children with language disorders into subcategories is that approaches to language intervention have little to do with subtypes of disorders. There is a danger in thinking that one intervention technique is right for one kind of syndrome or that a given child may be representative of that syndrome. There are many intervention techniques that work well with children whose language disorders result from quite different factors. Regardless of the cause or causes of a child's language disorder, clinicians should plan intervention that is appropriate for the child's developmental level, that matches his or her interests, and that provides him or her with the kind of language needed to function better in everyday environments.

Age Groups

Language disorders may be characterized somewhat differently for infants and toddlers in comparison to preschoolers. Age distinctions matter because children have different communication abilities and needs as they develop. A language disorder may manifest itself one way at one point in development and another way at a later point.

At or near the time of birth, there are few overt communication behaviors that can be assessed. Nonetheless, some infants are eligible for services and receive them. Clinicians who work with infants often base their decisions to provide treatment on the presence or absence of conditions such as prenatal (before birth) or perinatal (at birth) infections that are known to lead to language impairment and other developmental disorders.

As the infant develops during the first year of life, clinicians can attend to behavioral risk factors that are closely tied to communication. These include lack of eye contact, lack of consistent responsiveness to the environment, or slow development of speech and motor milestones (Billeaud, 1995). At present, we do not have precise ways to identify children at risk for language impairment in the first year of life unless they are severely involved.

Infants' comprehension of language form, content, and use grows dramatically during the second year of life (ages 12 months to 24 months) as they begin to understand more about the environment that surrounds them and begin to exhibit language-based communication. Between the ages of 12 and 24 months there are many communication, vocabulary, and speech behaviors that develop, which provide more skills for clinicians to look for during assessments. By the time children are 3 years old (the beginning of the preschool period), clinicians can look for a full range of language abilities (phonology, morphology, semantics, syntax, and pragmatics).

We believe careful description of children's language difficulties, their level of development, and their personal interests are necessary for identifying language disorders and planning intervention. A description of a child's language strengths and needs in the areas of language form, content, and use helps clinicians consider individual components of language as well as the ways components interact together.

DISORDERS OF FORM, CONTENT, AND USE

As noted in Chapters 2 and 16, speech-language pathologists typically examine three aspects of language development: form, content, and use (Bloom & Lahey, 1968). **Form** refers to the structure of language including syntax, morphology, and phonology. **Content** refers to the meaning of language, known as semantics. **Use** refers to the social aspects of language, known as pragmatics.

Comprehension and **expression** are additional facets of description that are important in understanding language disorders in children. Comprehension relates to the child's understanding of the world. For an infant, comprehension may be restricted to understanding that you look at something when Dad points to it. As children grow and develop, they begin to understand language at more finely grained levels. For example, 2-year-old children usually understand questions such as, *What is that?* Four-year-old children can understand questions like, *What is he doing with that?*

Language also involves expression; children must learn to produce language that integrates the dimensions of form, content, and use. Infants may not be able to produce words, but they may cry in certain ways to indicate

 CD-ROM

"I Drive the Car"

CD-ROM segment Ch.17.01 shows a 5-year-old girl playing with cars. She is pretending she is a 15-year-old boy who is learning to drive. She makes agreement errors as she interacts with her clinician. She says, "I drive the car," using the present instead of the past tense. Next, she says, "I didn't got yours," using the past tense instead of the present tense. In addition, in this sentence, she uses the more general verb "get" instead of "drive," which is a content-based error.

hunger or pain. Thus, different cry patterns are a form of communication that convey meanings to familiar communication partners. As they get older, children think more complex thoughts, and they learn the words and sentence structures that are needed for conveying those thoughts to others.

Language Disorders Related to Form

Infants/Toddlers

The earliest prelinguistic communication forms include visual regard (looking at something that is wanted), vocalization, body movements and orientation, and gestures. By 2 months of age, children express themselves by crying and by using other sounds. As they mature, vocalization becomes more important and body gestures may become more intentional. By 9 months, children use pointing reliably, and gesture use grows until words begin to overtake gestures as the preferred form for communication at approximately 12–15 months of age (Bates, 1976). Children use and combine words before they produce complete sentences. Although infants and toddlers may still use gestures or nonverbal acts, most of their communication will likely consist of words.

Two risk factors that are predictive of later language disorders in infants and toddlers include low frequency of vocalization and lack of syllable productions in babbling (Roberts, Rescorla, Girous, & Stevens, 1998). Extensive use of gesture in the absence of vocalization is also considered an important signal of potential risk for language disorder. It is important to remember there is a great deal of individual variability in normal development during this period, and risk factors for later communication disorders are not well established. However, we do know that infants and toddlers with overt medical conditions such as prenatal (before birth) or perinatal (at birth) infections, low birthweight, pulmonary (breathing) difficulties, intracranial hemorrhage (bleeding from the blood vessels in the brain), and other birth defects often present communication disorders later in life (Tomblin, Hardy, & Hein, 1991).

Preschool Children

There is rapid growth in aspects of language form (phonology, morphology, and syntax) during the preschool period. We expect the typical preschool-age child to be able to produce most speech sounds and to use them in a variety of words. They are able to be understood most of the time, although some of the more difficult sounds such as /r, s, and l/ may be mispronounced, and they may make some errors producing long words like *hippopotamus*. Preschoolers also learn inflections for nouns and verbs (for example, -ed and -s), and how to create simple and complex sentences. Review Chapter 2 for more information on typical language development.

Every child with a language disorder presents a different language profile. However, there are some aspects of grammar that are likely to be omitted or used incorrectly. For example, bound morphemes such as -*ed* or -*s*, may be problematic for children with language impairments. These children are likely to omit or use the wrong "be" verb forms (e.g., am, is, are, was, were). Certain classes of morphemes such as articles and pronouns can also be difficult to learn. Similar to the situation with the "be" verbs, children with language disorders often omit or misuse articles and pronouns. For example, a 4-year-old might say, *Hims got ball*. Finally, children with form difficulties often produce sounds and sequences of sounds incorrectly. Children may have trouble actually making all the sounds of their language or they may be able to produce all the sounds but not use them correctly in a variety of words. Chapter 10 details ways in which preschoolers may manifest form-based articulatory and phonological disorders.

Language Disorders Related to Content

Infants/Toddlers

Early joint attention between infants and their caregivers is a crucial precursor for beginning to build an understanding of the world. In earliest development, infants show visual attention and postural orientation to people and objects in the environment (Adamson & Chance, 1998), particularly to novel or changing events. By approximately 5 months of age, infants show preferences for faces, which is crucial to establish emotional bonding. Later, their preferences switch to objects (learning about how the world works). Naturally available motor reflexes associated with feeding (e.g., sucking and rooting) are also available at birth, and these reflexes serve to connect the infant with caregivers through establishment of consistent feeding routines.

As infants' motor abilities develop, they gain more sophisticated means to establish and maintain contact with those around them and to learn about the world through exploration. They reach for objects and people and point to what they want. Most infants "coo" and "goo" and use speech-like sounds before they are 1 year of age. Routines for feeding and dressing and games such as "peek a boo" (Bruner, 1977) are pleasurable events that promote interactions with communication partners and objects. Within these routine events, infants and toddlers begin to understand the world around them. This understanding is the basis for the "content" or semantic aspect of symbolic language. Turn-taking, balance of initiation, and vocal responses may emerge in these shared and pleasurable events. These are essential components of later language-based communication. At around 12–15 months, infants begin to develop triadic joint attention where the infant can simultaneously engage a person and a desired object or action. This phase of development is thought to be a seminal event for the infant in the transition to symbolic language from prelinguistic communication. The infant learns to engage a communication partner in a joint event that involves the meaning of objects and actions in the world. For example, the 12 month old who plays a game of roll the ball with an adult has to understand the nature of the ball and to engage a communication partner in acting on the ball in a consistent fashion.

Disorders related to content during the infant/toddler phase usually concern difficulties establishing consistent contact with communication partners. Additional risk factors include poor turn-taking or lack of balanced initiation and response in interactions with their caregivers. Impediments to this process may be sensory (hearing or vision deficits), motor (cerebral palsy or low muscle tone), cognitive (mental retardation), or social-emotional (effects of neglect). The effect of these impediments is to render either the child or the environment unable to maintain the consistent contact necessary for the development of meaning.

Preschool Children

Semantic knowledge and use are important aspects of language content. For children who are producing about one to two words per utterance (between the ages of 18 and 36 months), Brown (1973) suggests examining the use of relational categories. These categories account for most of what children at this stage of development are producing (see Table 17–1).

At more advanced stages of development, it is important to observe children's knowledge of different word classes. For example, preschool children should be able to respond to questions that begin with what, where, whose, why, how many, how, and when. They should have knowledge of concepts such as colors and spatial terms. They should be able to categorize objects, and they should be able to describe and understand similarities and differences among objects.

 CD-ROM

"Touch and Feel" Book

CD-ROM segment Ch.17.02 shows a 3-year old girl looking through a "touch and feel" book with an examiner. Each page in the book has a picture of an object. The child's attention is focused on concepts such as texture, color, and functions. This child has some difficulty understanding the content of the book. Although she is able to understand language in context, she has difficulty understanding and expressing concepts such as colors, descriptions (soft/scratchy), and actions (What's he doing?).

Table 17–1. Examples of Semantic Categories (Brown, 1973)

Semantic Category	Subcategories	Examples
Basic Concepts	Spatial terms	up, down, in
	Temporal terms	when, before
	Deictic terms	this/that
	Kinship terms	dad, sister, aunt
	Relational terms—physical	thick/thin
	Relational terms—interrogatives	who, which, what
	Colors	blue, green, red
Semantic relations	Possessor + possession	Mom shoe
	Recurrence + X	Cracker more
	Attribute + entity	sock stink
	Nonexistence or disappearance	Bye-bye juice
	Rejection or negation	No
	Demonstrative + entity	This juice
	X + locative	Sit down
	X + dative	Ten (take this) mom
	Agent + action	Daddy eat
	Action + object	Throw ball
	Agent + object	Dog ball
Embedding and conjoining	Sequential	And then, First . . . next
	Causal	Because
	Conditional	If . . . then
	Temporal	When, before, after, then
	Disjunctive	But, or

Semantic difficulties that preschool children with language impairments exhibit include restricted vocabulary size and reduced comprehension of basic concepts (spatial terms, temporal terms, deictic terms, kinship terms,

 CD-ROM

"Doctor, Doctor"

CD-ROM segment Ch.17.03 shows a 5-year-old girl playing with a giraffe and a doctor's kit. She pretends to examine the giraffe. The child uses nonspecific language. The toys are used as props that provide context for listener understanding. Children with content-based difficulties often use more "general" language in interaction. In one case she says, "How about if I do this" to indicate tapping

(continued)

the giraffe's legs with the hammer. Later, the clinician asks the child, "Why did the giraffe say ouch?" Notice that the child acts out the response and says, "Because this was going like this." Children with language impairment often use nonspecific words in the place of specific vocabulary and explanations.

A little later, the child reaches for the otoscope, and the clinician asks her what it's for. Note the amount of time that it takes for her to respond and the nonspecific response, "It's for checking something." It's important to note that previously in the interaction, the child has said she was going to check the giraffe's ears, so she has the vocabulary and knowledge of the function. However, she does not recall words at the moment they are needed to answer the question.

color terms, etc.). They may have a limited range of semantic relations that are expressed within sentences such as possession, recurrence, and location, or between clauses such as sequential, causal, and conditional. Finally, preschoolers with language impairment may have problems using a range of conjunctions (e.g., but, so).

Language Disorders Related to Use

Infants/Toddlers

Prelinguistic precursors of language use are present in the range of ways in which infants gain what they want from those around them. Infants have a need to be fed and to make emotional connections with their caregivers. They use visual regard (looking at mother), body orientation (moving toward an object or person), and motor movements (reaching up to be held) to gain these early needs. Familiar partners understand the communication of hunger from infants, which is usually expressed by crying. Infants may convey negation by averting their eyes or by spitting out food.

As they mature, infants develop intentional and varied means to use their bodies or voices to convey messages such as requesting objects (grabbing a toy away), negating (sticking out a tongue), or commenting about events (shrieking with pleasure at a balloon). Infants' use of their bodies may be quite individualized and only recognizable to a familiar partner (the child who scratches his leg if he wants to go to the bathroom). Typically developing children at the one-word stage begin to use words and phrases to interact in addition to or instead of gestures. Children will still request objects or actions, reject, protest, or comment, but they begin to use words and symbolic language beginning at about 12–15 months for these pragmatic uses.

Children with impairments in prelinguistic aspects of language use may not use their bodies for varied types of communication with those around them. The most consistent manifestation of use impairments is found in children older than 6 months of age who fail to engage in intentional actions related to the world around them. These children appear to be passive observers in life rather than active participants. Later, these children may not point at objects they want, and they may use words to express a restricted range of meanings. For example, a typically developing 14-month-old child may use the word *Daddy* in a variety of contexts (indicating surprise when Daddy walks into a room, asking for help, telling who a pair of shoes belong to, and naming a person in a picture). The same age child with a language disorder may only use the word *Daddy* when his mother points to his father and asks, "Who's that?" These differences show a restricted range of communicative functions and lack of communicative initiation.

Preschool Children

By the time they are between 3 and 5 years old, typically developing children take turns for three to five exchanges, adjust their speech style to the listener, and make revisions during turn-taking. During conversations with their peers, preschoolers are able to use phrases and sentences to both initiate and to respond in conversation (Fey, 1986). Social initiations include making requests, comments, statements, disagreements, and performatives (claims, jokes, teasing, protests). Responsive acts include responses to requests for information, action, clarification, attention, assertives, performatives, and imitations. Additionally, preschoolers can select, introduce, maintain, and change topics quite readily.

Problems affecting the area of pragmatics may include limited verbal communication and a lack of a variety of language forms. Preschoolers may

 CD-ROM

Pragmatics

CD-ROM segment Ch.17.04 shows a 3-year-old girl interacting with the examiner while playing with a set of food and dishes. She uses a few words, typically in one-word utterances. Her low level of language output suggests difficulties in the area of expressive language. She does understand quite a bit of contextualized language and demonstrates appropriate social pragmatic responses to adult requests. In this example, she understood and responded to the request, "Would you pour me some milk?" She selected a cup, got the milk bottle, poured pretend milk, and handed it to the examiner. She then responded affirmatively to the question, "Do you want some milk?" by pouring herself pretend milk and drinking it.

have difficulty initiating and maintaining communication. For example, they may not know how to ask for clarifications when they don't understand something, or they may not know how to restate something they have said (a conversational repair) when someone does not understand them. They may also express their meanings in appropriate ways. Most preschoolers learn their teachers' names quickly, and they know how to ask for something politely. In the preschool classroom, they might say something like, *Miss Jones, can I have some crayons please?* The child with a language disorder might say something like, *Teacher, want colors.*

SERVICE DELIVERY

Language intervention is usually conducted in two types of settings: educational service delivery and medical service delivery. Educational service delivery settings are those affiliated in some way with an educational institution such as a public or private school. Medical service delivery settings are affiliated with a hospital or rehabilitation unit. In both settings, the SLP operates in concert with the family to make decisions regarding assessment and treatment of the preschooler with language disorders. There are differences in the kinds of services that are routinely provided in these settings. Let's explore the differences between the two types of service delivery settings in greater detail.

Educational Settings

There are laws that affect the way intervention is provided to infants and toddlers in educational settings. Two federal statutes, PL 99-457 and the Individuals With Disabilities Education Act (IDEA), require early identification and intervention services for children from birth to 36 months of age. PL 99-457 emphasizes the provision of services that are designed to help families address children's special needs within the context of the family. An important part of working with infants and toddlers in educational settings is a focus on family-centered prctice. **Family-centered practice** means working with families to identify, describe, and develop an appropriate intervention plan for each child. The family has the ultimate choice in the kinds of services that are provided and in the extent they want to participate in the process. It is important for professionals to seek the family's perspective on the child's strengths and needs. Because the emphasis is on working in the context of the family, assessment and intervention decisions should be consistent with the family's culture. The primary concerns of the family may be different from those of professionals, but the family should be allowed to make final decisions about the nature and the extent of the services that are provided. Professionals should serve as a support and resource for family decision making.

For children birth to 3 years of age, IDEA mandates service provision in the "least restrictive environment." In many states, the "least restrictive environment" is interpreted to mean the child's own home. This setting allows the family to be involved in the implementation of the treatment plan to the fullest extent possible. There are times, however, when the home may not be the best place for intervention. For example, some families may not want strangers in their home, preferring instead to take their child to a service delivery center for intervention.

IDEA states that parents should be part of the assessment process from the onset. Parents must be notified about any services or evaluation for their child. They must be told about their right to view any records or reports regarding their child. Parents also have the right to seek an evaluation outside the local educational agency. Thus, the law requires that parents are integrally involved in assessment and intervention decisions.

Speech-language pathologists (SLPs) often work collaboratively with preschool teachers and early childhood special educators to provide intervention within preschool classrooms. The SLP may suggest ways the teacher can help the child participate in the daily classroom activities. For example, a child who has difficulty with *why* questions may need to be asked simpler *what* questions during circle time, while the teacher and other children model ways of responding to *why* questions. This way, the child can participate during circle time with a high level of success.

Medical Settings

In medical settings, assessment and intervention practices are often driven by insurance company requirements. This is an unfortunate consequence of the way medical services are funded in the United States right now. The active involvement of parents and families is optional based on the rules and procedures of each medical setting. The child is viewed as an individual for purposes of service reimbursement, and assessment and treatment are much more likely to be conducted in individual sessions. Clinicians who are delivering services for insurance reimbursement rarely provide intervention in the child's everyday environment.

Reimbursement for assessment and treatment in both public and private medical settings is in a state of transition as both government and private insurers deal with changes in Medicare, Medicaid, and managed health care. Speech-language pathologists will need to remain flexible in the near term in medical service delivery settings to continue to develop and maintain best clinical practices in a changing field.

ASSESSMENT

Infants/Toddlers

Assessment of language disorder in infants and toddlers is related to the issue of prediction (van Kleeck, Gillam, & Davis, 1997). Clinicians must collect the kinds of information about the child's language development that will help them predict which children with delays will eventually develop normally and which children will continue to show speech and language impairments. The most severe infants and toddlers with known etiologies for their impairment are the easiest to diagnose. Infants and toddlers with less overt developmental delays (i.e., those who may show only language impairment) are not easily diagnosed, as their differences may be at the lower end of the range of normal variation for a period of time.

Often, assessment with this population is conducted simultaneously by professionals from different disciplines. In educational settings, the Individuals With Disabilities Act mandates assessment teams comprised of professionals from a variety of disciplines. As a result, the SLP will likely work closely with occupational therapists, physical therapists, social workers, and educational professionals. The most common model of assessment and team collaboration is termed **transdisciplinary assessment** (Briggs, 1993). Transdisciplinary assessment involves collaboration and consensus building among professionals from many disciplines. One professional is usually designated as the coordinator of care to reduce the number of professionals handling the young child and to decrease the amount of intrusion into a family's life. The team is headed by different professionals depending on the most crucial problem for the child.

In medical settings, infants and toddlers are likely to be evaluated and diagnosed by a **multidisciplinary assessment** team, which usually includes a physician, an occupational therapist, a physical therapist, a social worker, and an SLP plus other medical specialists as needed. In the multidisciplinary approach, professionals conduct their own independent evaluations and then share their results in a team meeting. There is likely to be more limited exchange of information across disciplines than is typical of the transdisciplinary model. The physician, as the head of each team, has the final say over which professionals see the child and what recommendations result from the assessment process.

Test instruments and analyses are more likely to be broad-based assessments of general development than to be focused on communication or language development alone. One reason for this broad focus is the criteria for entry into educational intervention programs as well as the likelihood of multiple areas of impairment in medical settings. Although criteria vary from state to state within the United States, three types of diagnostic categories are typical: developmental delay (delay in one or more areas including motor, cognitive, sensory, social-emotional), atypical development (development in one or more areas listed above that is not typical of normally developing children at any stage), or medical risk factor (known risk factors for developmental delay such as severe mental retardation or cleft palate). With such broad criteria, assessment instruments are needed that will qualify children for services and indicate directions for intervention in a number of areas.

Two types of tests are available for this population: **standardized assessment** instruments and **criterion-referenced assessment** instruments. Standardized tests compare the child to other children the same chronological age in a given area (e.g., motor development). An example of a standardized test is the *Battelle Developmental Inventory* (Newborg, Stock, Wenk, Gruidubaldi, & Svinicki, 1988). The *Battelle Developmental Inventory* is a test that can be used to obtain developmental age scores in the following areas: personal-social skills, adaptive behaviors, motor skills, communication, and cognition.

Criterion-referenced tests outline patterns of strength and areas that need intervention within a single child (e.g., child is not sitting up at 15 months, needs help with muscle strength). The *Rosetti Infant Toddler Language Scale* (Rosetti, 1990) is a criterion-referenced scale most often used to plan intervention rather than to compare toddlers to others their age. It has items in the areas of interaction-attachment, pragmatics, gesture, play, language comprehension, and language expression. Most instruments for prelinguistic children include a direct child response format (ask questions and wait for responses), an observational format (watch the child play), and a parent report format (ask the parent questions) in order to provide as many ways as possible for the child's skills to be explored. In addition, informal observation and sampling are important, as the infant or toddler may not be able to cooperate with a test procedure due to age or extreme disability.

Preschool Children

Preschool children who are suspected of having language impairment should undergo a complete language evaluation. Generally, assessment questions take two forms: "Does this child have language impairment?" and "What should be done about it?" Most of the time, both questions should be answered with an assessment of language abilities related to expectations for the child's chronological age. The first question is one of identification. The child is compared to typically developing peers to find out whether language development is significantly delayed in comparison to children who are the same chronological age. This comparison can answer whether the child's language is impaired. Next, the child's language is analyzed to determine the level of language development. Intervention often focuses on language skills that are lacking in the child with a language disorder, but usually appear in younger, typically developing children who are functioning at the same language level. In other words, the clinician looks for aspects of language that make the child with a language disorder different from most children.

A combination of assessment tools and analyses are appropriate for understanding the difference between the child's developmental and chronological age level. These include use of standardized testing, criterion-referenced testing, and **interactive assessment.**

Standardized assessment can be used to determine how a child compares to peers. Some of the tests used for this age and purpose include the *Preschool Language Scale-3* (PLS-3; Zimmerman, Steiner, & Pond, 1991), *Clinical Evaluation of Language Fundamentals-Preschool* (CELF-P; Wiig, Secord, & Semel, 1992), and the *Test of Language Development-Primary* (TOLD-P:3; Newcomer & Hammill, 1997). These tests evaluate many areas of language form and content and provide a score of general language performance that is used to compare the child to his or her same age peers. The kinds of items that appear on these tests include asking the child to point to colored blocks in response to an examiner's question (as on the PLS-2), questions about a story (as on the CELF-P), or sentences the child is asked to repeat (as on the TOLD-P:3). Some tests are specific to one area of language. For example, the *Expressive One-Word Picture Vocabulary Test-Revised* (Gardner, 1983) provides information about expressive vocabulary by asking the child to name pictures presented on test plates.

Criterion-referenced nonstandardized approaches to assessment are used to help clinicians develop better descriptions of performance and to plan intervention. Examples of criterion-referenced procedures include checklists of language behaviors, inventories, and language sampling. For example, language sampling provides useful information about a child's level of syntactic or grammatical performance. The examiner video- or audiotape records a play session or a conversation with the child. These sessions usually last about 20 minutes. The conversation is transcribed (written out), and at least 50 sequential utterances are analyzed and coded. Clinicians usually determine the mean length of utterance (MLU), which is the average number of morphemes in each utterance. They also look for the types of syntactic structures that are used, and they assess the types of meanings that are expressed. These measures are compared to what we know about language development to determine where the child is in the language development process. Incorrect forms or missing forms may become targets for intervention, depending on when they are expected to develop.

For vocabulary development, a standardized test may tell us if the child is performing below their chronological age level. However, it does not tell us what kinds of words or word classes the child is having difficulty with. Further observation of vocabulary knowledge and use using structured probes may provide this information. For example, we can devise a list of question types, prepositions, or attributes (color, size, shape) that the child may need for preschool success. Then we can systematically test these through play to see what the child can express or understand. One example of such a probe would be to devise a "hiding game." With a puppet or stuffed animal, the clinician hides a ball in various places (in, under, on top), and the child helps the puppet find the ball. The clinician may ask the child to help the puppet find the ball that is under the bed to test comprehension of spatial prepositions or to tell the puppet where the ball is to test expression of spatial terms.

Pragmatics or use is best assessed through observation of interaction. Again, the clinician may have a predetermined checklist of pragmatic behaviors to look for. One possibility is to examine children's interactions with peers during a specific time period using Fey's (1986) model of assertiveness and responsiveness (see Figure 17–1). Here, the clinician writes down what the child says and does to initiate conversation (assertive acts) and to respond to others' initiations (responsive acts) during a predetermined length of time (for example, 10 minutes). A tally of assertive verses responsive acts is completed. Also, the clinician may note the percentage of communicative acts that were verbal or nonverbal and whether they were appropriate or inappropriate. The summary provides a picture of the types of interaction the child prefers and how the child performs these acts.

Nonbiased Assessment

Speech-language pathologists should make sure their assessment is culturally and linguistically appropriate. This is especially important for infants, toddlers, and preschoolers. Not all children learn English as a first (or second) language. The developmental course of other languages is not necessarily like that of English. In addition, not all families share the same set of interaction styles or beliefs about the nature and role of children. The possibility of a mismatch between parental and SLP expectations and beliefs makes it important to understand variation in language learning and in socialization practices (refer to Chapter 3 for more information on these topics).

Historically, children from non–English-speaking backgrounds have been assessed in English. This nearly always leads to misdiagnosis. Think about how well you would do on an intelligence test administered in Russian. You probably would not appear to be very smart, would you? Unfortunately, assessments conducted in children's second language can lead to misdiagnoses such as language impairment or mental retardation. Even though it seems obvious that children cannot be assessed in a language that is not their own, problems continue to persist. Some of these problems occur because the process of learning a second language or dialect variations may not be well understood. Other problems may occur because interaction styles reflective of different cultures do not match mainstream expectations for test-taking behavior. For example, in some cultures, parents emphasize single-word labels during interactions with their children. These children are well prepared for taking a single-word expressive vocabulary test that requires a naming response. In other cultures, parents may not label objects for their children as

Transcription/Description of Communicative Act	Assertive	Responsive

Figure 17–1. Observation of child interaction.

often. A single-word expressive vocabulary test would be an unusual experience for these children, and it is likely their performance would be a reflection of their lack of experience with this type of task.

Testing the Limits

Interactive assessment of form, content, and use allows us to test beyond the limits of the behaviors that the child displays in nonteaching (e.g., testing) situations. In interactive assessment, the clinician evaluates how easily or well a child learns something that is specifically taught. It is like turning intervention into assessment. This type of assessment helps us to rule out whether poor test performance is due to little or limited exposure to the types of questions that are being asked or to not understanding the test task itself. For children from culturally and linguistically diverse backgrounds, this step is particularly important. Many times, these children are misdiagnosed because they may not know the rules of testing and language, and they may be in the process of learning English as a second language. Furthermore, interactive assessment helps to guide intervention. We believe there are differences between children who quickly and easily learn something new and those for whom new learning is difficult.

Interactive assessment is guided by several principles. First, there is intent to purposefully teach new information or new strategies (based on standardized and nonstandardized procedures). Second, the examiner observes what the child does as a result of the teaching. Third, this information helps the examiner to make a judgment about how much change the child is able to make given adult support.

The general procedure for utilizing interactive assessment is to examine the results of standardized or criterion-referenced assessment to determine where the child may be having difficulty. Typically, one or two specific areas are then targeted in a short intervention. The intervention is guided by principles of mediated learning that focus on helping children understand the goal of teaching, helping them hypothesize, and helping them develop strategies that will lead to success in the identified area of weakness. For example, if a child had trouble with vocabulary, the examiner would help him or her understand that the goal of the task was to think about names for things. The examiner might also help the child talk about what might happen if we didn't have specific names for things and to think of different ways that vocabulary is used.

After a short mediation (typically two 20–30 minute sessions), the child is retested on what was taught to assess what changes occurred with teaching. We would also observe the approach and strategies the child used in completing the test task. For example, if the focus was on vocabulary because the child scored low on an expressive vocabulary test, we might see if he or she was able to respond to more items. We may also see whether the error types differed from pre- to posttest. For example, children may make more attempts at naming or may move from using descriptions at the time of the pretest to using more nouns at the time of the posttest. Children who are able to make great changes in a short amount of time may have had limited experience with the task and may not need intervention. Children who make moderate changes or few changes from pre- to posttest may require therapy. It is likely those children who made moderate changes would make more rapid progress in therapy than children who made almost no change.

INTERVENTION

According to Fey (1986), intervention approaches with young children with language impairment generally fall along a continuum of clinician-centered approaches to child-centered approaches. **Clinician-centered approaches** are those in which the clinician controls the intervention context, goals, and materials. **Child-centered approaches** often use less structured settings and stimulate language development indirectly in concert with the family. We discuss each of these in more detail in the following section.

Clinician-centered approaches are based on behavioral principles of learning in which the stimulus (clinician input) is designed to produce a correct response (child output). When the child produces the desired response, the clinician systematically provides reinforcement to increase the likelihood that the correct response will occur again. Advantages of this approach are that we can provide lots of practice, and the child receives immediate feedback. On the other hand, these approaches are often criticized for being too dissimilar to the situations in which language is actually used. Unfortunately, the unnaturalness of this kind of intervention reduces the likelihood that children will use the forms they learn in everyday conversations and interactions.

Child-centered approaches focus on facilitating language through more indirect means. The clinician is there to facilitate language through play or a whole language approach, but does not direct the activity. Similarly, family-centered approaches, especially in the case of early intervention, focus on the family as the primary unit of intervention. So, child-centered therapy looks much like play. The key is to have a clinician who is maximally responsive to the child and responds in ways that are known to facilitate language development. Rather than focusing on specific language structures (i.e., auxiliary verbs), the clinician focuses on overall communication. The role of the clinician is to respond to communication attempts consistently and to provide linguistic models for the child to learn from. Facilitative techniques include self- and parallel talk by the clinician in which running commentaries about the clinician's actions (self-talk) or the child's actions (parallel talk) are provided. Imitating the child may increase the probability that the child will, in turn, imitate the imitation. We can expand a child's utterance to provide a more complete or complex model for the child, increasing the possibility that the child will realize the relationship between the meanings he or she wanted to express and the language forms that can express those meanings. Extensions provide additional content to what the child says. Again, this technique increases the possibility that children will use longer utterances.

There is a third intervention approach that is somewhat in the middle of the two endpoints of the continuum that we have presented. This is referred to as a **hybrid approach.** Hybrid approaches focus on one or two specific language goals. The clinician selects the activities and materials rather than following the child's lead and responds to the child's communication to model and highlight the specific forms targeted for intervention. One example of a hybrid approach is *focused stimulation,* in which the clinician designs the materials and activities in a way the child is likely to produce utterances for the targeted language form. Furthermore, the clinician provides lots of models within this context without requiring the child to produce the form. This technique helps children improve comprehension as well as production skills.

There are several language stimulation techniques that have been shown to be helpful for children with language impairment. On the more clinician-centered side are techniques such as drill and drill-play. More child-centered techniques include indirect stimulation and whole language approaches. Table 17–2 provides some examples of these language stimulation techniques.

Regardless of which type of approch SLPs use, they need to think about the following parameters in order to select appropriate intervention targets:

Prior knowledge. Clinicians need to think carefully about the child's level of conceptual and linguistic development. Selected language goals need to be slightly more advanced than the abilities the child has and those that are likely to occur next in development.

Information processing. Clinicians need to take maximum advantage of the child's information processing system. For maximum attention, memory, and perception provide slow-paced input, stress important words, give repeated examples, and vary the examples given.

Motivation. Clinicians should think about what the child finds interesting. Play-based intervention that takes the child's interests, needs, and cultural values into consideration should be incorporated into the treatment plan.

SUMMARY

Working with young children with language impairment is one of the many roles of an SLP. The SLP needs to know the laws and the professional guidelines that govern intervention with infants, toddlers, and preschoolers. The SLP works to improve the language of young children either directly through the assessment and intervention process or indirectly by working with families and others who interact with the child, such as parents and teachers. It is important that SLPs who work with young children have an understanding

Table 17–2. Language Stimulation Techniques

Stimulation Technique	Focus	Example
Drill	Clinician-centered	Phonology—contrastive drills. The clinician models word pairs that differ by one (target) phoneme, and the child repeats the pairs, for example, *cap/tap* (for targeting /k/.
Drill play	Clinician-centered	Syntax—sentence completion tasks given in a play situation. For example, when children produce the syntactic target in response to picture cards they can move forward on a game board.
Self-talk	Child-centered	Clinicians talk about what they themselves are doing, seeing, and feeling as they play with children in an unstructured setting. This technique is especially appropriate for children whose language is emerging.
Parallel talk	Child-centered	Clinicians talk about what children are doing or looking at as they play in an unstructured setting. Again, this technique is appropriate with children who are beginning to use language to communicate.
Expansion	Child-centered	Clinicians repeat back the child's utterance, adding grammatical and/or semantic information to make it complete. For example, the child might say, "Daddy walking home," and the clinician then says, "Daddy *is* walking home."
Extension	Child-centered	Clinicians add information to what the child has said. For example, if the child says, "Daddy orange," the clinician might add, "Yes, daddy peels the orange."
Recast	Child-centered	This is similar to expansions, but here the clinician changes the voice of the original orange. In the example above, where the child says, "Daddy orange," the clinician might recast the utterance as a question, "Is daddy peeling the orange?"
Build-ups and breakdowns	Child-centered	Clinicians expand the child's utterance (build-up), then break it down into its components, then build it up again. Continuing with our example of the child saying, "Daddy orange" the clinician might then say, "Daddy is peeling the orange. Daddy is peeling. Peel the orange, Daddy. Daddy is peeling the orange."

of normal as well as disordered language development and have a wide range of approaches for identification and intervention with this population. In this chapter, we have given you a broad overview of language impairments and some of the options we have for working with this population.

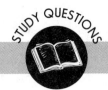

STUDY QUESTIONS

1 What is a language disorder?

2 Define chronological and developmental age.

3 Name and give an example of the three components of language.

4 What are similarities and differences in working with children 0–3 years old and 3–5 years old?

5 Why is the development of language use important?

6 How do you think language form and language content interact with language use?

7 How does the setting in which SLPs work with children affect service delivery?

8 What kinds of assessments are appropriate for young children?

9 What do different types of assessment contribute to the total picture of the child?

10 What are advantages and disadvantages of child-centered, clinician-centered, and hybrid intervention approaches?

REFERENCES

Adamson, L. B., & Chance, S. E. (1998). Coordinating attention to people, objects, and language. In A. Wetherby, S. F. Warren, & J. Reichle (Eds.), *Transitions in prelinguistic communication.* Baltimore: Paul H. Brookes.

American Speech-Language-Hearing Association. (1982). *Committee on language, speech, and hearing services in schools. Definitions: Communication disorders and variations.* Rockville, MD: Author.

Bates, E. (1976). *Language and context: The acquisition of pragmatics.* New York: Academic Press.

Billeaud, F. (1995). *Communication disorder in infants and toddlers: Assessment and intervention.* Boston: Andover Medical Publishers.

Bloom, L., & Lahey, M. (1968). *Language development and language disorders.* New York: John Wiley & Sons.

Briggs, M. H. (1993). Team talk: communication skills for early intervention teams. *Journal of Childhood Communication Disorders, 15,* 33–40.

Brown, R. (1973). *A first language: The early stages.* Cambridge, MA: Harvard University Press.

Bruner, J. (1977). Early social interaction and language acquisition. In H. R. Schaffer (Ed.), *Studies in mother-infant interaction* (pp. 271–289). New York: Academic Press.

Fey, M. (1986). *Language intervention with young children.* Austin, TX: Pro-Ed.

Gardner, M. (1983). *Expressive One-Word Picture Vocabulary Test.* Novato, CA: Academic Therapy Publications.

Nelson, N. W. (1998). *Childhood language disorders in context: Infancy through adolescence,* (2nd ed.). New York: Merrill.

Newborg, J., Stock, J.,Wenk, L., Guidubaldi, J., & Svinicki, J. (1988). *Battelle Developmental Inventory.* Allen, TX: DLM Teaching Resources.

Newcomer, P., & Hammill, D. (1997). *Test of Language Development-Primary* (3rd ed.). Austin, TX: Pro-Ed.

Paul, R. (1995). *Language disorders: From infancy through adolescence.* St. Louis: Mosby.

Roberts, J., Rescorla, L., Girous, J., & Stevens, L. (1998). Phonological skills of children with specific expressive language impairment (SLI-E): Outcomes at age 3. *Journal of Speech, Language and Hearing Research, 41,* 374–384.

Rossetti, L. (1990). *The Rossetti Infant-Toddler Language Scale: A measure of communication and interaction.* East Moline, IL: LinguiSystems.

Tomblin, B., Hardy, J. C., & Hein, H. (1991). Predicting poor communication status in risk factors present at birth. *Journal of Speech and Hearing Research, 34,* 1096–1105.

van Kleeck, A., Gillam, R. B., & Davis, B. (1997). When is "watch and see" warranted? A response to Paul's 1996 article, "Clinical implications of the natural history of slow expressive language development." *American Journal of Speech Language Pathology, 6,* 34–39.

Wiig, E., Secord, W., & Semel, E. (1992). *Clinical Evaluation of Language Fundamentals-Preschool.* San Antonio, TX: Psychological Corporation.

Zimmerman, I., Steiner, V., & Pond, R. (1991). *Preschool Language Scale-3.* San Antonio, TX: Psychological Corporation.

SUGGESTED READINGS

Fey, M. (1986). *Language intervention with young children.* Boston, MA: Allyn & Bacon.

McCormick, L., Loeb, D. F., & Schiefelbusch, R. L. (1997). *Supporting children with communcation difficulties in inclusive settings: School-based language intervention.* Boston, MA: Allyn & Bacon.

Nelson, N. W. (1998). *Childhood language disorders in context: Infancy through adolescence* (2nd ed.). Boston: Allyn and Bacon.

Paul, R. (1995). *Language Disorders: From infancy through adolescence.* St. Louis, MO: Mosby.

Rossetti, L. (1994). *Communication intervention: Birth to three.* San Diego: Singular Publishing Group.

GLOSSARY

Child-centered approaches: Child-centered approaches are those in which the clinician follows the child's lead with respect to the activities, the topics of discussion, and the toys that are played with.

Chronological age: We typically use years and months (e.g., 2;3 means 2 years, 3 months) to determine a child's age and to compare him or her to other children of the same age.

Clinician-centered approaches: Clinician-centered approaches are those in which the clinician controls the intervention context, goals, and materials.

Comprehension: The ability to understand language (the opposite of expression).

Content: Language content refers to the meaning of language (semantics).

Criterion-referenced assessment: Criterion-referenced, nonstandardized approaches to assessment provide descriptive information about tasks children routinely encounter in their environment. Unlike norm-referenced measures, scores on criterion-referenced measures are not compared to the average scores of same-age peers.

Developmental age: Developmental age refers to the child's level of development in a given area, in this case language. The developmental age is the age of most typically developing children at the time their language is simi-lar to the language of the child being tested.

Developmental language disorder: When a child has problems acquiring language even though there is no obvious cause. *See* Specific language impairment.

Expression: The ability to produce language (the opposite of comprehension).

Family-centered practice: Family-centered practice incorporates families into the assessment and treatment process. This construct is designed to recognize the importance of connections with family members in communication development.

Form: Language form refers to the structure of language including syntax, morphology, and phonology.

Hybrid approaches: Hybrid approaches focus on one or two specific language goals. The clinician selects the activities and materials rather than following the child's lead and responds to the child's communication to model and highlight the specific forms that are being targeted for intervention.

Interactive assessment: Interactive assessment allows speech-language pathologists (SLPs) to test beyond the limits of the behaviors the child displays in nonteaching (e.g., testing) situations. This type of testing helps clinicians decide whether poor test performance is due to language learning difficulties, lack of understanding the test task, or limited exposure to the types of questions that are being asked.

Multidisciplinary assessment: Members of an assessment team conduct their own independent assessments of the child's abilities that relate to their own interest areas (i.e., speech-language pathologists evaluate speech and language only, physical therapists evaluate motor abilities only, etc.). In a summary meeting, each member of the team shares their findings and recommends treatment. The emphasis is on the parts of the child rather than the whole child.

Neutralist approach: An approach to identifying language disorders in which clinicians base their diagnostic decisions on test scores without taking social norms into consideration.

Normativist approach: An approach to identifying language disorders in which clinicians account for social norms and potential social, educational, vocational, and economic consequences of the child's language abilities in the decision-making process.

Prelinguistic communication: Prelinguistic development of communication occurs before children use words. Prelinguistic communication includes gestures and nonword vocalizations.

Production: The use of speech or writing to express meaning.

Specific language impairment: Difficulties acquiring language in the absence of any other mental, sensory, motoric, emotional, or experiential deficits.

Standardized assessment: Administration of formal tests to determine how a child's performance on an aspect of language compares to the average performance of children who are the same chronological age.

Transdisciplinary assessment: A team of professionals works together to evaluate a child. Members of the team are not limited to the evaluation of any single area of development.

Use: Language use refers to the social aspects of language, which are also called pragmatics.

18

Language Disorders in School–Age Children

Ronald B. Gillam

LEARNING OBJECTIVES

1 To understand the nature and consequences of language disorders in school-age children.

2 To differentiate between language disorder, learning disability, and dyslexia.

3 To learn aspects of language development that are especially difficult for school-age children with language disorders in the primary and secondary grades.

4 To know the three laws that directly affect the way services are delivered to school-age children with language disorders.

5 To learn about assessment procedures that are commonly used to evaluate language disorders in students in the primary and secondary grades.

6 To learn about typical intervention procedures that are used by speech-language pathologists who treat school-age children with language disorders.

INTRODUCTION

Approximately 7% of all school-age children have unusual difficulties learning and using language, and more than 1 million children receive language intervention services in public schools each year (U.S. Department of Education, 1997). Many more children receive treatment for language disorders in hospitals, rehabilitation agencies, and private clinics. Clearly, language intervention comprises a large proportion of the health and education services that are provided to children with disabilities.

You know from Chapters 2 and 17 that some children are relatively poor language learners. There are numerous causes of language disorders in school-age children including mental retardation, problems processing information (deficits in attention, perception, and memory), hearing loss, emotional disorders, and neglect. Recall that in most cases of language disorders, the cause or causes of the child's language-learning difficulties are not known.

A variety of causes of language disorders can have the same effects on language development. Regardless of the cause (mental retardation, traumatic brain injury, autism, auditory processing deficits, etc.), many children with language disorders present similar clusters of problems. Frequently, these children do not attend well to what their parents and teachers say, do not mentally process and represent multiple pieces of language information at once, do not readily relate new information to what they already know, and/ or do not retain new information in a manner that permits easy retrieval. These kinds of problems interfere with children's ability to take maximum advantage of the language-learning opportunities that exist in primary and secondary school classrooms. That is why children with language disorders usually need specialized assistance beyond the education that is routinely provided by classroom teachers.

This chapter provides information about language disorders in school-age children. We divide the school-age years into two periods, the primary grades (K–5) and the secondary grades (6–12). We begin by explaining how laws affect public education, and we describe the contexts in which language

 CD-ROM

CD-ROM Summary

Volume 2 of the CD-ROM that accompanies this text contains four video segments that accompany this chapter. The first segment shows an 8-year-old girl who has been diagnosed as having specific language impairment, central auditory processing disorder, and learning disabilities. This segment was included to demonstrate some of the language difficulties that these children present. The second and third segments demonstrate formal tests of receptive and expressive language. The fourth segment shows part of a language intervention session with an 11-year-old boy with autism.

Segments

Ch.18.01. The clinician, LaVae, is collecting a language sample from Jennifer, age 8. Jennifer tells LaVae about an incident that happened with her bird. Jennifer's language includes lots of mazes (false starts, repetitions, and revisions). Notice that the mazes occur when she is unsure of the correct grammatical structure to use and when she is constructing longer, more complex sentences.

Ch.18.02. LaVae is administering the Grammatic Understanding subtest of the *Test of Language Development–Primary: 3rd Edition* (TOLD-P:3) to Jennifer. This is a test of receptive language. Jennifer points to one of four pictures on a page that LaVae names.

Ch.18.03. LaVae is administering the Grammatic Completion subtest of the TOLD-P:3 to Jennifer. This is a test of grammatical morphology. LaVae says part of a sentence. Jennifer provides the last word, which must contain a certain grammatical marker (plural, past tense, present progressive, etc.) to be correct.

Ch. 18.04. Trey, an 11-year-old boy with autism, is participating in a language intervention activity with his clinician. This activity was designed to help Trey improve his problem solving and his explanatory language.

intervention is delivered in school settings. The second section of the chapter concerns issues related to delivering services to school-age children with language disorders. We review critical aspects of language development and language disorders during the primary grades (K–5) and the secondary grades (6–12), and we summarize basic assessment and intervention principles that relate to these areas of language development.

SERVICES FOR SCHOOL-AGE CHILDREN

Recall from Chapter 17 that there are a number of laws that affect the way language intervention services are provided to preschoolers. There are also laws that affect the assessment and treatment of language disorders in school-age children. In 1973, the U.S. Congress passed a law, commonly referred to simply as **Section 504,** that prohibited any agency receiving federal funding from discriminating against individuals with disabilities. The term *discrimination* has been interpreted very broadly with respect to educational opportunities. Basically, a child is the subject of discrimination if, as a result of a disability, he or she cannot benefit from the same kinds of educational experiences that are routinely available for nondisabled students. As a result of Section 504, all public schools are required by law to ensure that, to the fullest extent possible, children with disabilities can profit from the instruction that is offered in classrooms. This is done by providing appropriate accommodations to the curriculum and/or modifying the way the curriculum is taught. Children with language disorders fall under the umbrella of Section 504 protection.

The requirements of Section 504 have been specified in greater detail over the years, and Congress has passed a number of bills that provide federal funding for special education. **Public Law 94-142, the Education of All Handicapped Children Act of 1975,** guaranteed a free appropriate public education in the least restrictive environment to all children with disabilities. The concept of least restrictive environment is important. It means that, to the extent possible, children with disabilities need to receive educational assistance in a manner that permits access to regular educational experiences. There was a time when children with severe forms of mental retardation, cerebral palsy, deafness, blindness, and other disabilities were sent to special schools. Many times, these children were not allowed to attend the schools in their neighborhood. In some states, parents were told if they wanted their children to receive treatment, they had to send them away from home to live in residential institutions. This was unfair to parents and children. In essence, it amounted to discrimination against children with disabilities. The requirement in PL 94-142 that services must be provided in the least restrictive environment has resulted in an increase in the number of special education services that are provided in neighborhood schools and in regular classroom settings. As a result, there are far fewer residential schools for children with disabilities. Children are only sent to institutions like a state residential school for the deaf and blind when their parents and school district representatives agree it is the most appropriate educational placement.

Recently, the name of the Education of All Handicapped Children Act was changed to the **Individuals With Disabilities Education Act (IDEA).** Some of the key provisions of this act are listed in Table 18–1. As part of the budget process each year, Congress must reauthorize the funding mechanisms that make it possible for school districts to provide a free appropriate public education in the least restrictive environment for all children. Parents can request a hearing with a state-appointed officer when they believe the school district has not met the requirements of IDEA (the Individuals with Disabilities Education Act). Either side (parents or school districts) can appeal a hearing decision to a higher court. Students in communication sciences and disorders need to understand the requirements of IDEA so they can be certain they always provide services to children in a manner that is consistent with the laws that regulate special education and related services in the schools.

To retain the advances that have been made in special education and related services to children with disabilities, including children with language disorders, it is important for students and professionals in communication sciences and disorders to stay informed about congressional actions related to IDEA. Most of us enter this profession because we are advocates for children

Table 18–1. Important Requirements of the Individuals With Disabilities Education Act (IDEA)

Parent Notification: Parent consent is required before children can be referred for special testing and again before they can be tested

Comprehensive Evaluation: Children must receive a full and individual evaluation by a team of professionals in order to determine whether they have disability. This evaluation must be conducted in the child's native language unless it is clearly not feasible to do so.

Determination of Disability: Following their assessment, professionals must meet with the child's parents to report their results and to determine whether the child has a disability. A "disability" is defined as a child "with mental retardation, hearing impairments (including deafness), speech or language impairments, visual impairments (including blindness), serious emotional disturbance, orthopedic impairments, autism, traumatic brain injury, other health impairments, or specific learning disabilities." For children between the ages of 3 and 9 years, a disability can also mean a child who is "experiencing developmental delays in physical development, cognitive development, communication development, social or emotional development or adaptive development."

Individualized Education Program (IEP): If it is determined that a child has a disability, school personnel must meet with the parents to develop an Individualized Education Plan (IEP). This program is a written statement that specifies the child's strengths and weaknesses, the child's levels of educational performance, the goals and objectives that the child needs to meet in order to profit from instruction, the type of services the child will receive, and the amount of time each week that services will be provided.

Review of Placement and Services: Each year, members of the IEP team and the child's parents must meet to review the child's progress, to determine whether the child is still eligible for special education services, and to create a new IEP (if needed).

Due Process: Parents have the right to review all records related to their child's education, to have their children evaluated by an independent professional, and to request a hearing if they are not satisfied with the type or amount of services that are being recommended for their child.

with disabilities. We want to provide the best possible services to these children, and we want these children to receive as much help as they need to succeed socially, academically, and vocationally. With that goal in mind, many professionals in communication sciences and disorders strongly support increased funding for special education programs across the nation. The Individuals With Disabilities Education Act (IDEA) is the primary mechanism by which continued or increased funding for special services to students with disabilities will occur.

LANGUAGE DISORDERS

We know there are many preschool-age children who have significant limitations in their ability to learn and use language. These children's development in areas of language form (morphology and syntax), content (size of the lexicon and semantic relations), and/or use (pragmatics and socialization) lags behind that of their same age peers. Some of these children benefit from early intervention and have language growth spurts that enable them to catch up to their age peers in language development by the time they are 5 years old (Paul, Hernandez, Taylor, & Johnson, 1996). Those children whose language disorders do not resolve by the age of 5 years frequently have difficulties with social and academic language during the elementary school years (Aram & Hall, 1989; Paul, Murray, Clancy, & Andrews, 1997). Often, these same children continue to exhibit social, academic, and vocational difficulties well into the secondary grades (Bishop, 1997; Stothard, Snowling, Bishop, Chipchase, & Kaplan, 1998) and even into adulthood (Records, Tomblin, & Buckwalter, 1995). For this reason, professionals need to be diligent in their efforts to identify children with language disorders as early as possible and to provide them with the kinds of intervention they need to succeed.

Language Disorder, Learning Disability, or Dyslexia?

Reading and writing are language-based skills. When children enter kindergarten, they usually have a great deal of knowledge about the vocabulary, grammar, and use of their language. This knowledge is based on their experiences with listening to and speaking the language that surrounds them. To learn how to read and write, children must organize their knowledge of language on a new level. They need to figure out how to use sequences of letters to represent the phonemes, words, sentences, and stories that have been part of their oral language for some time. To read, children must decode sequences of letters into language. To write, they must encode their language into sequences of letters. It only makes sense that children who have difficulty comprehending and producing spoken language are at a significant disadvantage when they begin to learn how to read and write. Therefore, it should not be surprising that most children with language disorders have significant difficulties with the development of literacy.

Children with learning disabilities and children with dyslexia have difficulties learning how to read and write. We have just learned that children with language disorders have the same kinds of problems. One question that naturally arises with school-age children is, "What is the difference between a language disorder, a learning disability, and dyslexia?"

Children with language disorders have difficulty with the comprehension and/or the expression of language form, content, or use, and these difficulties place them at risk for social, educational, or vocational difficulties. Students with learning disabilities sometimes have difficulties learning and using language as well. **Learning disability** is a general term used to refer to children who have significant difficulties in the acquisition and use of listening, speaking, reading, writing, reasoning, or mathematical abilities. We believe that learning disabilities in the areas of speaking and listening are, in fact, language disorders. Earlier, we discovered that reading and writing are language-based skills. Therefore, difficulties learning to read and write are often symptoms of language disorders.

Dyslexia is quite similar. Many researchers believe dyslexia is a neurologically based phonological processing disorder that interferes with single word decoding (Lyon, 1995). According to Catts and Kamhi (1999), dyslexia is one type of a developmental language disorder in which the child's specific difficulties are in the area of phonological processing skills that relate to reading.

What is the difference between a language disorder, a learning disability, and dyslexia? In theory, there is no difference. They are all manifestations of language-learning difficulties. However, theory and practice are two different things. Children with similar symptoms are often labeled differently because different procedures are used to diagnose language disorders, learning disabilities, and dyslexia.

Children are diagnosed as language disordered when they have difficulties with language form, content, and use that are unexpected given their chronological age. That is, they are poorer at comprehending or producing language than other children their same age. Clinicians make this determination by comparing children's performance on standardized tests to the norms for children who are their same age. They also make this determination by analyzing the level of language and the patterns of form, content, and use errors in conversational and narrative language samples. Comparing a child's language abilities to the abilities of typically achieving children the same age is referred to as **chronological age referencing.** That is, the expected language ability for a particular age is the reference on which a determination of a language disorder is based.

The criteria for diagnosing a learning disability are a little different. A learning disability is defined by law as a significant discrepancy between a child's ability and his or her achievement in one or more of the following areas: listening, speaking, reading, writing, reasoning, mathematical computation, and mathematical problem solving. To determine whether a child has a learning disability, professionals first assess their intelligence using an IQ test. The resulting score is thought to reflect their *ability*. Then, professionals assess the child's *achievement* in the areas of speaking, listening, reading, writing, reasoning, and/or mathematics using formal and informal tests. If there is a significant difference (usually considered to be 15 standard score points) between their *ability* as reflected by their score on an IQ test and their level of *achievement* in the areas of speaking, listening, reading, writing, reasoning, and/or mathematics, a child can be diagnosed with a learning disability. This identification procedure is referred to as **discrepancy modeling.**

The primary problem with discrepancy modeling is that children with higher-level skills sometimes qualify for special assistance in school while children with lower-level skills do not. For example, a child with an IQ score of 100 (right at the average) and a standard score of 85 on a test of reading could be identified as having a learning disability in the area of reading because there was a 15-point discrepancy between his standard scores on an IQ test and his standard scores on a reading test. Consider a child who is the same age and has a lower standard score (80) on a reading test. However, imagine that the second child earned a standard score of 90 on an IQ test. This second child would not be labeled as learning disabled and would not qualify for special education services because he did not present a significant discrepancy between ability and achievement. The problem with discrepancy modeling is that two children with similar difficulties with reading and with similar needs for extra assistance do not always receive the same help.

Dyslexia is diagnosed by examining children's reading ability. In the past 10 years, dyslexia has come to mean a difficulty decoding print due to phonological processing (phonological awareness) problems. Most professionals test for dyslexia by administering reading tests and tests of phonological processing skills like the ability to blend sounds together to make words or the ability to listen to a word and then make a new word by removing the first or last sound. The diagnosis of dyslexia is rarely based on discrepancy criteria.

There are some children who have difficulties in the areas of speaking, listening, reading, and writing who happen to have a discrepancy between intellectual ability and achievement in one or more of these areas and who have phonological processing problems that adversely affect their reading. These children could be labeled as language disordered, learning disabled, or dyslexic. There are other children who have the same kinds of speaking, listening, reading, and writing problems, but they do *not* have a significant discrepancy between their intellectual ability and their achievement in speaking, listening, reading, or writing. Given the current reliance on discrepancy modeling, these children could be called language disordered or dyslexic but not learning disabled. Finally, there are some children who have unusual difficulty reading words, but their spoken language and listening are within normal limits for their age. If they have a discrepancy between measure of intellectual ability and achievement, they can be diagnosed as learning disabled or dyslexic. If they do not have a significant discrepancy between ability and achievement, they can only be diagnosed as dyslexic. The important message is that language disorders; learning disabilities in speaking, listening, reading and writing; and dyslexia are all language-based problems. Because these terms have somewhat different diagnostic criteria, children with quite similar language abilities and disabilities can sometimes be classified with different labels.

CRITICAL AREAS OF LANGUAGE DEVELOPMENT DURING THE SCHOOL-AGE YEARS

Recall from Chapter 2 that many aspects of language form, content, and use continue to develop during the school-age years. For the purposes of this chapter, we focus on three critical aspects of language development during the primary grades (complex sentences, narration, and literacy) and three different aspects of development during the secondary grades (subject specific vocabulary, expository texts, and metacognitive strategies). Although there are many types of language disorders and many different kinds of language needs, these are the skills most often assessed and treated during the school-age years.

Primary Grades (K–5)

Complex Sentences

Most children use more complex sentences and a greater variety of complex sentence forms during the school-age years (see Table 18–2 for a list of different types of complex sentences). As children have more complex things to talk about, they need to have a command of various kinds of complex language forms that can express their ideas. Children experiment with the kinds of syntactic devices that are required for "literate" language, and they discover when and how to use these complex structures. Unfortunately, complex sentences pose unusual difficulties for many children with language disorders, and these difficulties are especially evident when children are reading and writing (Gillam & Carlile, 1997; Gillam & Johnston, 1992).

Table 18–2. Examples of Complex Sentences

Sentence Type	Example
Simple sentence	I saw the girl.
Compound sentence (and, but, so, or)	I saw the girl, and I said, "hello." I saw the girl but she didn't see me.
Complex Sentences	
Adverbial clauses	If you see the girl, call me.
Relative clauses	I'll call her because she is my friend.
Subjective	The girl who had brown eyes, was walking with my sister.
Objective	My sister was walking with the girl who had brown eyes.
Infinitive (with second subject stated)	I want you to play with me.
Clausal Complements	I saw the elephant run away. I heard the band playing its new song.
Multiple embedded clauses	He said, I hope you remember who you are supposed to talk to because I'm going to be mad if you say this to the wrong person.

Note: Main verbs are italicized.

Often, children with language disorders use more **mazes** when they are producing complex sentences. A maze is a repetition, a false start, or a reformulation of a sentence. For example, in the CD-ROM video segment Ch.18.01, Jennifer says, "But one time, when I had a b-, when uh, I uh, when last Christmas, I, uh uh, my aunt Mary Ann, my aunt, she gave me a bird, and her, and I called him Tweetie Bird." What Jennifer is trying to say is, *Last Christmas my aunt Mary Ann gave me a bird named Tweetie.* Jennifer has difficulties with pronouns and with adverbial phrases, and these difficulties get in the way of her ability to formulate and organize what she wants to say about her bird. These are not unusual problems for many school-age children with language disorders.

 CD-ROM

Mazes and Complex Sentences

Play CD-ROM segment Ch.18.02 on Volume 2 of the CD-ROM set. Jennifer is talking to LaVae, who is a certified and licensed SLP. Can you identify how many complex sentences there are? Note the number of mazes in her language and where they occur in her sentences. The mazes are clues to aspects of language that are difficult for her. Mazes are noted in parentheses in the transcript.

Conversation: "Bird"

Context: Jennifer is telling the examiner about her pet bird

Note: < > indicates overlap between speakers
     x indicates an unintelligible word

J: Jennifer

E: Examiner

> J: (But one time, when I had a b-) (when uh) (I uh) (when) last Christmas (x uh uh) aunt Mary Ann) my aunt, she gave me a bird (and her) and I called him Tweetie Bird.
> E: A real bird?
> J: Uh-huh.
> E: She gave you a real bird?
> J: Yeah.
> J: And uh and one time, Tweetie pooped on my head by accident.
> J: <Poop!>
> E: <Oh, not> really.
> J: Oh, yes he did.
> E: How did that happen?
> J: Because, when he was climbing up here, he pooped by accident.

E: You would let him climb on you?

J: Yeah, and he climbed right up here, then climbed right up here, then he pooped.

E: Oh, my goodness.

E: But you don't think he really meant to do it.

J: M-m.

E: So, sometimes you would let him go out of his cage?

J: No, (I let x) (I) I x x x.

J: (Uh) one time (when I was) (when I) (when I was uh) when I was playing, I stepped on Tweetie by accident, like this.

J: Then, he said, "Tweet tweet tweet tweet tweet tweet."

J: Then we had to take him to the vet.

E: Is that really true that you *stepped on* him?

J: <Uh-huh>

J: M-hm.

J: (It was very acci-) it was a accident.

J: Then I said, "I hope Tweetie doesn't die."

J: And Mom said, "(I hope he wasn't) (I hope he didn't) I hope he doesn't."

E: What happened when you took him to the vet?

J: (Oh we uh) I took Tweetie (and, and) and then I took Tweetie out, then the man said, "Well, that's a fine-looking bird."

J: "Maybe someday you will be a doctor (uh) when you grow up."

J: And I, and Mom laughed.

E: She did?

J: Uh-huh.

E: Yeah.

J: My sister cried when she wanted a turn.

E: Do you think you would like to be a veterinarian when you grow up?

J: No, I would like to be a artist from Walt Disney.

Narration

Narration is a critical aspect of language development during the school-age years. Children socialize by telling each other stories about their lives, they use stories as mental tools for remembering events, and they learn to read and write stories. Children's narratives become longer and more complex during the primary grades as they learn how to create more elaborate episodes (see Chapter 2). They also develop the ability to weave multiple episodes into their stories.

If children with language disorders have trouble creating complex sentences, it should not be surprising that they also have trouble combining groups of sentences into stories. Studies of the narrative abilities of children with language disorders have shown they routinely tell shorter stories that contain fewer story grammar elements and that are less coherent than the stories of typically developing children. As you might imagine, difficulties with narration interfere with socialization and with the development of literacy.

Literacy

Learning how to read is probably the most important achievement during the primary grade years. Children are taught how to decode words in kindergarten and first grade. Instruction in second grade is usually designed to make decoding skills more automatic. Beginning in third grade, the primary emphasis of instruction changes to the ability to use reading as a tool for learning. As we noted earlier, reading and writing are language tasks. Many school-age children with language disorders have literacy-learning problems.

Recall that children begin to think about their own language at about the time they enter kindergarten. This ability is called **metalinguistic awareness.** One aspect of metalinguistic awareness, called **phonological awareness,** has been shown to be critical for literacy development. Phonological awareness is the ability to identify the phoneme structure of words. For example, children can tell you that the word *light* starts with the sound /l/. Unfortunately, many children with language disorders have difficulties with phonological awareness, and these difficulties interfere with their ability to learn to read.

Secondary Grades (6–12)

Subject-Specific Vocabulary

We explained in Chapter 2 that children's vocabularies expand dramatically during the school-age years. Much of this expansion relates to the acquisition of subject-specific vocabulary in subject areas such as mathematics, social studies, and the sciences. Many students with language disorders have difficulty understanding and remembering subject-specific vocabulary, and this difficulty contributes to school failure. Therefore, SLPs who work with adolescents with language disorders often help these children acquire the vocabulary they need in order to succeed in their courses.

Expository Texts

Adolescents become adept at the rhetorical conventions of argument and persuasion. These skills require them to present information about persons, facts, and dates, and to provide specific details, generalizations, and conclusions. Children encounter these same forms of discourse, called **expository texts,** in their academic textbooks. Students with language disorders frequently have difficulties understanding the expository texts they must read for their courses. They also have difficulties creating the kinds of expository texts that are needed to complete assignments for class such as book reports, essays, and term papers. These difficulties often contribute to school failure.

Metacognitive Strategies

Adolescents learn to employ strategies for learning school subjects. Throughout the elementary school years, teachers support students as they learn the fundamentals of reading, writing, and mathematical computation. During the middle and high school years, there is a greater expectation for independence in academic learning. To be academically successful, adolescents must know how to acquire, store, recall, and use knowledge from assignments that are completed outside of class.

Metacognitive strategies are effortful actions that are used to accomplish specific learning goals. For example, students may reread passages they do not understand completely, take extra notes, memorize their notes by saying them out loud, or create their own practice tests. Adolescents with language disorders often demonstrate inefficiency or even reluctance in applying these kinds of effortful learning strategies.

ASSESSMENT

The Individuals With Disabilities Education Act (IDEA) requires clinicians to follow a sequence of steps when they conduct language assessments with school-age children. When classroom teachers have concerns about a child's language ability, they must do their best to help the child in the classroom before they refer the child for special education testing. Table 18–3 lists a number of strategies that teachers can use to facilitate language development in the classroom.

If a classroom teacher tries these facilitative strategies with little success, she can refer the child for a speech and language assessment. Before any testing can begin, the child's parents must be informed of the reasons why the child was referred and the tests that will be administered. The actual assessment can only begin after the child's parents give their permission for testing.

The assessment practices for school-age children are much like the preschool language assessment practices discussed in Chapter 17. As was the case with preschoolers, the assessment of school-age children is usually conducted by a multidisciplinary assessment team. Language assessment usually includes a review of the child's records, observation of the child in the classroom setting, administration of one or two standardized tests, and the collection and analysis of language samples.

Table 18–3. Alternative Strategies That May Be Used by Classroom Teachers and Speech-Language Pathologists in Classroom Settings

Strategies

1. Simplify teacher questions.
2. Shorten teacher directions.
3. Require the child to restate teacher directions.
4. Give the child extra time to organize thoughts.
5. Give cues to assist the child in word retrieval.
6. Explain questions and instructions in greater detail.
7. Repeat the child's statements, adding grammatical markers to make them complete.
8. Ask questions that encourage the child to explain his or her answers in more detail.
9. Explain concepts in greater detail.
10. Respond positively to any verbal output from the child.
11. Provide a "buddy" to assist the child when he or she is confused.
12. Show the child how to ask for assistance and/or clarification.
13. Provide minilessons on using descriptive language.
14. Ask questions that encourage the child to make connections between new and previously taught information.
15. Teach the child to make semantic maps of stories and expository texts he or she reads.
16. Use pictures and objects while you are giving directions or explaining concepts.

Most SLPs in elementary school settings give one of two standardized tests: the *Test of Language Development–Primary: 3rd Edition* (TOLD-P:3) (Newcomer & Hammill, 1997) (there is also a version of this test for adolescents) or the *Clinical Evaluation of Language Fundamentals: 3rd Edition* (CELF-3) (Semel, Wilig, & Secord, 1996). Recall from Chapters 2 and 17 that SLPs usually evaluate language comprehension and language expression. Volume 2 of the CD-ROM that accompanies this book contains examples of two subtests from the TOLD-P:3 *(Test of Language Development–Primary: 3rd Edition)* that are used for assessing comprehension and production.

 CD-ROM

Standardized Testing

Volume 2 of the CD-ROM contains two segments that show standardized testing. In segment Ch.18.02, a speech-language pathologist (SLP) is administering the Grammatic Understanding subtest of the TOLD-P:3 to an 8-year-old girl. The task requires the child to listen to the sentence that LaVae says and then point to the picture on the page that best represents the sentence. This is a test of the ability to comprehend and remember sentences (an aspect of language form).

Segment Ch.18.03 shows the same SLP administering the Grammatic Completion subtest of the TOLD-P:3. In this task, the SLP says a sentence or two but leaves off the last word. This is called a **cloze** task. For example, she says, "Carla has a dress. Denise has a dress. They have two _____." If the child knows the plural morpheme -*s*, she should answer, "dresses." This task assesses language production (expressive language).

By far, the most critical aspect of a speech and language evaluation is the language sample. When they are assessing a school-age child, SLPs usually converse with the child for about 20 minutes, then they have the child tell a story. One common procedure for collecting a narrative sample is to ask children to narrate a wordless picture book like Mayer's (1969) *Frog Where Are You?* The child tells a story that corresponds to a series of pictures. This sampling procedure is useful for eliciting complex sentences and literate language forms from children.

The CD-ROM video segment Ch.18.01 shows part of a language sample that was collected from Jennifer, an 8-year-old girl with specific language impairment. Video segment Ch.02.01 (contained on CD-ROM Volume 1) shows five children who are narrating *Frog Where Are You?* Clinicians record the samples of conversation and narration and write down everything the child says. This written record is called a **transcript.** A transcript of a conversation is provided in the CD box "Mazes and Complex Sentences." The transcript of the narration is provided in Chapter 2 in CD-ROM box "Speech Sound Acquisition." Clinicians can tell where children are in the language development process by analyzing the length and types of their utterances. Clinicians also look for patterns of language form, content, and use errors.

Assessment practices with adolescents are similar. In their language evaluations of adolescents, most clinicians administer at least one standardized test and collect a language sample. Formal tests usually provide a gross estimate of general language functioning in comparison to other children who are the same age as the child who is being assessed. Informal assessments are usually more informative for evaluating the adolescent's content-specific vocabulary knowledge, use of expository texts, and metacognitive strategies.

In addition to our testing and language sampling, we often include an interactive assessment procedure in our evaluations of adolescents. In our interactive assessment, we attempt to teach the child a history or science lesson. For example, we recently taught one student about the Santa Fe Expedition. We read a passage from a textbook aloud, asked the student to summarize it aloud, then conversed with the student about what we just read and how she might go about studying this information on her own. After we asked a few questions about the content of the material that was read, we reread the passage and asked the child to summarize it again. We evaluated the amount of content-specific vocabulary that was used, the amount of change in the child's ability to elaborate on details during her summary, and the child's ability to plan an effective study strategy.

INTERVENTION

Over the years, clinicians have used a variety of procedures to promote language development in children with language disorders. Recall from Chapter 17 that some of the primary types of facilitative interactions with preschoolers include imitation, modeling, expansion, focused stimulation (including milieu teaching), and growth-relevant recasts. These types of facilitative interactions can be used to teach different kinds of intervention targets to school-age children as well. However, there are two types of language intervention that are used quite often with children in the primary and secondary grades. These intervention procedures are called **literature-based language intervention** and **classroom collaboration.** We will discuss some general principles of language intervention with school-age children, then we will describe literature-based language intervention and classroom collaboration.

General Principles of Language Intervention With School-Age Children

Language intervention with school-age children can be conducted individually or in groups. In school settings, most language intervention is provided in groups. There are theoretical and practical reasons for intervening in group contexts. Theoretically, there may be a benefit to socially mediated peer interactions. On a practical level, groups are scheduled simply to accommodate the need to see a greater number of children.

The clinician's primary job is to mediate language learning through social interaction. The idea is that children who experience cognitive and linguistic activities in social situations will come to internalize them gradually over time. First, the child and the clinician work together, with the clinician doing most of the work and serving as a model. As the child acquires some degree of skill, the clinician cedes the child responsibility for the activity. Gradually, the child takes more of the initiative, and the adult serves primarily to provide support and help when the child experiences problems. Eventually, the child internalizes the language that is necessary to complete the activity successfully and becomes capable of performing the activities independently. Gillam and van Kleeck (1996) suggested that intervention should primarily focus on social-interactive and academic uses of language in pragmatically relevant situations. There are many intervention activities that benefit both memory and language. New clinicians should keep the following language intervention principles in mind as they plan and conduct activities.

Promote Attention

Recall from Chapter 16 that individuals with various kinds of language disorders evidence difficulties with attention. Learners process information more quickly after they have activated relevant information in long-term memory. Second, language learning is enhanced when learners selectively attend to the most critical information. Clinicians can mediate preparatory attention in adolescents by explaining what they plan to work on and why it is important. Clinicians can mediate selective attention by making the intervention models as clear as possible and by limiting distractions. For example, Ellis Weismer and Hesketh (1998) reported that children learned to produce novel words that clinicians had emphatically stressed better than novel words that had been produced with regular stress. These authors concluded that the emphatic stress helped direct the children's selective attention to new information to be learned.

Speak Clearly and Slowly

Speech perception and speed of cognitive processing contribute to learning language. Some children with developmental language disorders have difficulties perceiving and understanding rapidly produced speech. As noted by Ellis Weismer (1996), when clinicians slow their rates of speech, they provide learners with more time for processing, encoding, storage, and retrieval.

Plan Activities Around Topics or Concepts That Are Familiar to the Learner

Greater prior knowledge enables learners to attend more carefully to new information, which leads to better language learning. Clinicians who want to teach new language forms or new communicative functions should make optimal use of the learner's prior knowledge. For example, an 8-year-old boy with a language impairment might be interested in the World Wrestling Federation, and he might know a great deal about the wrestlers. If he had trouble with subject-verb agreement, it would make sense for the SLP to use growth-relevant recasts while talking to this child about wrestling and to work on writing and revising sentences contained in stories or reports on wrestling events.

Help Learners Organize New Knowledge

Learners can remember much more information when they have organized their knowledge meaningfully. For example, people struggle to recall 20 randomly presented letters, but they can easily remember sixty or eighty letters when the letters are part of words that comprise sentences. Following the same logic, it makes sense to help learners organize new knowledge in ways that facilitate recall. Practice with paraphrasing sentences and paragraphs from expository texts can help learners in the elementary grades use their own prior knowledge, vocabulary, and language structures to organize new information. Adolescents can be taught learning strategies that help them organize and recall information contained in their textbooks.

Provide Learners With Retention Cues

Clinicians need to build bridges between what they are teaching and learners' knowledge and expectations. Clinician questions, summaries, drawings, and pictures can be internalized by learners as recall cues. Recall cues provided by clinicians, parents, or teachers can be powerful. Children who are given retention cues during language intervention activities learn more than children who do not receive extra cues.

We have just discussed some general suggestions for conducting language intervention activities with school-age children. We now turn to an explanation of two specific language intervention approaches that are often used with children in the primary and secondary grades.

 CD-ROM

Language Intervention

CD-ROM segment Ch.18.04 shows an SLP conducting a langauge intervention lesson with an 11-year-old boy named Trey. Trey has been diagnosed with autism. The clinician and Trey are working on an activity that has been designed to promote problem solving and explanatory language. What types of language facilitation techniques does the clinician use to assist Trey when he encounters difficulty?

Literature-Based Language Intervention

Many clinicians use book discussions as the primary context for intervention. This type of intervention has been shown to be helpful for spoken language, listening, reading, and writing (Gillam, 1995; Gillam, McFadden, & van Kleeck, 1995). In this approach, activities that facilitate semantics, syntax, morphology, narration, and phonological awareness are centered around a common theme that is introduced in a story. Activities usually include pre-reading discussions about concepts that are contained in the books, reading and rereading the story on a number of occasions, retelling the story, and conducting various language activities, called minilessons, that are related to the story that was read, writing parallel stories, and discussing related books. Clinicians who believe that children need to learn language within natural contexts tend to use facilitative interactions (focused stimulation, modeling, recasting, and others listed in Chapter 17) as part of all their interactions with children.

Classroom Collaboration

Many SLPs who work in public school settings are beginning to conduct language intervention in the regular classroom. Usually, clinicians try to integrate their language-learning goals (complex sentence usage, narrative abilities, phonological awareness, vocabulary, expository texts, learning strategies, etc.) into the curriculum. This is done to make language intervention more functional for children. Sometimes, SLPs and classroom teachers work together to plan and carry out language-learning activities with the whole class. For example, some SLPs conduct minilessons on creating narratives with the whole class. The SLP will put up an overhead that contains a story like, "Once there was a whale. He swam. Then he got sick. Then he got better." The SLP and the class might work together to make this kind of story more complex and complete. Children suggest changes, and the SLP writes them on the overhead. Then, the class votes on the changes they like best, and they construct new sentences with the SLP's help. The SLP may repeat this overhead editing process two or three times until the class has a story they are all proud of.

Some SLPs work with small groups of students in the classroom. For example, van Kleeck, Gillam, and McFadden (1998) described a language intervention procedure in which they conducted phonological awareness activities with small groups of prekindergarten and kindergarten children as part of their center time. Children worked on rhyming and phoneme awareness activities in their "sound center" three times each week for 10-minute periods. The whole class rotated through the sound center on the same schedule that they rotated through other centers that were available in the classroom. At the end of the year, these children were better at phonological awareness activities than a comparison group of first graders who had been in these same classrooms 1 or 2 years before.

Finally, SLPs often consult with teachers about language intervention activities that can be conducted in the classroom. They might suggest language intervention procedures that the teacher can carry out as part of the regular classroom day. The teacher is responsible for actually conducting the activities. Classroom teachers have many responsibilities that they need to worry about. Asking them to act as a "speech and language clinician" in addition to their other duties is asking a lot. For this reason, collaborative teaching or small group activities within classrooms are usually preferred over consultation approaches.

SUMMARY

This chapter was about language disorders and language intervention with school-age children. The Individuals With Disabilities Act requires states to provide children with a free, appropriate public education in the least restrictive environment. Parents must be notified whenever children are to be tested for a language disorder, and they must be part of the decision-making team after testing.

Children with language disorders who are in the primary grades often have difficulties understanding and producing complex sentences, with narrative development, and with the phonological awareness abilities that support literacy development. Children with language disorders who are in the secondary grades often have difficulties with content-specific vocabulary, expository texts, and metacognitive learning strategies.

Speech-language pathologists (SLPs) assess these language abilities with the use of standardized tests and informal assessment procedures such as language sample analysis, narrative analysis, and interactive learning assessment practices. They use many of the same language-facilitation techniques that were explained in Chapter 17 in intervention with school-age children. Clinicians who work with school-age children also use literature-based intervention procedures and classroom collaboration.

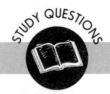

STUDY QUESTIONS

---

1 What aspects of language development are especially difficult for school-age children with language disorders in the primary and secondary grades?

---

2 What is the difference between a learning disability, a language disorder, and dyslexia?

---

3 Describe what a maze is. Give an example of a series of mazes within a complex sentence.

---

4 What is the difference between Section 504 and IDEA?

---

5 What is an IEP?

6 What procedures are commonly used to assess language disorders in school-age children?

7 What are three types of classroom collaboration?

REFERENCES

Aram, D. M., & Hall, N. E. (1989). Longitudinal follow-up of children with preschool communication disorders: Treatment implications. *School Psychology Review, 18*(4), 487–501.

Bishop, D. V. M. (1997). *Uncommon understanding: Development and disorders of language comprehension in children.* Hove, England: Psychology Press/Erlbaum (UK) Taylor & Francis.

Catts, H. W., & Kamhi, A. G. (1999). *Language and reading disabilities.* Needham Heights, MA: Allyn & Bacon.

Ellis Weismer, S. (1996). Capacity limitations in working memory: The impact on lexical and morphological learning by children with language impairment. *Topics in Language Disorders, 17*(1), 33–44.

Ellis Weismer, S., & Hesketh, L. (1998). The impact of emphatic stress on novel word learning by children with specific language impairment. *Journal of Speech, Language, and Hearing Research, 41,* 1444–1458.

Gillam, R. B. (1995). Whole language principles at work in language intervention. In D. Tibbits (Ed.), *Language intervention: Beyond the primary grades* (pp. 219–256). Austin, TX: Pro-Ed.

Gillam, R. B., & Carlile, R. M. (1997). Oral reading and story retelling of students with specific language impairment. *Language, Speech, and Hearing Services in Schools, 28,* 30–42.

Gillam, R. B., & Johnston, J. R. (1992). Spoken and written language relationships in language/learning-impaired and normally achieving school-age children. *Journal of Speech & Hearing Research, 35*(6), 1303–1315.

Gillam, R. B., McFadden, T., & van Kleeck, A. (1995). Improving the narrative abilities of children with language disorders: Whole language and language skills approaches. In M. Fey, J. Windsor, & J. Reichle (Eds.), *Communication intervention for school-age children* (pp. 145–182). Baltimore, MD: Paul H. Brookes.

Gillam, R.B., & van Kleeck, A. (1996). Phonological awareness training and short-term working memory: Clinical implications. *Topics in Language Disorders, 17*(1), 72–81.

Lyon, R. (1995). Toward a definition of dyslexia. *Annals of Dyslexia, 4,* 3–30.

Mayer, M. (1969). *Frog, where are you?* New York: Penguin Books.

Newcomer, P. L., & Hammill, D. D. (1997). *Test of Language Development–Primary* (3rd ed.). Austin, TX: Pro-Ed.

Paul, R., Hernandez, R., Taylor, L., & Johnson, K. (1996). Narrative development in late talkers: Early school age. *Journal of Speech & Hearing Research, 39,* 1295–1303.

Paul, R., Murray, C., Clancy, K., & Andrews, D. (1997). Reading and metaphonological outcomes in late talkers.

Journal of Speech Language & Hearing Research, 40, 1037–1047.

Records, N. L., Tomblin, J. B., & Buckwalter, P. R. (1995). Auditory verbal learning and memory in young adults with specific language impairment. *Clinical Neuropsychologist, 9,* 187–193.

Semel, E., Wiig, E., & Secord, W. (1996). *Clinical evaluation of language fundamentals.* (3rd ed.). San Antonio: TX: Psychological Corporation.

Stothard, S. E., Snowling, M. J., Bishop, D. V. M., Chipchase, B. B., & Kaplan, C. A. (1998). Language-impaired preschoolers: A follow-up into adolescence. *Journal of Speech Language & Hearing Research, 41,* 407–418.

U.S. Department of Education. (1997). *To assure the free appropriate public education of all Americans: Nineteenth annual report to Congress on the implementation of the Individuals with Disabilities Education Act.* (Publication No. 1997-616-188/90444). Washington, DC: U. S. Government Printing Office.

van Kleeck, A., Gillam, R., & McFadden, T. U. (1998). A study of classroom-based phonological awareness training for preschoolers with speech and/or language disorders. *American Journal of Speech-Language Pathology, 7,* 66–77.

SUGGESTED READINGS

Catts, H. W., & Kamhi, A. G. (Eds.). (1999). *Language and reading disabilities.* Boston, MA: Allyn and Bacon.

Duchan, J. F. (1995). *Supporting language learning in everyday life.* San Diego: Singular Publishing Group.

Fey, M. E., Windsor, J., & Warren, S. F. (Eds.). (1995). *Language intervention: Preschool through the elementary years.* Baltimore, MD: Paul H. Brookes.

Leonard, L. B. (1998). *Children with specific language impairment.* Cambridge, MA: MIT Press.

Naremore, R. C., Densmore, A. E., & Harman, D. R. (1995). *Language intervention with school-age children: Conversation, narrative, and text.* San Diego: Singular Publishing Group.

Nelson, N. W. (1993). *Childhood language disorders in context: Infancy through adolescence* (2nd ed.). Needham Heights, MA: Allyn and Bacon.

Nippold, M. A. (1998). *Later language development: The school-age and adolescent years* (2nd ed.). Austin, TX: Pro-Ed. Paul, R. (1995). *Language disorders: From infancy through adolescence.* St. Louis, MO: Mosby.

Wallach, G. P., & Butler, K. G. (Eds.). (1994). *Language learning disabilities in school-age children and adolescents: Some principles and applications.* New York: Merrill.

Chronological age referencing: The diagnosis of language disorder is accomplished by comparing a child's language ability to the language abilities that are expected for children his or her chronological age.

Classroom collaboration: Speech-language pathologists and classroom teachers work together to provide language intervention within the regular classroom setting.

Discrepancy modeling: The determination of a learning disability is based on a significant discrepancy between a child's IQ score (a measure of ability) and their scores on measures of achievement in the areas of speaking, listening, reading, writing, reasoning, and/or mathematics.

Dyslexia: A language-based disorder characterized by difficulties in decoding words during reading. The child's reading problems usually reflect insufficient phonological processing.

Expository texts: The language of academic textbooks. This type of language is used to teach or explain new information.

Individuals With Disabilities Education Act (IDEA): The federal law that provides federal funding for special education and regulates special education procedures.

Learning disability: A significant difficulty with the acquisition and use of one or more of the following abilities: listening, speaking, reading, writing, reasoning, mathematical computation or mathematical problem solving.

Literature-based language intervention: An approach to language intervention in which all the language therapy activities are related to a children's book.

Maze: A repetition, a false start, or a reformulation of a sentence.

Metacognitive strategies: Effortful actions that are used to learn new information (e.g., reading something twice, highlighting information in a textbook, making outlines that coincide with your notes from class, etc.).

Metalinguistic awareness: Overt thinking about one's language knowledge. One aspect of metalinguistic awareness, called phonological awareness, has been shown to be critical for literacy development.

Phonological awareness: A type of metalinguistic awareness. Phonological awareness is the ability to identify the phoneme structure of words (e.g., *ball* begins with a /b/).

Public Law 94-142, the Education of All Handicapped Children Act of 1975: The first law that guaranteed a free appropriate public education in the least restrictive environment to all children with disabilities and that provided funding for special education activities.

Transcript: A written record of the language that was used during a language sample.

Section 504: A law passed in 1973 that prohibited public schools from discriminating against children with disabilities in any way.

19

Acquired Neurogenic Language Disorders

Thomas P. Marquardt

LEARNING OBJECTIVES

1 To learn the primary causes of brain damage that result in communication disorders in adults.

---

2 To learn why the site of brain damage influences the type of language disorder.

---

3 To understand the social and emotional consequences of neurogenic communication disorders.

---

4 To learn differences between types of aphasia.

---

5 To understand the recovery of the brain after if has been damaged.

INTRODUCTION

As we explained in Chapter 2, there are some speech, language, and cognitive disorders that result from damage to the nervous system. The anatomy and functions of the nervous system that relate to language were described in Chapters 9 and 16. The disorders considered in this chapter are called neurogenic because they involve impairment of the nervous system. Damage to the nervous system results in different types of communication disorders depending on the site and extent of the lesion and the underlying cause. The disorders are termed *acquired* because they result from brain injury that disrupts otherwise normal communicative skills.

Although we will focus primarily on neurogenic communication disorders, it is important to note that injury to the nervous system frequently affects every aspect of the individual's life. The combined impact of paralysis of one side of the body, vision problems, and communication difficulties make everyday activities difficult and frustrating. Showering, dressing, and brushing teeth, once carried out with ease, become challenging obstacles to be conquered each day. A communication disorder is only one consequence of damage to the nervous system that the individual must face. In this chapter, we discuss the causes of brain injury, the consequences of the damage, and the role of the speech-language pathologist (SLP) in helping the individual regain success in everyday communication situations.

Causes of Brain Damage

There are four primary causes of brain damage that can affect communication: stroke, head injury, infections and growths, and progressive degeneration of the central nervous system. The effects of these disease processes on communication will depend on whether the left, right, or both sides of the brain are involved.

The most frequent cause of brain damage is a **cerebrovascular accident (CVA)** or stroke. Strokes can result from an **embolus,** a moving clot from another part of body that lodges in the artery, or a **thrombosis,** which occurs when an artery has gradually filled in with plaque. Both types of stroke result in the closing of an artery, which leads to the deprivation of oxygen **(anoxia)** to an area of the brain, with subsequent death of the tissue **(infarct).** A stroke may be preceded by a **transient ischemic attack (TIA),** a temporary closing of the artery with symptoms that generally disappear within 24 hours. **Hemorrhages** are another type of stroke that involves bleeding in the brain. A common cause of a hemorrhage is a ruptured **aneurysm,** a weakening in the artery that bulges and eventually breaks, interrupting blood flow to tissues fed by the artery.

The prevalence and morbidity vary for each of the etiologies of stroke. Thromboses occur more frequently than hemorrhages, but individuals with thrombosis are more likely to survive the stroke. Strokes occur most often in the elderly as the blood vessels of the brain become blocked and brittle due to arteriosclerosis.

The effects of a stroke are immediate. The individual may lose consciousness, have difficulty speaking, and be paralyzed on the side of the body opposite the hemisphere of the brain that was damaged. Typically, these effects are most prominent during the first 3 to 5 days after the stroke and are related to swelling of brain tissue **(edema)** and reductions in blood flow. After this period, there is a recovery of function **(spontaneous recovery)** associated with a reduction in edema, a return to more normal blood flow, and a reorganization of nervous system processes. Recovery generally is better if the brain damage is small and the stroke occurs at a young age.

A second cause of brain damage is head injury, which can result from any significant blow to the head. Injuries to the head that cause brain trauma occur most often in the young (16–24 years old) who are involved in motor vehicle accidents. Other causes include falls and being struck on the head. Head injuries are generally classified as open brain trauma or closed head injury. In open brain trauma, the integrity of the skull is damaged and underlying brain tissue is destroyed. For example, a gunshot wound to the head damages the skull and the underlying brain tissue through which the bullet has passed.

Nervous system damage occurs as a result of closed head injury when the force of the blow causes the brain to twist, turn, and push against the skull. Several types of damage may occur when the skull is struck but not penetrated. The surface of the cortex is bruised **(contusion)**, with disruption of mental functions **(concussion)**, pathways connecting different parts of the central nervous system are torn, and a twisting of the head results in damage to the brainstem. The contusion may involve both sides of the brain because, when struck, the brain surface is deflected off the interior of the skull on the opposite side. Coupled to this damage may be hemorrhages within the brain (intracerebral) or within the tissue coverings (meninges) that form **hematomas** (areas of encapsulated blood).

Head injuries can range from mild to severe depending on the force of the impact and the amount of brain tissue affected. Missile wounds, such as gunshots, may affect a very specific area of the brain. Damage sustained in a motorcycle accident will generally affect many different parts. The greater the severity and extent of the injury, the more that motoric, cognitive, and communication skills will be affected. In severe head injury, the individual may be comatose and not remember the incident at all when he or she recovers. The length of time the person is in a coma varies, but it is usually longer when the brain trauma is more severe.

Additional causes of damage to the nervous system are space-occupying growths within the skull and infections. **Neoplasms** (new growths) and tumors, which can be malignant or benign, can occur within the interior of the brain or on the surface within the tissue coverings. These growths take up space and, depending on their type, cause destruction of brain tissue and increased pressure in the skull. When their primary effect is to take up space, the symptoms reported are dizziness, headache, memory deficits, and generalized sensory and/or motor problems. Infections, when treatable with antibiotics, may produce temporary effects, but also may produce permanent damage because they destroy areas of brain tissue.

A final cause of brain damage is progressive deterioration. The host of progressive processes that affect the nervous system include, for example, disorders such as multiple sclerosis, Parkinson's disease, and amyotrophic lateral sclerosis as well as degenerative changes in the nervous system associated with dementing diseases such as Alzheimer's disease. Progressive and ultimately global deterioration of cells in the brain lead to impaired cognitive, communicative, and motor functioning. The effects will vary depending on the rate of degeneration and the order in which specific neural structures are affected.

The types of speech, language, or cognitive disorder produced by nervous system damage are dependent on the location and size of the damage or injury. Damage to the left (dominant) hemisphere is the cause of aphasia, the primary focus of this chapter. However, significant communication disorders also result from right hemisphere lesions and from the involvement of both hemispheres in traumatic brain injury and **dementia** (the deterioration of intellectual abilities due to organic disease or brain damage).

APHASIA

Aphasia is a language disorder due to left hemisphere damage, typically resulting from a stroke. Auditory comprehension, verbal expression, and reading and writing deficits are common characteristics of the disorder. Phonology, syntax, semantics, and pragmatics can all be affected. Typically, there are some aspects of language that are more or less impaired than others. Different patterns of language deficit have led to the identification of specific types of aphasia, and the type of aphasia is generally associated with the site of lesion. For example, damage to the frontal lobe causes difficulty with language expression; lesions to the posterior portion of the hemisphere result in auditory comprehension problems. One system in wide use is based on the premise that patterns of impairment are related to the site in the brain where the lesion occurred (Goodglass & Kaplan, 1983). I will use this system to organize the overview of aphasia (see Table 19–1 later in the chapter).

Patterns of Communication Performance in Aphasia

The *Boston Diagnostic Aphasia Examination* (Goodglass & Kaplan, 1983) is used to identify patterns of impairment for this classification system. This test includes items such as picture naming, sentence repetition, yes/no questions, rhythm, writing, and repetitive movements of the speech production structures at maximum rates. Performance on the test items reflects abilities in four primary language areas: naming, fluency, auditory comprehension, and repetition. Patterns of strengths and weaknesses in these areas of communication are used to classify the type of aphasia.

 CD-ROM

A Woman With Aphasia

A woman with aphasia is shown on Volume 2 of the CD-ROM. Included are a brain scan (segment Ch.19.01) and segments that show her talking (Ch.19.02 and Ch.19.03), following instructions (Ch.19.04), and repeating phrases (Ch.19.05 and Ch.19.06). These tasks allow classification of the patient into one of the types of aphasia.

Naming

Naming is the process of knowing and retrieving the label for an object, picture, or concept. If someone were to ask you "What are you reading?" The ability to respond "A *book*" involves a complex process to identify and say the label for the object you are holding. First you access the conceptual store that identifies the item as something with a cover, lots of pages, and that you read. Next you identify a semantic label that best fits the concept you established, in this case "book." In the third step, you develop a phonological form for the label, for example, b-oo-k. Finally, your brain programs the speech movements needed to say the word.

 CD-ROM

Word-Finding Problems

CD-ROM segment Ch.19.01 is a CAT scan showing a lesion to the left frontal area of the brain. In segment Ch.19.02, Mrs. L is describing moving to Arizona. Word-finding problems are evident, but she uses compensatory strategies including describing the location of the city, gesturing, and shifting some of the communicative burden to the listener. Notice that Mrs. L's speech is nonfluent but not agrammatic. She uses fully grammatical sentences, but they are produced slowly and with some struggle.

Naming deficits can result from a problem at any stage of the process. Individuals with naming problems have difficulty naming a concept and will instead say the wrong name, say a word that is phonologically or semantically similar, use a nonsense word, or avoid giving a name. **Neologisms** are new words such as the use of *gabot* for *table*. When a nonsense word of this type is produced, there may be no awareness that it is not meaningful to the listener. Selection of an alternate for an intended word in a category, such as *lion* for *tiger,* is an example of a **verbal paraphasia;** substitution of one or more sounds in the phonological realization of the word (*gable* for *cable*) or transpositions of sound elements are called **literal paraphasias,** both of which are relatively common in aphasia. At times, the individual uses strategies to locate and produce the word **(circumlocution).** The individual describes the characteristics of the item, how it is used, and in what circumstances, but cannot name it.

Although the errors provide information on the type of naming problem, there are times when the individual may indicate that he does not know the name of the item. In this case, failure to name does not provide information on why the task cannot be carried out. It could be due to a failure in recognizing the item, difficulty retrieving the label, or an inability to access the motor program for its production.

 CD-ROM

Word Retrieval

In CD-ROM segment Ch.19.03, Mrs. L is trying to say the word *Missouri.* She retrieves the name of *Kansas City,* but she begins saying the word *Arizona.* This is an example of a perseverative response since she has just finished talking about that state. She realizes the error and chooses the strategy of orally spelling the word until the clinician produces the word *Missouri* for her.

Clinicians use various tasks to assess naming. For example, the individual is shown a picture of a chair, cactus, or spoon and is asked to name the item. He also might be asked to name all the jungle animals he can think of and words beginning with the letter *s*. The kinds of errors made on the tasks allow the clinician to determine the severity of the naming impairment and make predictions about the stage(s) in the process that have been affected by the brain damage. Naming is a complex process that may have more than a single level at which it is impaired. Naming deficits are a universally expected feature of aphasia regardless of the lesion site. Because damage to the right hemisphere and progressive global deterioration of the brain also may cause naming problems, the deficit is an indicator of a neurogenic communication disorder rather than a specific type of aphasia.

Fluency

In fluent speech, syllables are produced rhythmically, and speakers use pitch and stress variations that are appropriate to the intended meaning of the utterance. In aphasia, speech output may be nonfluent with hesitations and stops and starts, slow and effortful production, and the absence of normal pitch and stress variation. Generally, lesions to the left front area of the brain produce nonfluent speech. Lesions to the left back area (posterior to the central fissure) do not routinely interfere with speech fluency. Therefore, fluency is used as an indicator of aphasia type, tending to differentiate anterior and posterior lesion sites. There is no absolute way to decide when speech is fluent or nonfluent. Clinicians listen for unusual patterns of rhythm, rate, ease of production, and intonation (variations in pitch and stress) as individuals engage in conversation, describe pictures, give directions, and tell stories.

Auditory Comprehension

Auditory comprehension is the ability to understand spoken language, that is, words, commands, questions, or groups of utterances. Auditory comprehension is a complex process that involves being able to segment the sounds heard into meaningful phonemes, understanding the meaning of the words within the sentence, and retaining the message in memory long enough to understand it and formulate a response. The ability to understand language interacts with the ability to discriminate between words and to remember instructions. Therefore, nonperformance on a comprehension task may indicate a deficit but it does not necessarily provide an understanding of the underlying reason for the problem. Damage to areas of the left hemisphere that are posterior to the central fissure typically cause significant deficits in auditory processing. Comprehension is usually more intact in lesions in front of this landmark.

Clinicians assess auditory comprehension by asking questions, making statements, or giving commands, to which the individual must provide a

 CD-ROM

Simple and Complex Commands

CD-ROM segment Ch.19.04 demonstrates Mrs. L's ability to perform simple and complex commands without error.

response. Responses can be nonverbal in order to ensure that the individual is not limited by an inability to produce language. The individual with aphasia can be asked to point to the door or ceiling, to follow complex instructions such as placing a pencil between a cup and a spoon, and to respond to questions such as "Does a stone float?"

Repetition

Repetition of words and phrases assesses the integrity of connecting pathways between Wernicke's area of the temporal lobe and Broca's area of the frontal lobe. When asked to repeat a phrase, the task requires the individual to hear the phrase (Wernicke's area) and then organize the output for repetition (Broca's area). Damage to Broca's area or Wernicke's area will affect spontaneous production as well as repetition. However, when the major pathway (the arcuate fasciculus) between the two areas has been damaged, there is usually a marked difficulty repeating words and phrases but minimal problems with auditory comprehension or fluency.

 CD-ROM

Repetition of Short Phrases

In CD-ROM segment Ch.19.05, Mrs. L repeats short phrases with only minor articulation errors. Notice in CD-ROM segment Ch.19.06 that Mrs. L has difficulty with longer and more unusual phrases. There also is evidence of a verbal paraphasic response with a self-correction.

Classification of Aphasia

The categories of naming, fluency, auditory comprehension, and repetition provide a method for describing the symptoms of aphasia. The classification of aphasia type can be based on differences in relative impairment of naming, fluency, auditory comprehension, and repetition. We review the different types of aphasia in the next section. The system for classifying aphasia does not work for every case. A significant portion of the aphasic population (approximately 25%) cannot be reliably assigned to a specific category because their disorder includes patterns that are indicative of more than one type of aphasia. Descriptions of the different types of aphasia are listed in Table 19–1.

Broca's Aphasia

Damage to Broca's area on the posterior inferior frontal lobe (see Figure 19–1) causes a type of aphasia that is marked by difficulty with fluency. The lesion

Table 19-1. Classification of Aphasia

Type	Lesion Site	Characteristics
Broca's	Broca's area Left posterior/inferior	Nonfluent awkward verbal expression with reduced phrase length, agrammatism, and prosodic disturbance. Auditory comprehension is relatively preserved.
Wernicke's	Wernicke's area Left posterior/superior temporal	Impaired auditory comprehension with fluently produced speech marked by paraphasic errors. Reading and writing are usually severely impaired.
Conduction	Supramarginal gyrus deep to arcuate fasciculus	Repetition disproportionately impaired relative to auditory comprehension and verbal fluency. Verbal expression may be circumlocutionary with numerous literal paraphasias.
Anomic	Inferior pareital/posterior temporal	Major feature is word-finding problems in the context of fluently articulated speech and relatively preserved auditory comprehension.
Transcortical Sensory	Pareital with preservation of Wernicke's area	Severely impaired auditory comprehension and reading with spared repetition. Verbal xpression is fluent but includes paraphasias and neologisms. Severe naming problems.
Transcortical Motor	Superior frontal lobe with preservation of Broca's area	Marked absence of spontaneous speech and writing. Preserved repetition and auditory comprehension.
Global	Large area extending from frontal to temporal	Severely impaired naming, repetition, and auditory comprehension with nonfluent verbal expression that may be limited to jargon and a few words.

most frequently involves surrounding areas of the frontal lobe, including the insula, in addition to Broca's area, but may also occur below the surface of the brain in this area. Broca's aphasia is characterized by nonfluent, effortful speech and **agrammatism.** Oral expression is slow with very short sentences (3–4 words in length) that contain mostly content words (nouns and verbs). Function words such as articles, prepositions, and conjunctions are frequently omitted. The speaker's prosody is usually quite flat, meaning there is little change in stress or rate. In response to a question about what happened to cause his aphasia, a 42-year-old man responded "Shot in head. Communicate hard. Me zero talk." This type of agrammatic verbal expression is also observed in phrase repetition and in writing. Patients are usually aware of their struggle to produce speech, and they make repeated efforts to correct their errors. Auditory comprehension is relatively intact, although not entirely spared. When they are asked to follow directions that require comprehension of function words ("Put the ball *under* the box") or grammatically

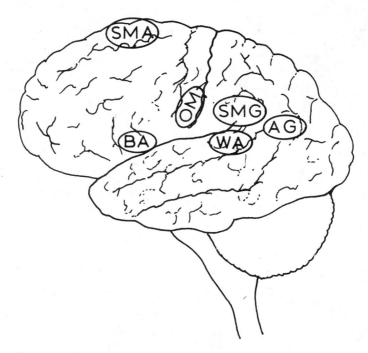

Figure 19–1. Lateral aspect of the left cerebral hemisphere, with major speech-language areas labeled. BA = Broca's area, WA = Wernicke's area, AG = angular gyrus, SMG = supramarginal gyrus, SMA = supplementary motor area, and OM = orofacial motor cortex. (From R. Kent [1977] *Speech sciences,* Figure 7-48, p. 285. San Diego: Singular Publishing Group. Used with permission.)

complex sentences ("Point to the boy who is pushing the girl"), comprehension errors are more frequent.

Wernicke's Aphasia

Damage to Wernicke's area and tissue surrounding the superior posterior temporal lobe causes a type of aphasia that is marked by deficits in auditory comprehension and fluent oral expression. Individuals with Wernicke's aphasia have marked difficulty in comprehending language, spoken or written. Sometimes, the deficit in auditory comprehension is so severe that patients cannot even identify single words. Speech output has normal intonation and stress. However, speech production is filled with verbal paraphasias (mixing up sounds in words) and neologisms (making up new words). This kind of speech may seem "empty" due to the lack of intelligible content words. Some patients are not aware their speech is not understandable, and they show little obvious concern about their problems with communication. The use of meaningless neologisms may be so frequent that speech sounds like jargon (these sequences of phonemes that sound like words were discussed in Chapter 2). For this reason, the individual is described as having **jargon aphasia.** In addition to problems with speech, reading and writing abilities are significantly affected. Repetition is impaired, and writing mirrors oral expression with the production of neologisms and paraphasias.

Conduction Aphasia

Recall from Chapter 9 that there is a group of fibers (the arcuate fasciculus) that connects Broca's area to Wernicke's area and the supramarginal gyrus. Damage to this pathway results in a type of aphasia where there is an impaired ability to "conduct" information from one part of the nervous system to another. This disconnection results in the ability to comprehend what is heard and to produce spontaneous speech, but an inability to repeat what was heard because the auditory input cannot be transmitted to the area of the brain where speech output is organized. Individuals with conduction aphasia have marked problems with repeating phrases in the context of normal auditory comprehension. Their oral expression is fluent, but it often includes frequent literal paraphasias (transpositions of sounds) due to a deficit in the ability to select and order phonological elements of words. The literal paraphasias, such as *cake* for *take,* appear in their speech and in their writing. These patients often try to correct their phonemic errors by saying the word repeatedly.

Anomic Aphasia

Anomia literally translated means "without words." The primary deficit of patients with anomic aphasia is a difficulty in retrieving the names of objects, pictures, or concepts. Auditory comprehension, verbal expression, and repetition are otherwise relatively unimpaired. Their connected speech is characterized by an absence of nouns. Patients will produce paraphasias and circumlocutions in an attempt to convey meaningful information. The site of lesion cannot be reliably inferred from these behaviors, although most physicians and clinicians suspect that the patient has suffered a posterior lesion in the temporal-parietal area. In some cases lesions elsewhere in the left hemisphere have also resulted in similar symptoms.

Transcortical Aphasia

Widespread "watershed" lesions of the frontal and temporal-parietal areas interrupt the ability to process sensory information and to program sequential skilled movements. Generally, there is widespread damage to these areas of association cortex. Wernicke's area, the arcuate fasciculus, and Broca's area are usually left intact. Transcortical aphasias are found most often in older individuals, because the nervous system damage that causes this type of aphasia results from a gradual deterioration of the blood supply at the periphery of the major arteries to the brain.

There are two types of transcortical aphasia. When the damage involves the frontal lobe, a type of aphasia termed "transcortical motor" results. Patients with this type of aphasia often have good auditory comprehension and repetition, but they have significant difficulty initiating speech production. When you ask a patient with transcortical motor aphasia a question, you will likely get a grammatically complete response. However, the response will be nonfluent. Even though this type of patient responds to questions, he or she is not assertive. That is, the patient does not ask many questions and does not add information to a conversation unless specifically asked.

When the damage involves areas of the posterior part of the brain around Wernicke's area, a type of aphasia termed "transcortical sensory" results. Patients with transcortical sensory aphasia have severe deficits in auditory comprehension. However, their speech is usually fluent and they can repeat words and sentences that are spoken to them. This combination of good repetition ability and poor comprehension results in an unusual pattern of behavior. These patients are able to repeat commands verbally, but they are unable to understand or carry them out.

Global Aphasia

When the damage to the left hemisphere is extensive enough to involve a wide area of the lateral aspect, all parts of language processing are severely impaired. Patients with global aphasia have nonfluent verbal expression, poor auditory comprehension, and difficulty repeating words and sentences. In the most severe form of global aphasia, the patient's lexicon (their bank of available vocabulary items) is reduced to a few words that are used repeatedly to respond to questions. These patients cannot even follow one-stage commands or repeat single words. Their speech output may be accompanied by gestures that are not meaningfully employed for communication.

ASSESSMENT AND DIAGNOSIS OF APHASIA

Immediately following brain injury, when language ability is most impaired and variable, the speech-language pathologist (SLP) observes and interacts with the patient to determine the level of impairment in verbal expression, auditory comprehension, repeating, reading, and naming. This assessment is usually conducted while the patient is recovering in the hospital. When conducting the assessment, the SLP usually employs informal tasks to evaluate language skill, such as engaging the patient in conversation, asking the patient to name items located in the hospital room, and asking the patient to follow simple commands. During the first few weeks following brain injury, there is a period referred to as "spontaneous recovery." This is a period of significant changes that occur from day to day as the nervous system recovers and reorganizes. The patient's communication during this period is variable and is affected by fatigue, medical complications, and medications. The SLP's role is to make a preliminary determination of the type and extent of aphasia and to serve as a resource for the patient and the family. Of particular importance at this point is the provision of information to the patient and family about the effects of stroke and the development of a functional communication system for the patient.

A more formal assessment that includes administration of an aphasia test battery is conducted when the patient becomes more stable. The *Boston Diagnostic Aphasia Examination* (Goodglass & Kaplan, 1983), the *Porch Index of Communicative Ability* (Porch, 1967), and the *Western Aphasia Examination* (Kertesz, 1982) are three examples of comprehensive aphasia batteries. Each test contains tasks that assess reading, writing, auditory comprehension, naming and other language abilities. The batteries are supplemented by informal procedures that are developed by the SLP to provide a more complete picture of the patient's language processing abilities. Results from these assessment tasks are placed in the context of other information about the patient's medical, educational, and family history to arrive at a differential diagnosis, that is, a labeling of the language deficit pattern. The diagnosis is valuable to the extent that there are treatment programs proven to be most effective for particular disorders.

The SLP also assesses functional communication skills or the ability to communicate meaning in familiar contexts regardless of the quality of the spoken language. It has been long observed that individuals with aphasia communicate more effectively than one might expect given their poor performance on formal language tests. Aphasics often use compensatory skills like gesturing, intonation, facial expression, and writing to supplement residual verbal expression and to facilitate communication success. Functional measures like the *Functional Communication Scale* (Sarno, 1969) and assessments based on role-playing as in the *Communicative Abilities in Daily Living* (Holland, 1980) test are often used to estimate the individual's ability to communicate in everyday situations.

Motoric, visual, and cognitive deficits commonly associated with aphasia may complicate the assessment process. When there is damage to the frontal lobe, a **hemiplegia** (muscle weakness or paralysis) is often observed on the side of the body opposite from the side of the brain damage. A motoric impairment may make it difficult for a patient to follow commands. Vision may also be affected because of interruption in the visual pathways between the optic chiasm and the visual processing areas of the occipital lobe. An example of a visual problem that accompanies some aphasias is **homonymous hemianopsia,** which is a loss of one half of the visual field on the side opposite the brain hemisphere that was damaged. A homonymous hemianopia may make it difficult for a patient to see objects in order to name them or point to them, or it may impair reading. Cognitive deficits such as a decreased ability to remember or maintain attention can co-occur with aphasia. The ability to follow commands, answer questions, and repeat phrases are all dependent on the ability to attend to and remember what was heard. A clinician conducting a speech and language assessment must also be aware of how the patient's response is influenced by these nonlinguistic variables. An inability to follow a command because it cannot be remembered must be treated differently from an inability to remember a command because the words are not understood

 CD-ROM

Patterns of Performance

Review the brain scan and CD-ROM segments for Ms. L again. Note that her diagnosis is based on the pattern of communication abilities/disabilities.

Case Study: Mrs. L

Mrs. L, age 68 years, incurred a left hemisphere cerebrovascular accident when she was 65 years old (see Figure 19–2). Computerized transaxial tomog-

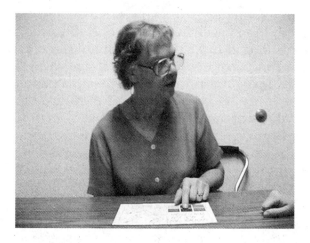

Figure 19–2. Patient with aphasia responding to pictures.

raphy (better known as a CT scan) revealed a subcortical lesion involving the left middle cerebral artery in the basal ganglia. As a result of the stroke, Mrs. L had a nonfluent aphasia, minimal comprehension deficits, and a right hemiparesis. Results from the *Boston Diagnostic Aphasia Examination* 3 years postonset of brain damage showed mild to moderate problems in auditory comprehension and repetition and in reading and writing skills. Mrs. L's word finding and articulation were the most impaired areas of communication. An SLP administered a measure of functional communication, the *Communicative Abilities in Daily Living* (Holland, 1980). This test revealed minimally reduced functional communication abilities with mild difficulty with memory, word finding, and interpreting nonliteral situations and incongruous language.

Based on the assessment, Mrs. L was diagnosed as having mild Broca's aphasia. Her auditory comprehension was minimally impaired, but her speech production was nonfluent, with word-finding problems and difficulty on more demanding repetition tasks. Mrs. L had an excellent recovery, which was anticipated because she was highly motivated, the lesion was small, and therapy for this type of aphasia is usually quite effective.

THE TREATMENT OF APHASIA

Assessment provides the basis for treatment by identifying the type and severity of aphasia and a general picture of the communication tasks the patient can perform. Speech-language pathologists may provide aphasia treatment in individual or group therapy sessions. The initial goal is to provide the patient with a reliable communication system. Just like language intervention with young children, intervention with adults who have aphasia must begin at the level of communication ability of the person. In the case of severe aphasia, intervention activities may target the production of single words or the use of some gestures. In the case of less severe aphasia, intervention activities may target oral expression abilities, reading, and/or writing. There are two primary goals in therapy: maximizing language abilities and developing compensatory communication strategies.

Individual and Group Therapy

Methods used in individual therapy for aphasia are based on the type and severity of aphasia, communication needs of the patient, associated medical problems, and the kind of environment the patient will return to after treatment. Treatment programs can be constructed specifically to meet particular problems in oral expression, auditory comprehension, reading, writing, and discourse. However, the most fundamental purpose of the intervention is to empower the patient to communicate successfully in everyday communication situations. Therefore, an early step in the process is to explore communication needs in everyday settings, such as making telephone calls, buying groceries, or communicating personal needs to a spouse. Treatment then focuses on improving the ability to communicate in those settings in which the patient has not been successful.

Communicative settings are complex, and a patient is unlikely to be initially successful at all aspects of the interaction. To help the patient learn the targeted communication skills, treatment programs for aphasics are usually constructed on a difficulty hierarchy. Treatment must be structured to allow the patient to be successful with one step of the process at a time, beginning with the easier steps. If the patient is anomic, an SLP may start with helping the patient develop strategies for saying concrete, single words *(drink, doctor)* because they are easier. The clinician will then help the patient apply the strategies for saying the words in phrases, then sentences, and finally in conversation. In addition to structuring therapy hierarchically, clinicians also use cues and prompts to foster successful responding. Cues and prompts are techniques that give the patient a clue to help access the target information without giving him the answer. For example, the patient is shown a picture of a banana and is asked to name it. The patient responds, "It's uhh it's uhhh, uhhh, umm, you eat it it's uhh yellow." The communication partner can then provide a cue or prompt. She may put her lips together to indicate that the word starts with a "b" (providing the first articulatory position), may say "b" (phonemic cue), say "It's a kind of fruit" (semantic cue), or say "This skinny yellow fruit you peel is a . . . ." (sentence cue). The clinician does not say "banana" but gives clues to help the patient find the word he is struggling to produce. Note that when cues and prompts are used by the clinician, she is taking some of the burden for communicating off the patient and is carrying an increased portion of the communication load. Reduction in the use of cues requires the patient to communicate with a greater degree of independence and returns the process to a more balanced interaction.

One goal of therapy is to fade the use of cues and prompts to facilitate independent and successful communication. The use and fading of cues and prompts can be used effectively regardless of the aspect of language targeted for intervention: naming, reading, auditory comprehension, articulation, and so forth.

Many SLPs teach compensatory communication strategies during aphasia therapy. Compensatory strategies involve the use of specific techniques to compensate for the communication deficit rather than changing a specific speech or language skill. Problem-solving strategies can be employed to communicate necessary information by use of alternative modalities (e.g., writing or gesturing) or finding ways to work around the specific problem. Devon, a young man with Broca's aphasia due to a gunshot wound to the head, provides a good example of a person who was taught communication strategies to compensate for his speech and language difficulties. Devon was unable to say is address. When someone asked him where he lived, he was taught to remove his wallet and to use his drivers license to provide the necessary information. Another strategy was to use related words when he could not think of the exact word that he wanted to say. For example, when Devon was asked where he had been on vacation, he said "Volcano. Diamond Head. Black sand." to which the interviewer responded with "Hawaii." Devon could spell words that he could not say, so he was encouraged to use spelling as a communication strategy. For example, in discussing his hobbies, Devon was not able to indicate verbally what he collected. He then spelled "s-t-a-m-p-s" in the air with his finger. In each of these cases, Devon used an alternative strategy for providing information. His communication was slower, but his alternative strategies enabled Devon to be a responsive communicator.

Improving communication skills can also be addressed in group therapy. Group sessions are often used for practicing communication skills in a non-threatening and supportive environment. When three or four individuals with aphasia meet together with an SLP, they have an opportunity to use their own regained communication skills and to observe the kinds of communication strategies that are used by other members of the group. Topics for discussion are chosen by the group, such as the best sites to visit in the city, how I met my spouse, hobbies, and places traveled to on vacations. Although an SLP leads the group, the focus is on helping individuals with aphasia to communicate with each other, demonstrating communication strategies in a supportive environment.

Family Participation in Therapy

Group therapy can also be an opportunity for individuals and their families to engage in open discussion of the consequences of stroke and positive strategies for dealing with everyday problems they encounter. Meetings of this type are helpful because aphasia affects the family as well as the patient and there are important changes in family responsibilities and interactions. Waisenen (1998), in interviews with wives of stroke patients about changes in their lives, reported the following comments:

> "I have to do everything that (my husband) used to do, because he really can't do much of anything around the house."

> "He's like three different people, like three personalities. He's his old self, he is childish, and at times he even acts retarded. But these things pass, and they're not him. Basically he's his sweet gentle self."

> "My circle of friends are the same, his are not. I learned early on that the men drop off. They don't come to see him; they don't check on him. I think they don't want to put themselves in his place."

There is a reorganizational change that takes place in the family. There are feelings of loss, anger, and grief as the patient and family recover from the changes caused by the stroke. Spouses who have not worked outside the home now may be the primary wage earners. Some old friendships wither, and new ones are made as the patient and family change to meet the challenges brought about by brain injury. One aspect of therapy directed by the clinician is to assist the family in developing new ways to communicate effectively and devising strategies for improving the patient's ability to communicate meaningfully.

RIGHT HEMISPHERE COMMUNICATION DEFICITS

Aphasia, as we discussed, results from neurological damage to the left hemisphere of the brain. The left hemisphere is generally considered to house the neuroanatomical structures associated with the form and content of language. Damage to the right hemisphere also affects the communication process in aspects related to language use rather than form or content. Aspects of communication dependent on the functioning of the right hemisphere can be broadly considered within the following areas, which will be addressed in detail: affective processing, comprehension of indirect meanings, and the structuring of conversational and narrative discourse.

An important aspect of communication is the ability to interpret the emotion that overlays the spoken word. Emotion is generally conveyed through facial expressions and changes in intonation. Patients with right hemisphere damage often have difficulty conveying emotion through facial expression and prosody. There is sometimes a reduced sensitivity to displays of emotion in others as well. An individual with right hemisphere damage will fail to understand the angry tone behind a statement like, "Thanks for forgetting to pick me up after work," and interpret it based on the words as a genuine expression of gratitude. An inability to interpret the underlying emotion can result in misinterpretation of the message.

The right hemisphere seems to be involved in the ability to produce the "big picture" from the details. Individuals with right hemisphere damage often see the details but are unable to understand the broader meaning they represent. They also have difficulty interpreting nonliteral meanings of phrases. They understand the individual meanings of the words but cannot put them together to grasp the figurative meaning. They have difficulty interpreting metaphors and analogies such as, "The man is a knight in shining armor" and, "He is big as a house." This kind of figurative language is usually interpreted in concrete terms. Coupled to the inability to use abstract interpretations of figurative language is a lack of appreciation of humor. This happens because humor is based on ambiguity and incongruities that do not make sense if they are interpreted literally.

Discourse in a communication context is difficult for the individual with right hemisphere brain damage. Narration and conversational discourse are marked by an overabundance of detailed information, with some of the information not directly relevant to the topic. Some individuals with right hemisphere damage begin to talk too much, even though they may have been somewhat reticent prior to experiencing a brain lesion. This results in inefficient communication, and the listener must infer how all the extra information that is provided relates to the topic of discussion. For example, Mr. P, a 72-year-old retired businessman with a history of right hemisphere brain damage, was asked to tell about what happened at the time of the stroke. He indicated that he was playing golf and noticed a tingling in his left leg. He then proceeded to describe the rules of golf, the best golf courses in Texas and Colorado, the brand names of golf equipment, and the merits of playing golf. He only returned to the topic of what happened at the time of the stroke after prompting from the examiner.

Stories told by these individuals often are poorly organized, making it difficult for listeners to tell exactly who did what to whom. Individual elements of a story may be described, but the description includes both important and unimportant information. These individuals suffer from an inability to isolate the most important facts, to integrate this information, and to interpret the main theme or underlying cause of events.

In conversations, individuals with right hemisphere damage demonstrate an inability to maintain the topic. Conversational interactions are complicated by deficits in turn-taking and by the patient's assumption that the listener has more shared knowledge about people, ideas, and events than the listener really does. When asked to provide information, patients often give listeners facts not related to the topic at hand. Sometimes, they continue talking in a rambling fashion.

Assessment for right hemisphere disorders focuses on the expected areas of deficit. Typically, SLPs administer a collection of tasks that focus on prosody, inference, discourse comprehension, and production. They also use conversation and narrative tasks to assess aspects of language pragmatics that are expected to be impaired. As with individuals with aphasia, treatment is geared toward developing compensatory strategies for problems the individual may be experiencing. Rather than focusing on basic language production issues, treatment goals for individuals with right hemisphere lesions usually focus on attention, memory, story interpretation, and the ability to make inferences.

Brain Trauma

As we discussed earlier, brain trauma involves neurological damage due to injury to the head. The trauma usually results in damage to multiple areas in the brain, as well as the connecting fibers within the brain. Because brain trauma tends to be diffuse, multiple motor, speech, language, and cognitive functions may be impaired. Some patients may exhibit symptoms characteristic of aphasia if language areas in the left hemisphere are damaged.

However, the majority of the characteristics of communication disorders resulting from brain trauma are most often associated with disrupted cognitive processes.

The effect of brain trauma on cognitive processes varies as a result of the extent and severity of injury. Immediately after the trauma, there is a period of "black-out" that may last just seconds but can extend as long as months. When the individual regains consciousness, there typically is a loss of memory about the accident. The effect of traumatic brain damage is usually disrupted orientation, attention, memory, visual processing, and executive functioning (see Chapter 16 for a review of these intellectual functions) that become more apparent as the patient recovers.

There are various scales such as the *Levels of Cognitive Functioning Scale* (Hagan, 1984) that have been developed to monitor the behavioral changes associated with recovery from traumatic brain injury. They are not objective tests. Rather, they are measures of tested or observed behavior that can be employed to monitor improved performance as the brain recovers. Initially, individuals who have experienced brain injury will open their eyes but will be severely confused (they know who they are but they are confused about where they are) and restless. This stage is followed by improved orientation and a reduction in confusion, but severe problems in attention, memory, and problem solving continue. Over time, these problems resolve, but even with rehabilitation, there are often lasting problems.

The course of these predictable changes is dependent primarily on the severity of the brain trauma. In mild brain trauma, cognitive processing deficits may be noticeable only when the individual must perform in a complex situational environment such as dealing with a computer crisis that arises at work. In severe trauma, recovery may be limited to the development of some self-help skills with required supervision in everyday situations.

Most communication deficits in brain trauma are cognitively based or due to dysarthria, an impairment in speech production due to motor-based problems, discussed in Chapter 14. Cognitively based communication deficits are associated with decreased attention, memory, problem solving, and executive function. It is difficult to identify how specific cognitive skills affect specific aspects of communication because they all interact. Researchers have shown that in many cases, reducing the dependence on attention or memory leads to fairly normal language comprehension. For example, adolescent boys with brain trauma were able to correctly determine if two complex sentences had the same meaning, but only if they compared two sentences (Turkstra & Holland, 1998). If they compared three sentences, the memory demands were too high, and they answered incorrectly. Cognitive processing deficits may lead to poor comprehension of written and auditorially presented information. Individuals with traumatic brain injury often miss social cues, have poor topic maintenance, have difficulty knowing when to take turns in communication, and have a reduced ability to make inferences. Coupled with these pragmatically based problems are difficulties in word-finding and excessive repetition of information (Brookshire, 1998).

Dementia

Recall that dementia is the loss of intellectual abilities due to organic disease or brain damage. Individuals with dementia often exhibit emotional problems and personality changes. The effects of **dementia** are insidious. At the beginning, dementia is difficult to separate from the normal effects of aging. As people get older, they often have difficulty recalling the names of items, and they forget where an item was left. Individuals in the early stages of dementia also exhibit the same memory and naming difficulties. As the disease progresses, they begin to experience more pronounced problems in working memory and orientation. There may be personality changes, problems in visuospatial processing, and reduced learning and reasoning ability. Language content is vulnerable and sometimes deteriorates quickly even when language form is preserved. Communication becomes more disjointed and incomplete, demonstrating a lack of informational content. In contrast, syntactic and phonological processing are well preserved until late in the disease. Also, information in long-term memory may continue to be retained.

There are several types of dementia. The disease may arise within the context of heredity such as in Huntington's chorea. Dementia may also result from advancing cerebrovascular disease or even from repeated trauma to the brain as sometimes happens in amateur and professional boxers. The largest group of individuals with dementia are diagnosed with dementia of an Alzheimer's type. The cause of Alzheimer's disease is unknown. While there are characteristic changes in the brain that are presumed to be associated with a diagnosis of Alzheimer's disease, the only definitive diagnosis can be made by a type of brain biopsy which is rarely performed. Most commonly, the disorder is identified by exclusion. That is, other conditions such as vitamin deficiency or hormonal imbalance are ruled out as causes of the changed behavior until Alzheimer's disease is left as the most reasonable explanation for the symptoms.

There are few test batteries for communication problems associated with dementia. The *Arizona Battery for Communication Disorders in Dementia* (Bayles & Tomoeda, 1993) includes a number of assessment tasks that are sensitive to deficits in dementia. Included are tasks such as naming, pantomime expression, oral description of objects, and oral and written discourse. The test battery includes normative data for normal elderly individuals and individuals with dementia.

The communication problems that are identified in individuals with dementia vary with the progression of the disease. Bayles (1986) observed that individuals in the early stages of dementia experience word omissions and trouble thinking of the correct word. They also have a reduced ability to comprehend new information, and they tend to drift from the topic. However, their grammar is generally intact. By the middle stages of the disease, vocabulary is noticeably diminished and there is difficulty comprehending grammatically complex sentences. In conversation, individuals with dementia may express ideas with little sensitivity to the communication partner. They may also fail to correct errors. By the late stages of the disease, severe anomia (inability to recall words) and jargon can be observed along with sentence fragments. These individuals produce few complex sentences, and their conversation is marked by meaningless content, repetition of words, and little meaningful use of language. By this stage patients may be dependent on assistance with most self-help skills, and they may need continuous monitoring and support.

Unfortunately, direct therapy for patients with dementia typically is not helpful. However, Bourgeois (1991), in a review of reports from fields such as psychology, nursing, and communication sciences and disorders, concluded that there are some positive outcomes from programs for dementia that focus on changing the communication environment, counseling caregivers, and providing group therapy.

SUMMARY

There are many variations in the kinds of communication disorders that result from brain injury. Where the injury occurred, how much of the brain is damaged, and the cause of the problem all influence the type of communication disorder that is observed. Communication disorders may involve all aspects of language (such as in aphasia), or they may be limited primarily to activities such as interpreting the emotion of the speaker or knowing when it is your turn to speak (as frequently happens following right hemisphere damage). The role of the SLP is to identify the type and severity of communication deficits and to implement a plan of remediation to address these problems.

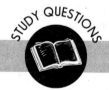

STUDY QUESTIONS

1 What are three types of brain damage that cause aphasia?

2 What are the primary differences between Broca's and Wernicke's aphasia?

3 What are three deficits associated with damage to the right hemisphere?

4 How are the cognitive deficits in dementia different from those found in brain trauma?

5 What are the expected emotional responses of the family to a family member who has had a stroke?

REFERENCES

Bayles, K. (1986). Management of neurogenic communication disorders associated with dementia. In R. Chapey (Ed.), *Language intervention strategies in adult aphasia* (2nd ed., pp. 462–473). Baltimore: Williams & Wilkins.

Bayles, K., & Tomoeda, C. (1993). *The Arizona Battery for Communication Disorders* (ABCD). Phoenix: Canyonland Publishing.

Bourgeois, M. (1991). Communication treatment for adults with dementia. *Journal of Speech and Hearing Research, 14,* 831–844.

Brookshire, R. (1998). *Introduction to neurogenic communication disorders* (5th ed.). St. Louis, MO: Mosby.

Goodglass, H., & Kaplan, H. (1983). *The assessment of aphasia and related disorders.* Philadelphia: Lea and Febiger.

Hagan, C. (1984). Language disorders in head trauma. In A. Holland (Ed.), *Language disorders in adults: Recent advances* (pp. 245–282). San Diego: College-Hill Press.

Holland, A. (1980). *Communicative Abilities in Daily Living.* Baltimore: University Park Press.

Kertesz, A. (1982). *Western Aphasia Battery.* New York: Grune & Stratton.

Porch, B. (1967). *The Porch Index of Communicative Ability.* Palo Alto, CA.: Consulting Psychologists Press.

Sarno, M. T. (1969). *Functional Communication Profile.* New York: University Medical Center.

Turkstra, L. S., & Holland, A. L. (1998). Assessment of syntax after adolescent brain injury: Effects of memory on test performance. *Journal of Speech, Language, and Hearing Research, 41,* 137–149.

Waisanen, S. (1998). Adjusting to life with aphasia: The partner's perspective. Unpublished manuscript, University of Texas, Austin.

SUGGESTED READINGS

Bayles, K. (1982). Language function in senile dementia. *Brain and Language, 16,* 265–280.

Coelho, C. (1997). Cognitive-communicative disorders following traumatic brain injury. In C. Ferrand & R. Bloom

(Eds.), *Introduction to organic and neurogenic disorders of communication* (pp. 110–133). Boston: Allyn & Bacon.

Damasio, A. (1992). Aphasia. *New England Journal of Medicine, 326,* 531–539.

Myers, P. (1997). Right hemisphere syndrome. In L. LaPointe (Ed.), *Aphasia and related language disorders* (2nd ed., pp. 201–225). New York: Thieme.

GLOSSARY

Agrammatism: Language characterized by predominance of content words (nouns, verbs) and absence of functors (articles, prepositions); characteristic of Broca's aphasia.

Aneurysm: Bulge in the wall of an artery due to weakness.

Anoxia: A lack of oxygen

Aphasia: Language disorder affecting phonology, grammar, semantics, and pragmatics as well as reading and writing due to focal brain damage.

Cerebrovascular accident: A stroke. Interruption of blood supply to an area of the brain.

Circumlocution: A circuitous description of a word that cannot be recalled.

Concussion: The effect of brain trauma with loss of consciousness.

Dementia: Deterioration of intellectual abilities such as memory, concentration, reasoning, and judgment due to organic disease or brain damage. Emotional disturbances and personality changes often accompany the intellectual deterioration.

Edema: Swelling.

Embolus: A moving clot from another part of the body that may lodge and interrupt the blood supply.

Hematoma: Encapsulated blood from a broken blood vessel.

Hemiplegia: Paralysis or weakness on one side of the body. Typically the side effected is opposite the side of the brain injury.

Hemorrhage: Bleeding from a broken artery or vein.

Homonymous hemianopsia: Loss of vision in part of the visual field due to brain injury.

Infarct: An area of dead tissue resulting from interruption of the blood supply.

Jargon aphasia: Meaningless words typical of Wernicke's aphasia

Literal paraphasia: Sounds and syllables of a word are articulated correctly but are substituted or transposed (i.e., *bork* for *fork*).

Neologism: A new word that may be meaningless.

Neoplasm (tumor): A new growth.

Spontaneous recovery: Recovery from stroke due to physiological and reorganizational changes in the brain and not attributable to rehabilitation.

Thrombosis: Accumulation of material within an artery. When complete, it causes a stroke.

Transient ischemic attack: Temporary interruption of blood flow to an area of the brain. The effects typically resolve within 24 hours.

Verbal paraphasia: Unintended substitution of one word for another, usually from the same category (e.g., *horse* for *cow*).

Index